Voice Training Programs for Professional Speakers

Global Outcomes

Voice Training Programs for Professional Speakers

Global Outcomes

Aliaa Khidr
MD, PhD, CCC/SLP

PLURAL PUBLISHING INC.

Plural Publishing Inc.

5521 Ruffin Road
San Diego, CA 92123

e-mail: info@pluralpublishing.com
Website: http://www.pluralpublishing.com

Typeset in 11/13 Adobe Garamond by Flanagan's Publishing Services, Inc.
Printed in the United States of America by McNaughton & Gunn, Inc.

Library of Congress Cataloging-in-Publication Data:
Names: Khidr, Aliaa, editor.
Title: Voice training programs for professional speakers : global outcomes / [edited by] Aliaa Khidr.
Description: San Diego, CA : Plural Publishing, [2017] | Includes bibliographical references and index.
Identifiers: LCCN 2017016565| ISBN 9781597569668 (alk. paper) | ISBN 1597569666 (alk. paper)
Subjects: | MESH: Voice Training | Voice Disorders--prevention & control | Voice Disorders--therapy | Cross-Cultural Comparison
Classification: LCC RF540 | NLM WV 500 | DDC 616.85/56--dc23
LC record available at https://lccn.loc.gov/2017016565

Contents

SECTION IV
Practices and Outcomes of Experts From South America

SECTION V
Practices and Outcomes of an Expert From North America

Introduction

The voice carries many rich unspoken messages that are readily perceived and appreciated, such as compassion, candidacy, self-confidence, and sincerity. When these messages are an authentic reflection of the psychological state of the speaker, the listener usually perceives them as genuine and true. Some speakers are able to intentionally convey these messages to their listeners in every communicative situation, regardless of the content. These are usually the ones that get naturally selected as professional speakers.

Speakers whose voices and communication styles convey trust, authority, and motivation may find themselves equipped for political, leadership, teaching, media, or sales positions. Speakers whose voices and communication styles convey comfort and sincerity may get self-selected for spiritual positions, and so forth.

Today, in this age of professionalism, individuals no more get self-selected based on their natural vocal and/or communicative skills. They self-select a career based on their interests, the cost of education, the job market, and so on. In addition, those interested in pursuing careers that typically require professional speaking skills must keep in consideration, the need to maintain a good and robust vocal quality to ensure the communication efficiency that is inherent to the nature of their jobs.

Future professional speakers, like all professionals, rely on academic institutions to prepare them for their selected careers. These institutions are expected to provide them with the information, resources, and skills they will need to be successful in their prospective job market. Unfortunately, the core vocal and communicative skills for professional speaking that should have been intuitively targeted are not even part of most of these programs. Graduates pursuing professional speaking jobs discover, years after graduation, the effect of their inexperience in commanding their voice and caring for it. This realization may come after paying the high price of failing to meet the vocal demands of their professional career and in many cases, their social life. Such problems could have been easily prevented if voice education, training and care have been addressed early in their education, as well as throughout their careers.

Professional speakers have to look hard to find a training program that fits their individual needs by trainers and/or clinical providers who have enough experience regarding the unique vocal demands and occupational challenges of their career. Fortunately, in the past decade, many voice professionals have not only started developing specialized career-specific professional vocal and communication training programs, but also have been actively lobbying to institutionalize these programs within the workforce in their countries.

This book contains the experiences, practices, and outcomes of the work of experts from all over the world in developing, implementing, and advocating for professional voice and communication skills education and training programs in their respective academic institutions, national associations, professional unions, service organizations, and workplaces. Our goal is to avail professional speakers, clinical practitioners, coaches, and policy makers with well-traveled road maps, evidence based programs and functional outcomes to guide our efforts in training and advocating for all the professional voices that enrich our world.

Foreword

When thinking of voice production, speech-language pathologists (SLPs) often describe voice as either being good or bad, normal or abnormal, thus limiting their attention to disability rehabilitation. This unique text reminds us that the disability view of voice production is shortsighted. In fact, there is a complete range of voice productions that should be represented on a wellness continuum where disordered/dysfunctional voice occupies only one end, and normal and superior voices comprise two thirds of the model as represented in the figure below.

Thinking in terms of a wellness continuum permits us to expand our concentration beyond voice rehabilitation, to other important areas such as how to prevent vocal problems, face vocal challenges in a healthy manner, and enhance the normal voice.

Voice Training Programs for Professional Speakers: Global Outcomes concentrates on the right two thirds of the wellness continuum, the normal to superior voice. The book provides a comprehensive discussion of the characteristics and vocal demands of professional speakers. These speakers include radio and television broadcasters, fitness professionals, teachers, telemarketers, and clergy, all individuals who, without functional voice, could not adequately perform their jobs, thus threatening employment.

Global experts from around the world share detailed education and training programs, practices, and outcomes related to educating, improving, and maintaining vocal health in this professional voice population. Most academic programs in speech-language pathology concentrate on rehabilitation of voice disorders. Core vocal and communicative skills for professional speakers are not often included in these educational programs. This book fills that gap. Each of the eight chapters provides a detailed description of a unique professional speaker population including the history of their professions, demographics, vocal challenges, and communicative demands.

In Chapter 1, the authors provide an excellent discussion on voice ergonomics of the professional speaker. While some books describe the importance of vocal health and lifestyle, this discussion includes details related to acoustic environment, air quality, posture, and specific employment-related voice demands. The chapter provides the reader with a practical guide for developing personal and environmental environments for maintaining vocal health.

Chapter 2 provides a detailed description of a training program specifically for radio broadcasters. The program involves making broadcast students aware of the characteristics of their own voices, basic vocal hygiene issues, and individual training in voice production.

Chapter 3 will be very interesting to academics responsible for teaching speech-

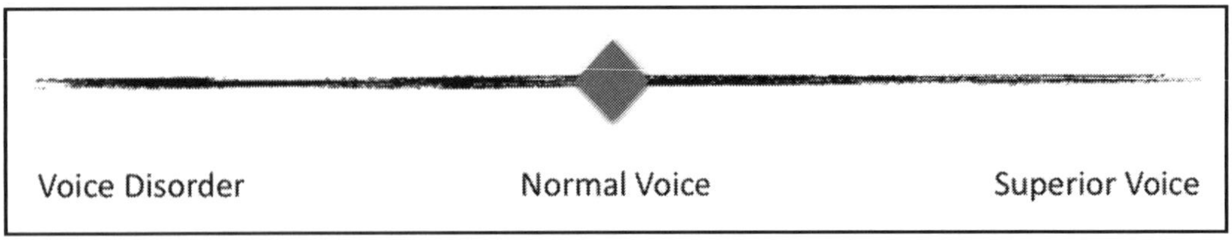

language pathologists (SLPs) courses in voice disorders. This chapter offers a detailed description of a voice education and training program for prospective SLPs. The authors of this chapter make the case that SLPs are professional voice users and as such, must know how to care for their own voices. This care, in turn, will make the students more aware of and sensitive to those they will eventually treat. The program includes topics such as personal vocal awareness, awareness of other voices, vocal hygiene issues, and general health education as related to voice. This chapter provided me with many ideas that will enrich the experiences of my own students in the graduate voice disorders class.

Chapter 4 is a detailed description of a specific voice education and training program for a group of professionals who often seek treatment in voice centers, fitness trainers. Speaking and shouting instructions while being physically active is a challenge. This educational program includes topics regarding the components of voice production, tips for keeping the voice healthy, signs and symptoms of voice problems, and should voice problems occur, where to seek help. Three delivery models are described including group seminars and workshops, small group practical sessions, and individualized training.

Chapter 5 discusses the challenges of professional television broadcasters, specifically television and Internet journalists, television hosts, and sports journalists. Beyond a clear, pleasing, and healthy voice, the authors explain that the good media professional must know how to use language to express his or her ideas, and how to synthesize and use the aspects of expressiveness of communication through voice, articulation, rate, prosody, breathing, posture, and facial expressions to communicate on video a sense of spontaneity and naturalness. The chapter precisely describes how SLPs may help broadcasters to attain these goals.

Chapters 6 and 7 provide detailed vocal health education and training sessions for two professionals who historically are presented with vocal challenges, teachers and telemarketers. Discussions for both professions include demographics, history of SLP involvement in vocal health training, and specific outlines of programs involving vocal ergonomics, health promotions, specific prevention recommendations, and communicative competence training.

Perhaps one of my favorite chapters, Chapter 8 describes the importance of "theater voice" and "text work" training for clergy. The following is a quote from the author:

> Aspiring clergy who have not been nourished with the meat-and-potatoes practical tools that are needed to speak from the soul, who have only been served bread-and-water public speaking techniques, or pie-in-the-sky homiletics training, can take heart.

Indeed, the quote left me hungry for more. And this chapter provides much more in a detailed description of the theater training methods used to permit this population to "speak from the soul."

In short, this book is unique. It fills that giant void where training to improve disordered voice leaves off, often at the expense of enhancing, improving, and maintaining the health of the normal voice. These authors have succeeded in encouraging this voice therapist to open his mind to a more "global" view of voice care. Enjoy!

—Joseph C. Stemple, PhD, CCC-SLP, ASHAF-H
Professor
Division of Communication Sciences and Disorders
Department of Rehabilitation Sciences
College of Health Sciences
University of Kentucky
Lexington, Kentucky

Contributors

Luiz Antonio Barbagli, BS
President, São Paulo Teachers Union
SinproSP
São Paulo, Brazil
Chapter 6

Mara Behlau, PhD, SLP
Director of Centro de Estudos da Voz, CEV
Permanent Professor of the Human Communication Graduate Program
Universidade Federal de São Paulo, UNIFESP
São Paulo, Brazil
Chapter 6

Mary K. (Kate) Burke, MFA
Head of Voice and Text Training
Associate Professor, Department of Drama
University of Virginia Master of Fine Arts Actor Training Program
Charlottesville, Virginia
Chapter 8

Marc De Bodt, MA, PhD
Visiting Professor, Ghent University
Director, University Rehabilitation Center for Communication Disorders
Antwerp University Hospital
Edegem, Belgium
Chapter 2

Ana Elisa Moreira-Ferreira, MD, SLP
Speech Pathologist, Communication Coach, Consultant in Human Communication
Executive Director at UNIVOZ
São Paulo, Brazil
Chapter 7

Michael Hull, PhD
Instructor, Educational Research, Statistics, and Program Evaluation
Department of Education Leadership, Foundations, and Policy
University of Virginia, Curry School of Education
Charlottesville, Virginia
Chapter 3

Aliaa Khidr, MD, PhD, CCC/SLP
Professor of Phoniatrics
Unit of Phoniatrics, Department of Otolaryngology, School of Medicine
Ain Shams University, Cairo, Egypt
Department of Communication Disorders
Curry School of Education (Retired)
University of Virginia, Charlottesville, USA
Chapter 3

Vanessa Pedrosa, PhD, SLP
Speech Pathologist, Communication Coach
Executive Director at Fonoevidence
Consultants in Human Communication
São Paulo, Brazil
Chapter 5

Leena Rantala, PhD
Senior Lecturer in Speech Language Pathology

Faculty of Social Sciences
University of Tampere
Tampere, Finland
Chapter 1

Meredith Roper, BSEd
MEd Speech-Language Pathology Candidate
Associate Clinician
Sheila C. Johnson Center for Human Services
University of Virginia
Charlottesville, Virginia
Chapter 3

Anna Rumbach, BSc, MSpPathSt, GCHEd, PhD
Lecturer in Speech Pathology
School of Health and Rehabilitation Sciences
The University of Queensland
St. Lucia, Brisbane, Australia
Chapter 4

Eeva Sala, MD, PhD
Docent in Phoniatrics
University of Turku
Secretary of the Finnish Voice Ergonomic Society
Turku, Finland
Chapter 1

Bernadette Timmermans, MA, PhD
Professor, SLP – Voice Coach
Docent, Royal Institute of Theatre, Screen and Sound
Erasmus University
Professor of the Free University of Brussels
Consultant VRT, Medialaan
Brussels, Belgium
Chapter 2

Fabiana Zambon, PhD, SLP
Teacher's Vocal Health Program Coordinator,
São Paulo Teachers Union, SinproSP
Professor, Centro de Estudos da Voz, CEV
São Paulo, Brazil
Chapter 6

I dedicate this book to

My father, Ali Khadr, for his amazing capacity to love, for always believing in me, and for showing me that teaching is a lifelong relationship that grows way beyond the classroom walls.

My mother, Alia Abdel Moty, for taking so much pride in her teaching skills, for boasting about her students' command of the subjects she teaches, and for planting in me the seeds of enthusiasm for developing engaging educational activities.

My mentor, Nasser Kotby, for fighting for what he believes in, for enjoying every small gift in life, and most importantly for making me realize that "Academia" is a big family of international best friends who have fun working together toward changing the world.

My husband, Emaad Abdel Rahman, for being my home, my beloved and my best friend, and for showing me every day what does it really mean to live in the presence of GOD.

My daughter, Rana, the peacemaker, and my son, Ali, the debater, for being my radiant sun and reflective moon.

All my loving family and friends, for keeping my heart warm.

For all my talented students, clients, and colleagues, for keeping me motivated to do more.

SECTION I

Practices and Outcomes of Experts From Europe

CHAPTER 1

Voice Ergonomics for Professional Speakers: Who Needs Them? Who Provides Them? What Do They Do?

Leena Rantala and Eeva Sala

Basic Concepts

Clear and well-functioning voice is part of the professional skills and ability to work. Voice should be under the control of a voice user so that he or she knows the possibilities and restrictions of the voice as well as the risks that may threaten it. Environment where voice is used should be conducive for that purpose. Noise and poor acoustics should not disturb those who are producing voice or listening to it.

Speech (voice) is the most important tool in communication between humans. Voice source is in the larynx that changes aerodynamic energy generated by exhalation into acoustic energy. Acoustic energy is worked up and amplified in the supraglottic tract into words and sentences. Voice propagates through air as the mechanical waves of pressure and meets the ear where it changes into mechanic and electroacoustic energy. A neural tract starting from the inner ear transfers signals to the brain for interpretation and understanding.

Voice ergonomics has been developed for improving voice and speech as a communication tool. It addresses all the measures that increase possibilities to good voice and speech production and their hearing (perception). Voice ergonomics contains personal and environmental factors. Its purpose is to make personal ergonomic measures such as taking care of the health of the voice organs and adopting less loading (loading-free) activities/working practices. It also contains environmental ergonomic measures such as observing and treating noise sources and acoustics, working/activity postures, and indoor air quality proper for voice and speech production. When voice ergonomics is taken more extensively, there also includes reduction of noise that is important for cognitive functions of listeners such as attention and memory. This chapter will cover voice ergonomics, its background, risks, and problems and solutions.

Voice disorder is a state in which voice does not function according to the needs of a speaker or in which voice quality is considered not proper/adequate for the purpose. Speakers often suffer from various symptoms related to voice use and/or injury of the voice organs. Voice disorder is a complex entity and has several levels to explore.

There are several risk factors behind a voice disorder, and they often occur at the same time. When vocal load increases over a tolerance, symptoms caused by voice dysfunction and/or voice organs appear. Vice versa when risk factors are picked up and deleted, voice function returns to its original or to a better functional state at least. Risk factors for a voice disorder can be found from issues related to person and from those related to the environment.

Box 1–1

Risk factors for a voice disorder can be found from issues related to a person and from those related to the environment.

Personal factors include

- the health of the voice organs,
- voice use skills and practices,
- personality,
- lifestyle,
- leisure time activities, and
- voice demands at work.

Environmental factors are

- noise and acoustic conditions,
- indoor air quality,
- possibilities to use good working postures, and
- access to aids (loudspeakers), if necessary.

When voice does not function according to a user's needs it may lead to the avoidance of voice use, to the selection of practices or work tasks with less/no voice demands, to the decrease of ability to be active or work, to the drop of outcomes, to be unable to work, and absence/absenteeism from work. At worst, a worker may even have to change his or her work and educate himself or herself to a new profession.

It is possible to prevent a voice disorder to a certain level at least. Ways to do this are to acquire good/excellent skills in voice production, to take care of the health of the vocal organs, to adopt light loading activity/working practices, and to keep good postures. To keep the voice production in a good state, voice exercises are recommended as a daily regular habit.

To treat a voice disorder successfully, underlying causes need to be examined carefully because the treatment is not the same for all voice disorders and a serious underlying condition may be present. There are several kinds of voice disorders: functional, organic, and neurologic. A physician (voice specialist) has the responsibility to assess and define (diagnose) a voice disorder, to explore a voice disorder type, and offer and outline the treatment.

The treatment of a voice usually contains the remedy of a disease, the elimination or decrement of risk and loading factors, checking the voice production manner, and if necessary correcting it.

Prevention of a voice disorder is based on the knowledge of the physiology of voice production and risk factors. Personal and environment risk factors are checked and deleted or decreased as effectively as possible. In addition, voice ergonomic information is given and exercises for health and economic voice use habits are taught.

Voice Ergonomics

The Development of Voice Ergonomics

The first research concerning occupational voice disorders was published in Germany in 1970; this was a monograph by Gunderman (1970). Fifteen years later a Finnish phoniatrician Erkki Vilkman started systematically to connect voice and environmental factors (Vilkman & Manninen, 1986). At the same time in Sweden Ann-Christine Ohlsson (1987) got interested in the same issues for her dissertation research and measured the prevalence of voice disorders among teachers (Ohlsson, Järvholm, & Löfqvist, 1987). Ohlsson also surveyed teachers' vocal behavior and created a method for measuring voice use at work (Ohlsson, Brink, & Löfqvist, 1989). After those studies, research regarding prevalence of voice disorders in occupations started to come out with increasing number in different countries, for example, in Finland (preschool teachers): Pekkarinen (Sala), Himberg, and Pentti, (1992); in Sweden (patients in phoniatric clinics): Fritzell, 1996; in Australia (teachers): Russell, Oates, and Greenwood (1998); in the United States: (teachers and other occupations) Smith, Gray, Dove, Kirchner, and Heras, (1997) and (teachers) Roy, Merrill, Thibeault, Parsa, Gray, and Smith (2004).

In addition, the number of studies assessing the consequences of voice risk factors also increased. The studies were mostly carried out in laboratory settings (e.g., Vilkman, Lauri, Alku, Sala, & Sihvo, 1997), in schools (e.g., Rantala, Vilkman, & Bloigu, 2002) or in preschools (e.g., Södersten, Granqvist, Hammarberg, & Szabo, 2002); sporadically also in other working places (in theater: Novak, Dlouha, Capkova, & Vohradnik, 1991; in call center customer service: Lehto, Alku, Bäckström, & Vilkman, 2005).

Voice ergonomics has gradually been included as part of a wide ergonomic field. The definition of ergonomics is "the theoretical and fundamental understanding of human behavior and performance in purposeful interacting sociotechnical systems, and the application of that understanding to the design of these interactions in the context of real settings" (Wilson, 2000).

The development of voice ergonomics as a part of general ergonomics has been a natural course because voice ergonomic studies have consistently shown that for workers in several occupations, voice is a main working tool and factors threatening vocal health originate from suboptimal working practices and environment.

Especially Nordic countries have been forerunners in developing and applying good voice ergonomic habits in working places. The Finnish Institute of Occupational Health (Työterveyslaitos) addressed this topic to their schooling program through which occupational health services got knowledge about the topic. Arbetsmiljöverket (Swedish Work Environment Authority) in Sweden also included voice ergonomics in their publicity program. Södersten and Lindhe (2011) wrote a scientific review on occupation-related voice disorders and voice ergonomics for Arbetsmiljöverket (Swedish Work Environment Authority). Arbetsmiljöverket (Swedish Work Environment Authority) also put information about voice and a simplified screening form of voice ergonomics in a working place on their web pages (retrieved December 5, 2016, from https://www.av.se/globalassets/filer/checklistor/rostergonomi-checklista.pdf).

Several articles in international publications are available. Of two books available, one concerning voice ergonomic risk factors in working places has been published in Finnish and Swedish. The book was written for the use of occupational and professional voice users and also for occupational health service personnel (Sala, Sihvo, & Laine, 2005, 2011). It has been used also as a textbook in logopedic education. The other book (Sala et al., 2009 in Finnish, 2011 in Swedish) was written for occupational health service personnel in order to help them to observe and measure the voice ergonomic risk factors in the environment. The book also contains suggestions on how to solve problems if found.

More information is still needed in the voice ergonomic field. For instance, there is no follow-up study on how occupational health personnel consider voice ergonomics when they visit workplaces. In spite of that, our clinical experience is, however, that risk factors found in the environment are more and more taken into account when evaluating and treating voice disorders. This means that the awareness has increased among voice experts and occupational health personnel as well as among voice users themselves.

Occupational and Professional Voice Users

There are several groups of voice users whose voice use is essential for managing their work. We differentiate those people into two groups depending on their voice skills and work situations where they use their voices.

Occupational voice users are those who need a lot of voice and often have to use loud voice in their work while speaking. They usually speak to groups and in the presence of noise. They have none or only a little guidance in voice and training for speech production. Typical occupational voice users are teachers.

Professional voice users are those who need a lot of voice in their work. They have got a lot of information concerning voice and had voice training during their studies. Typical professional voice users are actors and classical singers.

People who are also responsible for voice ergonomics are the planners of the buildings and rooms. They ought to take into account the special needs of voice users (occupational and professional voice users). The environment where voice is used should be proper for that purpose. Noise and poor acoustics should not disturb those who are producing voice and speech or listening to it. Voice users should also use proper postures while speaking. A good speech communication environment is quiet with proper acoustics, has fresh air without harmful impurities, has an environment that supports using good posture; and has aids (e.g., voice amplifiers) available, if needed.

Occupational, Professional, and Work-Related Voice Disorders

Definitions for occupational or professional voice disorders depend on the legislation of a country and terminology used in the school of the medical/scientific field.

An occupational voice disorder is often the functional correlation of a disease. In the most strict definition, occupational disease (tissue damage) is considered a disease that is most likely caused primarily by exposure at work. The exposure may be physical or chemical by nature. The definition also involves exposure in such an amount that it can cause a disease. Accordingly, occupational voice disorder is a disorder that is due to tissue damage that is most likely caused primarily by exposure at work.

A professional voice disorder is basically the same as an occupational voice disorder but lower exposure to poor ergonomic conditions may cause it.

A work-related voice disorder is due to tissue damage that is most likely caused primarily by exposure other than work, for example, tissue damage due to laryngopharyngeal reflux, which causes a disease, increases the risk for laryngitis, vocal fold cyst, polyp, pseudocyst, and so on, or if a speaker has a vocal fold paresis (viral infection or trauma). People with a work-related voice disorder mainly have symptoms at work because of the high demands of voice use needed there.

A voice disorder often causes a handicap mainly at work because of the high demands (amount and level) work sets for communication and vocal performance. The study of Sala, Laine, Simberg, Pentti, and Suonpää (2001) showed differences in vocal demands between work and free time: 38% of teachers experienced voice symptoms that complicated their communication and voice use at work, but only 4% of the same teachers reported similar problems during their leisure time.

Occupational Voice Ergonomic Risk Factors

Risk factors for voice disorders include several factors that a speaker is able to influence. Working practices in the field of voice ergonomics mean habits or practices a speaker uses while speaking. Box 1–2 presents the most typical factors threatening voice health in a workplace. There are several factors a speaker is able to regulate and influence. In many professions it is necessary to speak a lot, but to some degree this can be restricted if necessary. The same applies to some other voice use practices: using a loud voice, speaking with surrounding noise, or projecting the voice to a long distance.

Box 1–2

Working practices that may include a risk factor for an occupational voice disorder are

- speaking a lot,
- using a loud voice,
- speaking in noise,
- speaking to long distances,
- poor posture, and
- lack of aids.

Vocally harmful working practices increase voice handicap (measured with Voice Handicap Index, VHI; Rantala, Hakala, Holmqvist, & Sala, 2012) and also change acoustic features of voice in the course of a working day (Rantala, Hakala, Holmqvist, & Sala, 2015b). For instance, workers' voice levels are higher and voice quality more hypofunctional if they use voice loading practices. Several small changes in voice ergonomic factors may result in a significant improvement in the overall situation. It is often enough that a worker becomes conscious of his or her voice loading habits, and then he or she is able change them.

Working Practices

Speaking a Lot During a Working Day

In many occupations speech is the main or one of the most important working tools. Speaking is such an automatic process that speakers are usually not aware of how much they are speaking until they have voice or throat symptoms. There are differences between how much speakers tolerate speaking without symptoms. The differences can be found in the status of vocal organs, the environment, and vocal demands caused by an occupation.

There are many different methods to measure the amount of speaking during work. Teachers speak nearly twice as long as nurses during a working period. The average speaking time of teachers per work day was 40 ± 10%, and that of hospital nurses was 28 ± 12% (Sala et al., 2002). According to Durup, Shield, Dance, Sullivan, and Gomez-Agustina (2015), teachers speak around 24% of their working period, as measured with a voice dosimeter (APM, Ambulatory Phonation Monitor, KayPentax APM 3200) that measures a speaker's phonation time (the time when vocal folds are vibrating—note that phonation time is not a real speaking time but is much shorter).

Although the speaking rate may seem quite small it is not experienced that way by the speaker. A recent study showed that all the teachers who participated in the research (N = 39) reported that their voice use was excessive during work (Rantala & Sala, unpublished data). This study also revealed that those teachers not being able to decrease their speaking time reported the symptom "voice does not carry" more often than those who could regulate their speaking time.

Ergonomic recommendations include that the amount of speech can be decreased and the breaks for recovery increased since even short breaks allow vocal organs recover from loading strain. Workers may benefit even from short breaks from talking, during which vocal organs can recover from loading strain (Vintturi et al., 2001a). A voice ergonomic study also showed that if a voice rest is not possible for occupational voice users (teachers) they will experience quite serious voice symptoms such as "voice gets low or voice breaks occur during speaking" (Rantala & Sala, unpublished data).

Using Loud Voice, Speaking Against Noise and/or Across Long Distance

Loud voice is necessary for listeners to hear the speaker. It is necessary to increase speech loudness (level) when speaking across a long distance and when speaking over noise. Speech loudness is also a personal feature of people: Some people talk with a quiet voice, some talk with a loud voice, and some between these extremes, even in the same circumstances.

People raise their voices when speaking in a noisy environment. This happens from 0.22 to 1 dB per 1-dB increments in noise level (Lindstrom, Waye, Södersten, McAllister, & Ternström, 2011). Values depend on the details of the method used (study arrangements, the quality of background noise, measurement distance and unit). People also react individually to noise exposure: When one increases the voice level by 1 dB as noise level increases 1 dB, others do not increase the voice level at all (Lindstrom et al., 2011).

To control the noise it is possible to agree on different ways and methods. The easiest way is to avoid noisy speaking places or decrease all unnecessary activities that cause noise. An extremely loud activity noise can be controlled, for example, by installing a noise detector. A noise detector is a device that measures the sound level. It can also be set to give an alarm by flashing LED-light when the agreed-upon noise level is exceeded. In that way people get feedback on activities that are too noisy, which they can adjust to be quieter. Technical progress brings new solutions to this need.

Speaking Across a Long Distance

Speaking across a long distance is often necessary when speaking to a group or speaking outdoors. Outdoors the sound level decreases by 6 dB when a distance is doubled, because there are not as many reflecting surfaces. Indoors the walls and the ceiling reflect sound and attenuation is less. Sound attenuation depends on the acoustic properties of the room. In a room speech sound may decrease 3 dB when the distance is doubled (room volume 200 m^3, and reverberation time 0.5–0.6 s). This means that when, for example, a teacher speaks to a student across a distance of 1 m, a normal voice level (60 dBL_{A1m}, where A is A-frequency weighting and 1 m is measurement distance) is enough, but when he or she speaks to a 4-m distance, a raised voice is needed (the voice level should be 67 dBL_{A1m}) to reach a listener at the level he or she hears the message loud enough (60 dBL_{A1m}). It is wise to decrease the speaking distance. A speaking distance can often be decreased if the situation and furniture are organized in a new way.

When speaking to a group, there are several persons speaking at the same time. This causes noise while speaking and hence the need to increase the voice. Speaking to a group also means speaking to a long distance. This, too, necessitates speaking with a louder voice. It is advisable to arrange the situation so that only one person speaks at a time and group members are near a speaker.

Speaking to a person with a hearing loss, people usually speak with a loud voice, but hearing impaired individuals do not necessarily perceive and understand that kind of speech better. Speaking with a too loud voice makes the sound distort in the ear/hearing system because of the narrow dynamic range of hearing (narrow dynamic range means that a person does not hear quiet sounds, and loud sounds feel uncomfortable or distorted). Instead, it is best to go near to the listener, speak slower, and speak face to face so that the listener can see the lips and expressions of the speaker.

Speakers may also use a loud voice when they speak to elderly people. Elderly people have difficulties in speech identification due to their age per se and also due to presbyacusis (a hearing loss that exists in aged people). In addition, they may have difficulties in high-level speech processing. They should be spoken to in a similar manner as to people with a hearing loss: face to face, with normal voice level but slowly and with pauses. Speaking slowly with pauses is also less loading for a speaker.

Personal Factors: Working Postures

Good Speaking Posture

When speakers use good working postures, their muscles, joints, ligaments, nerves, and other body structures do not get loaded. Good postures (called also neutral or resting postures) are ergonomic and feel comfortable. Good postures allow optimal length-tension relationships between muscle groups (Arboleda & Frederick, 2008), the thoracic wall to move freely, and the larynx to situate approximately at its neutral—that is, resting—position.

The best posture for speaking is the standing position (Vintturi et al., 2001b). This permits internal abdominal organs to sink down making space for breathing movements with higher lung volume. High lung volume, in turn, lowers vertical laryngeal position caused by the tracheal pull (Iwarsson & Sundberg, 1998). The tracheal pull is the force that lowers the cricoid cartilage and,

Box 1–3

Voice ergonomic guidelines include the following:

- Be aware of the detrimental effects of noise on speech production.
- While speaking in noise, remember the right way to increase voice loudness.
- Lead and supervise situations and activities so that noise is avoided.
- Go near listeners.
- While speaking in a group, arrange so that one person is speaking at a time.
- Gather group members near the speaker.
- Avoid continuous and long-standing speaking in noise.
- Avoid speaking near equipment that emits noise.
- Keep discussions in quiet rooms.
- Choose and buy equipment that is quiet.
- Check if the noise levels of equipment can be lowered or moved to other rooms.
- Keep windows and doors closed if intrusive noise is audible and disturbing.
- Consider if a noise detector is of benefit to decrease noise.

consequently, the larynx (Vilkman, Sonninen, Hurme, & Körkkö, 1996). The downward movement (associated with tilt of the cricoid cartilage) shortens the vocal folds and, hence, lowers fundamental frequency. The vertical larynx position during phonation has been found to be higher in patients with muscle tension disorder than in people with healthy voices (Lowell, Kelley, Colton, Smith, & Portnoy, 2012).

Straight posture of the pelvis allows proper weight distribution and balance in the body and so upholds an ergonomic position. An upright position is also the most favorable posture for the head (Bonney & Corlett, 2002). When the head inclines forward the compressive load on the cervical disks increases as well as the relative weight of the head (see the section, Consequences of Poor Head Postures). More information about postures can be found in the article of Arboleda and Frederick (2008). Informative sites for good ergonomic postures can also be found on the Internet.

Effects of Poor Postures on Voice: Voice Production and Voice Symptoms

Poor postures make voice production difficult and increase vocal loading, thus leading to symptoms. Although there are sparse studies on relationships between voice and postures, the collected data are quite extensive though: it is from a survey of almost 1,900 elementary and secondary school teachers (Kooijman et al., 2006), from 25 dysphonic teachers (Kooijman et al., 2005), and from a voice ergonomic project regarding 40 elementary school teachers (e.g., Rantala et al., 2012; Rantala, Hakala, Holmqvist, & Sala, 2013). The results of these studies show that poor postural alignment increases the incidence of voice symptoms (Kooijman et al., 2005, 2006; Rantala et al., 2012) and affects voice production (Kooijman et al., 2005; Rantala et al., 2013). Results for different working postures are explained more specifically throughout this chapter.

Teachers use several postures that may load vocal organs while speaking. A voice ergonomic study revealed that over half of the teachers (58%; N = 40) used three or more poor postures during a working day (Rantala & Sala, unpublished data). The most typical poor working postures were turned head (55% of teachers) and hunched (55%) or raised up shoulders (48%). Only 10% of the teachers did not use any poor posture. The more poor working postures a teacher used, the higher the voice level he or she spoke with (Rantala et al., 2013). The increased voice level might result from worsened vocal organ function reflecting a teacher's attempt to compensate for deteriorated voice quality or uncomfortable sensations in the throat. Box 1–4 presents most typical poor working postures during talking that affect vocal organs.

Box 1–4

Working postures that may include a risk factor for an occupational voice disorder are as follows:

- Head
  - ☐ turned
  - ☐ thrust forward/ backward/ upward
  - ☐ tilted toward shoulder
  - ☐ poor posture (e.g., when using bifocals or progressive glasses)
- Shoulders
  - ☐ bent down/hunched
  - ☐ risen up
- Body
  - ☐ turned to side while speaking
- Arms
  - ☐ held up/picking up heavy things

A typical standing posture for dysphonic people is posterior weight-bearing (Figure 1–1; Kooijman et al., 2005). In this posture the pelvis is anteriorly relative to the torso, thoracic kyphosis is increased as is lumbar lordosis to some extent. In this posture, lumbopelvic stabilizing musculature is passive, while in erect and ergonomic posture, it works actively (O'Sullivan et al., 2002).

Furniture and Devices Affect Working Postures

Tables and chairs ought to be adjusted for each occupational voice user separately. Preschool staff members are at increased risk of low back pain due to activities that require awkward and static working postures, such as using child-sized furniture, sitting on the floor, or bending at the waist (Grant, Habes, & Tepper, 1995). People who work with toddlers and lift them with bent backs (e.g., over the side of a crib or from a floor) are especially at risk.

The use of certain devices may trigger poor speaking postures such as projectors reflecting slides on screens behind the teachers. Using projectors or smart boards, speakers easily twist their bodies and turn their heads back- and upward. In this way the lower part of a speaker's body faces listeners, but the head and the shoulders are turned to the board behind his or her back to see the content of his or her presentation. Over 40% of teachers ($N = 40$) in the voice ergonomic study of Rantala and Sala (unpublished data) twisted their body in this way during speaking in lessons.

Consequences of Poor Head Postures

If a speaker's head is in an unbalanced position, neck and upper limb muscles and vocal organs may be loaded. Many teachers (23%) speak with poor head postures (Rantala & Sala, unpublished data). Head thrust forward posture has been found to be connected with

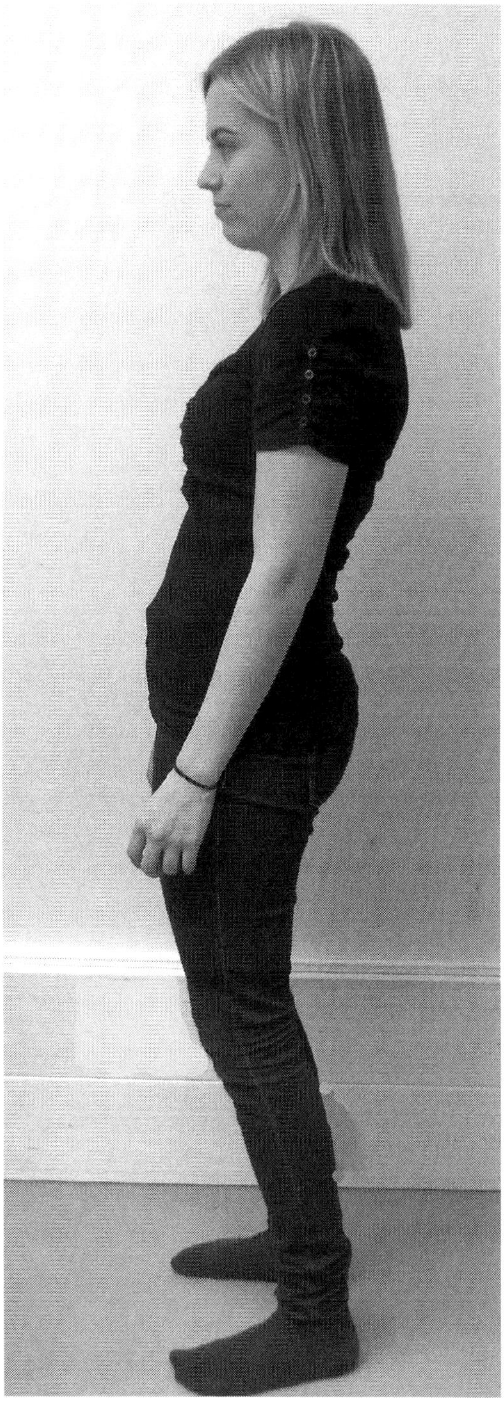

Figure 1–1. *In a posterior weight-bearing posture the pelvis is anteriorly relative to the torso and thoracic kyphosis and lumbar lordosis are increased. (Photo credit: L. Rantala.)*

voice disorders (Figure 1–2): about 75% of dysphonic teachers held their heads in this way (Kooijman et al., 2005). The forward head posture is the anterior positioning of the cervical spine that induces load on the posterior spine, burdening significantly non-contractile structures (e.g., posterior cervical structures; Bonney & Corlett, 2002; Chiu & Lam, 2007). One reason for this is the weight of the head. Namely, weight dramatically increases when the head is not in its neutral posture (Hansraj, 2014). The head weighs about 12 pounds (4–5 kg), but when the neck is at a 15-degree angle forward, the weight is about 27 pounds (12 kg), at 30 degrees it is 40 pounds (18 kg), at 45 degrees it is 49 pounds (22 kg), and at 60 degrees it is already 60 pounds (27 kg).

Computers, smartphones, and tablet computers provoke forward thrust of the head. The smaller the screen of a computer, the more tilted are the cervical and thoracic spines (Szeto & Lee, 2002). Further, when speaking using a phone, a worker easily tilts the head toward the shoulder; the head posture is even worse if a worker speaks and writes at the same time.

Rubin, Blake, and Mathieson (2007) have presented that the forward head posture shortens the suprahyoid musculature and thereby elevates the position of the larynx. This, in turn, changes the shape of the vocal cavity and, consequently, alters resonance of the voice. Furthermore, this kind of head posture may restrain forward movement of thyroid cartilage (Rubin et al., 2007) and impair the production of low pitches (Honda, Hirai, Masaki, & Shimada, 1999).

Forward head posture also loads body parts that may indirectly affect vocal organs. For instance, the effects of loading emerge as

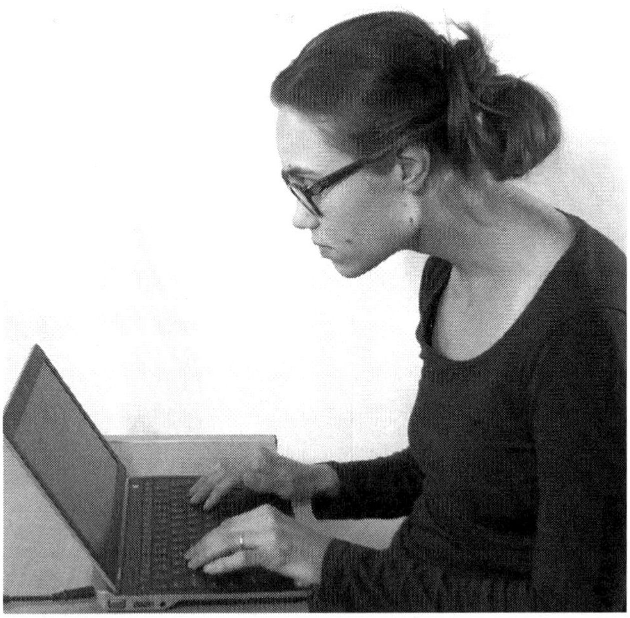

Figure 1–2. *A forward thrust head posture increases the weight of the head and induces load on the posterior spine, burdening significantly posterior cervical structures. (Photo credit: L Rantala.)*

neck pain (Chiu & Lam, 2007) and shrinkage of the cervical spine (about 1 mm over a 1-h period; Bonney & Corlett, 2002). The spine shortens because intervertebral disk fluid expels through the disk walls due to the stress being directed to the spine. The longer the time a speaker works in this posture, the higher the risk for neck or upper limb pain (Chiu & Lam, 2007). Even a small change from a neutral head posture may load organs, although it has been shown that the angle of the head tilt does not predict the severity of neck pain (Yip, Chiu, & Poon, 2008). Consequently, a clinician should also focus on head mobility, not only on its posture, when making a voice ergonomic assessment.

Consequences of Poor Shoulder Postures

Risen up shoulders and arms quickly strain muscles. Work tasks where a speaker may use these postures are writing on a board or showing pictures from a book to children while reading. Voice ergonomic study revealed that 48% of teachers (*N* = 40) spoke with raised up shoulders, which also increased the incidence of voice symptoms (Rantala & Sala, unpublished data). Teachers who talked with uplifted shoulders experienced symptoms of "voice gets low" or "the feeling of pain or lump in throat." Furthermore, the longer the time a speaker works with hands raised, the risk for neck or upper limb pain increases (Chiu & Lam, 2007).

Breaks Are for the Benefit of Voice

Taking breaks is essential for avoiding loading caused by static postures. At least this is true in elementary school teachers according to the study of Rantala and Sala (unpublished data): all the teachers (*N* = 40) were able to move around and rest and relax their bodies during work. At present and to our knowledge, there are no other field studies on the effects of short breaks among occupational voice users. In a laboratory setting, Vintturi et al. (2001a) found that during a break loading changes diminished in a speaker's voice and a phonation type became more economical. Many acoustic parameters also expressed these rest changes.

Similar information can be found from the field of general ergonomics. For instance, it has been shown that neck and upper-limb pains in computer workers were relieved if they had regular breaks (Van den Heuvel, de Looze, Hildebrandt, & Thé, 2003).

More General Perspective: Musculoskeletal Disorders in Neck, Upper Limbs, and Back

Most of all, awkward working postures or repetitive or loading movements threaten musculoskeletal well-being that, in turn, may play a part in the origin of voice disorders in many ways. Musculoskeletal disorder (MSD) also causes worries for voice care professionals, because it is one of the most frequent occupational health problems in the working-age population (Erick & Smith, 2011, review). Pain and impaired movements worsen the quality of life and incur an economic burden to society.

Teachers present an occupational group that has a high prevalence of MSD (Erick & Smith, 2011). According to a large study regarding teachers (*N* > 3,000), the 1-year prevalence of neck pain was 67%, upper limb pain was 33%, and both 30% (Chiu & Lam, 2007). Teachers also have reported pain in upper back (37% of teachers) and in lower back (44%) (Korkmaz, Cavlak, & Telci, 2011).

Some teachers, such as preschool teachers and music teachers, are more vulnerable to MSD than others (Erick & Smith, 2011). Long working hours and a large number of pupils in a class increase the incidence of MSD. Teachers working with younger children are also at an increased risk for MSD.

Although both genders experience MSD, it is more typical in females (Chiu & Lam, 2007; Korkmaz et al., 2011). Psychosocial factors are also involved in the origin of MSD, such as high workload, stress, low colleague support, low job satisfaction, and monotonous work (Chiu & Lam, 2007; Erick & Smith, 2011; Korkmaz et al., 2011).

Environmental Factors: Speaking Environment, Acoustics, Background and Activity Noise

Good acoustics support voice production and speaking but also speech hearing. In an acoustically good room, speech voice carries well to listeners without extra effort, a speaker gets feedback from his or her voice to conveniently adjust it for the situation. In quiet spaces speakers have no need to raise their voices due to noise. In an acoustically good room, the listener hears the speech loud enough and is able to identify the message clearly: he or she hears the message in the original and undistorted form.

In an acoustically poor room a speaker has to raise the voice. Using raised voice for long periods of time increases loading of the vocal organs. Listeners have difficulties in speech identification: they hear the speech but do not catch what is said. If a listener needs to put extra effort into listening, he or she gets tired and the attention escapes easily to things other than the message. When the listener hears the speech easily, he or she does not need to put so much effort into listening, and the energy is available for processing the message.

In large spaces the speaking distances are long. To overcome the effects of a speaking distance, a speaker has to use raised, loud, very loud, or shouting voice. It is nearly like speaking outdoors. Large spaces are often reverberant and noisy. If they are well attenuated, there may be a problem getting the speech voice to carry loud enough to the listener. In large spaces amplifiers are often used to overcome the speech attenuation due to distance. When using adequate speech amplifiers, it is possible to speak with a normal and comfortable voice level.

Open-plan learning environments are becoming more popular because of changes in pedagogic methods, which are progressive student-/child-centered methods. School buildings should be flexible to support different learning methods and changing trends in classroom practice (Shield, Greenland, & Dockrell, 2010).

Open-plan environments may be noisy. Noise comes from the activity of students within the group, intrusive noise from adjacent groups, background noise from sources associated with building services and utilities, or noise from traffic.

Average noise levels in open-plan school settings have been found to be from 55 to 72 dB(A) (Shield et al., 2010). According to Walsh (1975) the maximum acceptable background noise level in open-plan classrooms should fall between 55 and 65 dB(A).

It is possible to restrict noise and choose working practices appropriate for the occasion without neglecting the disadvantage with acoustic designs. Noise can be restricted by choosing quiet furniture and things and using less noisy working practices. Audiovisual equipment is adjusted to the minimum level so that they can be heard clearly but not to a higher level than that. When speaking to a group, a speaker should use a speech level loud enough but not higher, go near listeners or collect listeners near him or her. No loud nonverbal manners are favored, such as hand clapping or shouting while giving praise. Instead of this students can raise hands up or carry out other noiseless gestures that are settled before. It is also necessary to make an agreement about group working habits. If a group needs a quiet environment in order to concentrate to a task, a group leader informs a neighbor group for this.

Open-plan spaces need a special kind of acoustics. The most important target is an acoustic design that attenuates noise, because noise is the most disturbing feature in open-plan learning spaces (Shield et al., 2010). Sound support is not as important as attenuation, because group members sit near each other when speech does not need to carry to a long distance. Amplifiers may be installed and used in cases where speech sound should reach a big listener group.

Speaking outdoors lacks reflective surfaces that enhance the speech voice. Sound attenuates 6 dB as the distance is doubled. Speaking outdoors entails raising the voice in order to be heard. When a listener is at a 1-m distance from a speaker, a speaker's voice level has to be 60 dB (measured at 1-m distance) in order for a listener to hear what he or she says.

Box 1–5

Speaking outdoors a speaker has to raise the voice in order to be heard:

- At 1 m normal voice (60 dB)*
- At 2 m raised voice (66 dB)
- At 4 m loud voice (72 dB)
- At 8 m very loud voice (78 dB)
- At 16 m shouting voice (84 dB)

*Measured at a 1 m distance

Background and Activity Noise

Environmental noise is a handicap to a speaker and a listener. Two kinds of noises can be detected on the bases of their origins: (1) background noise (ambient noise) that consists of interior- and exterior-source background noise and (2) activity noise that is generated by people within the building or sound generated by temporary or permanent instructional equipment. These noises have been found to affect the voice use somewhat differently (Rantala, Hakala, Holmqvist, & Sala, 2015a, 2015b, see more precisely below). Furthermore, noise deteriorates speech perception. Some people groups are much more vulnerable to its effects than other people on average (Box 1–6).

Box 1–6

There are special groups who need quiet surroundings for acceptable speech perception:

- aged people,
- people with a hearing loss,
- people whose mother tongue is a foreign language,
- people who are bilingual,
- people who have specific language impairment,
- people who have short working memory capacity,
- those who have an attention problem, and
- people with noise sensitivity.

Background noise includes sounds from outdoor sources like traffic, playground activities, and building services and utilities like ventilation, air conditioning, heating, water pipes, elevators, and lamps (ANSI/ASA S12.60-2010).

The number of noise sources in a speaker's environment seems to have a cumulative effect on voice. A study made in elementary schools showed a positive relationship (= the more noise sources, the more voice symptoms in teachers) between the number of noise sources and voice symptoms (Rantala et al., 2012).

Because of many harmful effects of noise, recommendations have been set for regulating it. A low background noise level is especially important for learning spaces where the recommended level for noise has been set at 35 dBA (ANSI/ASA S12.60-2010). However, this level is exceeded in most classrooms (Kristiansen et al., 2014; Sato & Bradley, 2008). In big cities such as London, 86% of the schools were exposed to noise levels of 57 dBL_{Aeq} from road traffic (Shield & Dockrell, 2004).

Activity noise arises from the activity of the people in the building, noise from inside the space, and adjacent spaces. This noise source is people's activities resulting from normal daily activities such as talking, walking, moving furniture, and handling papers, educational materials, and temporary or permanent instructional equipment. Activity noise usually varies in pitch, loudness, and periodicity depending on the events.

Activity noise consists of a lot of speech. This kind of noise (speech babble) is a strong speech masker because it has the same spectrum as the target speech. Such noise impairs sound identification whenever the number of speakers rises as the speech-noise becomes more continuous (Lu & Cooke, 2008; Simpson & Cooke, 2005).

Activity noise levels and their effects on voice use have been studied most often in schools and in kindergartens. There were no large differences between the activity noise levels for class levels from one (6–7 years old) to six (11–12 years old). (Sato & Bradley, 2008). The younger and the more the children, the higher are the noise levels (Shield et al., 2015). Learning spaces for 5- and 6-year-old children are some of the noisiest (83 dB) (McAllister, Granqvist, Sjölander, & Sundberg, 2009), meaning that noise levels are highest when they should be lowest. The high activity noise levels are also measured in many schools (69–87 dB L_{Aeq}) (Kristiansen et al., 2014; Sala & Rantala, 2016; Shield & Dockrell, 2004; Wålinder, Gunnarsson, Runeson, & Smedje, 2007).

To overcome the effects of an interfering noise, a speaker has to use raised voice, which mostly happens unconsciously (ISO 9921–1). The phenomenon is known as the Lombard effect (Amazi & Garber, 1982; Lane & Tranel, 1971) and triggered in noise containing speech-similar frequencies (Stowe & Golop, 2013). The activity noise levels measured in schools and kindergartens indicate that teachers will have to increase their vocal effort to increase their voice SPL if they want to be heard (van Heusden, Plomp, & Pols, 1979). Speakers raise their voice level even up to 1 dB per 1 dB rising noise level (ISO 9921–1.1996). There is some variation in different studies and of course considerable individual variation (Lindstrom et al., 2011).

Besides voice level, noise also regulates other voice features. A speaker's F_0 increases (Aronsson, Bohman, Ternström, & Södersten, 2007; Garnier, Henrich, & Dubois, 2010) and changes can also be found in voice spectrum (energy shifts toward higher frequencies; Cooke & Lu, 2010). The spectral changes reflect voice quality becoming more hyperfunctional. Furthermore, noise affects speech prosody: Speech rate gets slower and expressions shorter (Van Summers, Pisoni, Bernacki, Pedlow, & Stokes, 1988). These alterations make speech easier for a listener to perceive. Speaking in noise may decrease speech capacity to code positive emotional information to the speech or the codes are incorrect (angry). Some reference for that has been found in preliminary studies by Lyberg-Åhlander (2016).

A recent study showed that speakers' (teachers') voices seem to react to some extent in different ways to the background noise versus the activity noise, probably due to their different qualities (Rantala et al., 2015a). In the study, teachers' voices were recorded before and after work. According to the results, the teachers working in louder background noise used higher voice levels already before work than those working in quieter classrooms. This may express the teachers' adaptations to use loud voice ("teacher's voice"); thus, it may also be a sign of chronic loading. Loud voice naturally causes a risk for a voice disorder.

Another finding was that background noise lowered F_0 of male teachers but did not affect females' F_0. A reason for this may be the quality of background noise containing typically low frequencies (Berglund, Hassmen, & Job, 1996) that are closer to men's voice pitches than those of women. Low-frequency noise has also been shown to be annoying, especially among sensitive people (Leventhall, 2004) and plausibly among young children, too. As a vocal reaction to pupils' restless behavior, male teachers lowered their voice pitch instead of increasing it as one could expect on the basis of the Lombard effect (Garnier et al., 2010). Namely, low voice expresses dominance (Hodges-Simeon, Gaulin, & Puts, 2010) that might have helped teachers to keep pupils calm. It is also possible that edema in the vocal fold mucosa due to loading may have caused lower F_0 in men.

In turn, under high activity noise, teachers' ability to react to loading seems to deteriorate (Rantala et al., 2015a), which becomes apparent in the finding that voice features generally changed less (more narrow dynamic range of voice variability) during work for teachers with higher activity noise than for teachers with quieter classes. Because the participants of the study were teachers who have worked years in the same conditions, one can assume that the findings may express the long-standing loading-induced effects of noise or compensation reactions to it.

Acoustics

Good acoustics support speaker's voice production and listener's speech perception. In a room with good acoustics, a speaker gets feedback from his or her voice and the voice carries to a long distance without extra effort in voice production. In an acoustically good room, acoustics do not change the acoustic structure of the speech so that it is available to the listener in its undistorted form. A listener hears the message loud enough without extra effort in listening, and energy is left for the processing of the message.

There are standards in which acceptable or recommended values of acoustics are given to several kinds of environments (ANSI/ASA S12.60-2010). Different nations have their own standards that, however, are near each other.

Poor acoustics in a classroom exacerbate the harmful effect of the noise by making it more continuous and restricting its attenuation (Pekkarinen (Sala) &Viljanen, 1991; Sala et al., 2002; Sala, Viljanen, & Honka, 1995). Worryingly, only in a few learning spaces do acoustics comply with the recommendations in the literature (Kristiansen et al., 2014; Sala et al., 2002; Sala & Rantala, 2016). Noise levels naturally depend on the numbers and the ages of pupils and the work they are engaged in, and likewise for the measurement method used in the studies and the period of observation.

Speaking in Vehicles

Speaking in a vehicle may be loading. In a car there is a lot of noise because of the running motor, tires, air flow, ventilation, and audio equipment. Noise levels depend on a car, but the level may rise up to around 70 dB(A) or even much higher. This means that when speaking in a car, a raised or even shouting voice is used. In cars, air quality may also cause a risk for voice. Air may be dry and contain impurities (pollution) from a car itself and from the road and nature.

Environmental Factors: Indoor Air Quality

Indoor air may affect vocal fold mucous membranes. When the mucous membranes of vocal folds are moist and pliable, they move easily, and the voice springs up effortlessly. At rest people inhale through the nose. This warms up and humidifies air, which keeps mucous membranes moist. Nose breathing moistens air up to over 90% relative humidity. There are, however, several situations when people take air through the mouth. The most typical situation is naturally when people speak and then the quality of indoor air affects immediately the mucous membranes.

Good indoor air is humid, and its temperature varies between 70°F and 73°F (21°C and 23°C). Air is not dusty or stuffy, and there are no unpleasant smells in a room. The idea of the ventilation is to change the air with different kinds of impurities to fresh air. The volume of ventilation is usually given in liters per second either per square meter or number of subjects in the room. When people work or spend time indoors with good air quality, their eyes do not become irritated, and they do not have other adverse effects.

Regrettably, indoor air quality has been shown to be poor in many schools both in Europe (Simoni et al., 2010) and in the United States (Godwin & Batterman, 2007). Visible mold has also been found in 14 to 39% of buildings according to a study made in 132 different areas of 12 countries (Antova et al., 2008). A most typical reason for mold formations is water damage. Moreover, in a cold climate when heating temperatures in classrooms tend to be higher than are the recommendations (Mumovic et al., 2009) or being even at recommended limits the humidity may drop below 20% relative humidity.

Indoor air affects voice. In poor indoor air people experience more voice symptoms and more often get laryngitis than those working in good conditions (Rantala et al., 2012). As a sign of this, it was found that their voice loudness (level) rises (Rantala et al., 2015b). This reaction may be due to changes in the mucous membranes of vocal folds (increment in viscoelasticity). To produce good voice, more power in voice production is needed, thus resulting in higher level (loudness). This means that louder voice may be a speaker's way to improve voice functioning and quality.

If the air is dry, the viscosity and stiffness of the mucosa of vocal folds increase (Hemler, Wieneke, Lebacq, & Dejonckere, 2001; Miri, Barthelat, & Mongeau, 2012), which raises the phonation threshold pressure (Vilkman et al., 1997) and changes the mucosal wave by decreasing its amplitude and frequency (Nakagawa, Fukuda, Kawaida, Shiotani, & Kanzaki, 1998; Witt, Taylor, Regner, & Jiang, 2011). These alterations make voice production more effortful. Dry and stiff mucosa needs more muscle power and subglottic pressure to get the mucosal wave to propagate, which, for its part, increases a risk for tissue damage. An experiment using excised canine larynges revealed that the direct effect of dry air on voice production is a slight decrease in sound pressure level when using the same flow (Jiang, Ng, & Hanson, 1999).

In a work environment, an impurity deteriorating indoor air quality is dust. Dustiness may arise from lack of cleaning and/or furnishing materials that collect dust. Dust inside a room contains skin epithelium and different kinds of cloth and textile fibers. As a hygroscopic material, dust also dehydrates air.

Exposure to organic dust has been shown to cause voice symptoms (Geneid et al., 2009), and further, respiratory allergies increase risks for getting voice symptoms (Simberg, Sala, Tuomainen, & Rönnemaa, 2009). Organic and chemical impurities trigger allergic or inflammatory reactions in the laryngeal mucous membranes (Roto & Sala, 1996; Sala, Hytönen, Tupasela, & Estlander, 1996). People with occupational asthma were found to develop asthma in the long term and as such confirm the primary asthma diagnosis. It is probable that laryngitis also results from occupational exposure. Namely, the same agents in indoor air that have been diagnosed to be the causes of occupational asthma have also been diagnosed as the causes of laryngitis. This same exposure agent in asthma and laryngitis supports the existence of occupational laryngitis (Hannu, Sala, & Toskala, 2009). Toxic substances emitted by mold may also cause voice (Patovirta, 2005) and upper respiratory symptoms (Hope & Simon, 2007). Although there is no evidence so far that toxic substances cause laryngitis and voice symptoms and thus, voice disorders, on the basis of clinical experience this kind of mechanism seems to be very presumable. If ventilation is poor in a room, the risks of acquiring a voice problem will multiply because fresh air does not replace impure air fast enough (Godwin & Batterman, 2007).

Coldness and draft are also voice ergonomic risk factors. They tend to increase muscle activity and tension since the body tries to increase body temperature by means of muscle activity. These reactions also occur to voice organs. Feeling of draft is due to a too intense local cooling of skin. Airflow velocity, turbulence, air temperature, and heat transfer by radiation (for example, cold window surfaces) are factors that affect feeling draft (Melikov, Popiolek, Silva, Care, & Sefker, 2007).

Personal Factors: Stress

Stress is a complex physiological reaction of an organism to a stressor that may be environmental, acute (affects an organism in the short term), or chronic (affects an organism over the longer term). Stress is a reaction of the sympathetic nervous system that interacts with the endocrine system and the parasympathetic nervous system. Everyone experiences some level of stress, but severe acute stress or chronic low-grade stress may induce abnormalities in body physiology and thus cause cognitive, emotional, physical, or behavioral symptoms.

Stress is a normal physiological response reaction, but it has also a pathological side. Stress or actually perception of stress is harmful and has detrimental effects on the human body. Psychological stress is given as an interpretation for many symptoms and diseases, including voice symptoms and voice disorders. Studies on association of voice symptoms and psychological stress have revealed the association to be true. The effect of psychological stress on voice has been found in a questionnaire study (N = 1,728) (Holmqvist, Santtila, Lindström, Sala, & Simberg, 2013). Stress also changes acoustic voice parameters (Mendoza & Carballo, 1998, 1999).

How stress increases the risk for a voice disorder is a complex cause and effect continuum or circle of events/acts. As a voice disorder affects the performance of a speaker (Sala et al., 2002), the voice disorder itself can be a stressor for an individual, which may create a circle: Stress is a risk factor of a voice disorder, and a voice disorder increases stress in the affected individual.

General anxiety or tension is known to be associated with increased muscle tension (Dahlström, Carlsson, Gale, & Jansson, 1985). Stress may increase even laryngeal muscle tension in association with emotional (and cardiovascular) arousal. Stress has also been mentioned to be a potential cause of muscle tension dysphonia (MTD) (Altman, Atkinson, & Lazarus, 2005; Dietrich, Abbott, Gartner-Schmidt, & Rosen, 2008). Stress affects upper and lower esophageal sphincters by relaxing them, thus increasing the possibility of stomach contents regurgitating into the esophagus (gullet) and larynx. As laryngeal mucous membranes do not tolerate stomach contents, they get inflamed. Inflamed mucous membranes are stiff and not as pliable as normal mucous membranes to make vocal fold waves. That causes a voice disorder. Muscle tension dysphonia may also develop via laryngitis. This may not be a direct consequence of stress (Morrison, Nichol, & Rammage, 1986), but many other factors are also probably involved.

Because of this manifold connection between stress and a voice disorder, the stress level of individuals with a voice disorder is worth exploring. By dealing with causes of stress, the voice disorder may get better, although stress seldom is a sole reason.

Environmental Factors: Sound Amplifiers

The most commonly used aids by occupational or professional voice users are amplifiers. Their use is standard in many situations. The speaker and singer get information about his or her voice production via internal and external channels. Internal feedback comes from the intention to produce a particular utterance and stored spatial-temporal voice patterns (central nervous system). Feedback is received from respiration, laryngeal and articulation muscle activity, and movements (articulatory contact and air pressure changes). The external feedback comes from a speaker's own voice as auditory feedback and listener reactions, which are verbal and nonverbal. The speaker gets information about his or her own voice through body-conduction, direct airborne sound from mouth, and reflected sound to his or her ear. Reflected (indirect) sound is radiated from the speaker, reflected from the environment surfaces, and returned back to the speaker's ear. The reflected sound of a speaker's own voice depends on the acoustic environment, but the reflected sound is usually lower in level than are body-conducted and direct airborne sounds. The reflected sound can be affected by using electroacoustic amplification systems (Pellegrin-Garcha, 2011). Another indication for using an amplifier is to amplify the sound to be better heard.

From the voice users point of view, using an amplifier decreases loading of vocal organs. Voice disorders are frequent among teachers (Pekkarinen (Sala) et al., 1992; Smith et al., 1997; Roy et al., 2004; Russel et al., 1998,) because of the high loading of voice production in learning environments (Sala et al., 2002). By using sound amplification the loading can be reduced. The subjective benefit of using a sound amplifier is less voice tiring and voice symptoms (Bovo, Trevisi, Emanuelli, & Martini, 2013; Jonsdottir, 2003; Jonsdottir, Laukkanen, & Vilkman, 2002; Jonsdottir, Rantala, Oskarsson, & Sala, 2015; Rosenberg, Blake-Rahter, Allen, & Redmond, 1994; Roy et al., 2004). In the study of Bovo et al. (2013), teachers' handicap due to vocal symptoms (VHI) decreased during 3 months follow-up using amplification. In addition, it is easier to speak and voice can be used for longer durations in speaking without fatigue (Jonsdottir, 2003). Particularly, teachers with a voice disorder benefit from using amplification. They report less symptoms and an improved voice quality, which means that their voice disorder may start recovering (Bovo et al., 2013; Roy et al., 2004)

Box 1–7

Benefits of sound amplifier on teachers' voice are as follows:

- easier to speak,
- decreased need to repeat instructions,
- voice that lasts a longer time,
- less voice tiring and symptoms,
- better voice quality,
- decreased voice symptoms, and
- easier recovery from a voice disorder.

From the listener's point of view, sound is at a level where it is possible to hear and identify the message. When the student hears the speech easily, it is not necessary to put so much effort into listening, and the energy is available for higher central processing. The sound-field amplification improves students' activity in many ways: The system had a positive effect on overall achievement of students (Edwards & Feun, 2005). According to teachers' observations, students concentrate better while the teacher is using sound amplification (Jonsdottir, 2003). Students perform better in language (Chelius, 2004)) and mathematical tests. Students also perform better in tests concerning reading skills (Chelius, 2004). According to a questionnaire study among teachers, students are more relaxed, behave better, understand instructions better, answer quicker, and perform better because concentration was improved (Jonsdottir, 2003).

Sound amplification may have detrimental effects, too. If the inconveniences are not eliminated, the use of the amplifier may decrease, and the possible improvement of student performance cannot be reached (Pinard, 2006). According to a questionnaire study, one-third of the students ($N = 528$) at schools felt the voice was too loud or annoying (Jonsdottir, 2003; Jonsdottir et al., 2015). They felt the sound was tiring (Jonsdottir et al., 2015) or annoying (Jonsdottir, 2003). In free comments of 528 students, some felt irritated because the teacher could not use the amplifier. The teacher did not remember to shut off the amplifier while making personal instructions (Jonsdottir, 2003) since the amplification should be used only when giving instructions to the whole class.

It is important to choose the right kind of amplifier for the purpose, to find out how the system works, to learn to use it, and to maintain it in good and working condition. It is best to consult an expert in the field. If there is an internal circulation problem, it will cause a whistling noise, which is very annoying/disturbing. That occurs when the amplification is set at too high a level and the microphone and the loudspeaker are too near each other. This can be avoided by adjusting the amplification to a proper level and/or increasing the distance between the microphone and loudspeaker. In spaces with poor acoustics, the use of an amplifier meets challenges because the use of it may increase noisiness. Although the advantages have been shown also in acoustically poor classrooms (Larsen, Vega, & Ribera, 2008), it is wise to make acoustic treatment if the acoustics of the room do not meet the recommended criteria.

References

Altman, K. W., Atkinson, C., & Lazarus, C. (2005). Current and emerging concepts in muscle tension dysphonia: A 30-month review. *Journal of Voice, 19*, 261–267.

Amazi, D. K., & Garber, S. R. (1982). The Lombard sign as a function of age and task. *Journal of Speech, Language, and Hearing Research, 25*(4), 581–585. Retrieved from http://dx.doi.org/10.1121/1.396660

ANSI/ASA S12.60. (2010). *Classroom acoustics, part 1: Permanent schools.* New York, NY: American National Standards Institute/Acoustical Society of America.

Antova, T., Pattenden, S., Brunekreef, B., Heinrich, J., Rudnai, P., Forastiere, F., . . . Nikiforov, B. (2008). Exposure to indoor mould and children's respiratory health in the PATY study. *Journal of Epidemiology and Community Health, 62*(8), 708–714.

Arboleda, B. M. W., & Frederick, A. L. (2008). Considerations for maintenance of postural alignment for voice production. *Journal of Voice, 22*(1), 90–99.

Aronsson, C., Bohman, M., Ternström, S., & Södersten, M. (2007). Loud voice during environmental noise exposure in patients with vocal nodules. *Logopedics Phoniatrics Vocology, 32*(2), 60–70.

Berglund, B., Hassmen, P., & Job, R. S. (1996). Sources and effects of low-frequency noise. *Journal of the Acoustical Society of America, 99*(5), 2985–3002.

Bonney, R. A., & Corlett, E. N. (2002). Head posture and loading of the cervical spine. *Applied Ergonomics, 33*(5), 415–417.

Bovo, R., Trevisi, P., Emanuelli, E., & Martini, A. (2013). Voice amplification for primary school teachers with voice disorders: A randomized clinical trial. *International Journal of Occupational Medicine and Environmental Health, 26*(3), 363–372.

Chelius, L. (2004). *Trost amplification study.* Canby, Oregon: Canby School District.

Chiu, T. T., & Lam, P. K. (2007). The prevalence of and risk factors for neck pain and upper limb pain among secondary school teachers in Hong Kong. *Journal of Occupational Rehabilitation, 17*(1), 19–32.

Cooke, M., & Lu, Y. (2010). Spectral and temporal changes to speech produced in the presence of energetic and informational maskers. *Journal of the Acoustical Society of America, 128*(4), 2059–2069.

Dahlström, L., Carlsson, S. G., Gale, E. N., & Jansson, T. G. (1985). Stress-induced muscular activity in mandibular dysfunction: Effects of biofeedback training. *Journal of Behavioral Medicine, 8*(2), 191–200.

Dietrich, M., Abbott, K. V., Gartner-Schmidt, J., & Rosen, C. A. (2008). The frequency of perceived stress, anxiety, and depression in patients with common pathologies affecting voice. *Journal of Voice, 22*(4), 472–488.

Durup, N., Shield, B., Dance, S., Sullivan, R., & Gomez-Agustina, L. (2015). How classroom acoustics affect the vocal load of teachers. *Energy Procedia, 78*, 3084–3089.

Edwarda, D., & Feun, L. (2005). A formative evaluation of sound-field amplification system across several grade levels in four schools. *Journal of Educational Audiology, 12*, 59–66.

Erick, P. N., & Smith, D. R. (2011). A systematic review of musculoskeletal disorders among school teachers. *BMC Musculoskeletal Disorders, 12*(1), 1.

Fritzell, B. (1996). Voice disorders and occupations. *Logopedics Phoniatrics Vocology, 2*, 7–12.

Garnier, M., Henrich, N., & Dubois, D. (2010). Influence of sound immersion and communicative interaction on the Lombard effect. *Journal of Speech, Language, and Hearing Research, 53*(3), 588–608.

Geneid, A., Rönkkö, M., Airaksinen, L., Voutilainen, R., Toskala, E., Alku, P., & Vilkman, E. (2009). Pilot study on acute voice and throat symptoms related to exposure to organic dust: Preliminary findings from a provocation test. *Logopedics Phoniatrics Vocology, 34*(2), 67–72.

Godwin, C., & Batterman, S. (2007). Indoor air quality in Michigan schools. *Indoor Air, 17*(2), 109–121.

Grant, K. A., Habes, D. J., & Tepper, A. L. (1995). Work activities and musculoskeletal complaints among preschool workers. *Applied Ergonomics, 26*(6), 405–410.

Gunderman, H. (1970). *Die berufsdysphonie.* Leipzig, Germany: Georg Thieme.

Hannu, T., Sala, E., & Toskala, E. (2009). Long-term prognosis of immediate hypersensitivity type of occupational laryngitis. *Respiratory Medicine, 103*(1), 130–135.

Hansraj, K. K. (2014). Assessment of stresses in the cervical spine caused by posture and position of the head. *Surgical Technology International, 25*, 277–279.

Hemler, R. J., Wieneke, G. H., Lebacq, J., & Dejonckere, P. H. (2001). Laryngeal mucosa elasticity and viscosity in high and low relative air humidity. *European Archives of Oto-rhino-laryngology, 258*(3), 125–129.

Hodges-Simeon, C. R., Gaulin, S. J., & Puts, D. A. (2010). Different vocal parameters predict perceptions of dominance and attractiveness. *Human Nature, 21*(4), 406–427.

Holmqvist, S., Santtila, P., Lindström, E., Sala, E., & Simberg, S. (2013). The association between possible stress markers and vocal symptoms. *Journal of Voice, 27*, 787.e1–787.e10. doi:10.1016/j.jvoice.2013.06.012

Honda, K., Hirai, H., Masaki, S., & Shimada, Y. (1999). Role of vertical larynx movement and cervical lordosis in F0 control. *Language and Speech, 42*(4), 401–411.

Hope, A. P., & Simon, R. A. (2007). Excess dampness and mold growth in homes: An evidence-based review of the aeroirritant effect and its potential causes. *Allergy and Asthma Proceedings, 28*(3), 262–270.

ISO 9921-1. (1996). *Ergonomic assessment of speech communication. Part 1: Speech interference level and communication distances for persons with normal hearing capacity in direct communication (SIL method).* Geneva, Switzerland: International Organization for Standardization.

Iwarsson, J., & Sundberg, J. (1998). Effects of lung volume on vertical larynx position during phonation. *Journal of Voice, 12*(2), 159–165.

Jiang, J., Ng, J., & Hanson, D. (1999). The effects of rehydration on phonation in excised canine larynges. *Journal of Voice, 13*(1), 51–59.

Jonsdottir, V. (2003). *The voice: An occupational tool. A study of teacher's classroom speech and effects of amplification* (Academic dissertation). Acta Universitas Tamperensis 969. Tampere, Finland: University of Tampere.

Jonsdottir, V., Laukkanen, A. M., & Vilkman, E. (2002). Changes in teachers' speech during a working day with and without electric sound amplification. *Folia Phoniatrica et Logopaedica, 54*(6), 282–287.

Jonsdottir, V., Rantala, L. M., Oskarsson, G. K., & Sala, E. (2015). Effects of pedagogical ideology on the perceived loudness and noise levels in preschools. *Noise and Health, 17*(78), 282–293.

Kooijman, P. G. C., De Jong, F. I. C. R. S., Oudes, M. J., Huinck, W., Van Acht, H., & Graamans, K. (2005). Muscular tension and body posture in relation to voice handicap and voice quality in teachers with persistent voice complaints. *Folia Phoniatrica et Logopaedica, 57*(3), 134–147.

Kooijman, P. G. C., De Jong, F. I. C. R. S., Thomas, G., Huinck, W., Donders, R., Graamans, K., & Schutte, H. K. (2006). Risk factors for voice problems in teachers. *Folia Phoniatrica et Logopaedica, 58*(3), 159–174.

Korkmaz, N. C., Cavlak, U., & Telci, E. A. (2011). Musculoskeletal pain, associated risk factors and coping strategies in school teachers. *Scientific Research and Essays, 6*(3), 649–657.

Kristiansen, J., Lund, S. P., Persson, R., Shibuya, H., Nielsen, P. M., & Scholz, M. (2014). A study of classroom acoustics and school teachers' noise exposure, voice load and speaking time during teaching, and the effects on vocal and mental fatigue development. *International Archives of Occupational and Environmental Health, 87*(8), 851–860.

Lane, H., & Tranel, B. (1971). The Lombard sign and the role of hearing in speech. *Journal of Speech, Language, and Hearing Research, 14*(4), 677–709.

Larsen, J. B., Vega, A., & Ribera, J. E. (2008). The effect of room acoustics and sound-field amplification on word recognition performance in young adult listeners in suboptimal listening conditions. *American Journal of Audiology, 17*(1), 50–59. doi:10.1044/1059-0889(2008/006).

Lehto, L., Alku, P., Bäckstöm, T., & Vilkman, E. (2005). Voice symptoms of call-centre customer service advisers experienced during a work-day and effects after a short vocal training course. *Logopedics Phoniatrics Vocology, 30*(1), 14–27.

Leventhall, H. G. (2004). Low frequency noise and annoyance. *Noise and Health, 6*(23), 59.

Lindstrom, F., Waye, K. P., Södersten, M., McAllister, A., & Ternström, S. (2011). Observations of the relationship between noise exposure and preschool teacher voice usage in day-care center environments. *Journal of Voice, 25*(2), 166–172. doi:10.1016/j.jvoice.2009.09.009

Lowell, S. Y., Kelley, R. T., Colton, R. H., Smith, P. B., & Portnoy, J. E. (2012). Position of the hyoid and larynx in people with muscle tension dysphonia. *Laryngoscope, 122*(2), 370–377.

Lu, Y., & Cooke, M. (2008). Speech production modifications produced by competing talkers, babble, and stationary noise. *Journal of the Acoustical Society of America, 124*(5), 3261–3275.

Lyberg-Åhlander, V. (2016, September 9). *The teacher voice in a noisy classroom: How does a hoarse teacher voice affect students' performance and attitudes?* Presented at the Fifth Symposium of the Finnish Society of Voice Ergonomics, Helsinki, Finland.

McAllister, A. M., Granqvist, S., Sjölander, P., & Sundberg, J. (2009). Child voice and noise: A pilot study of noise in day cares and the effects on 10 children's voice quality according to perceptual evaluation. *Journal of Voice, 23*(5), 587–593.

Melikov, A. K., Popiolek, Z., Silva, M. C. G., Care, I., & Sefker, T. (2007). Accuracy limitations for low-velocity measurements and draft assessment in rooms. *HVAC&R Research, 13*(6), 971–986.

Mendoza, E., & Carballo, G. (1998). Acoustic analysis of induced vocal stress by means of cognitive workload tasks. *Journal of Voice, 12*(3), 263–273.

Mendoza, E., & Carballo, G. (1999). Vocal tremor and psychological stress. *Journal of Voice, 13*(1), 105–112.

Miri, A. K., Barthelat, F., & Mongeau, L. (2012). Effects of dehydration on the viscoelastic properties of vocal folds in large deformations. *Journal of Voice, 26*(6), 688–697.

Morrison, M. D., Nichol, H., & Rammage, L. A. (1986). Diagnostic criteria in functional dysphonia. *Laryngoscope, 96*(1), 1–8.

Mumovic, D., Palmer, J., Davies, M., Orme, M., Ridley, I., Oreszczyn, T., . . . Way, P. (2009). Winter indoor air quality, thermal comfort and acoustic performance of newly built secondary schools in England. *Building and Environment, 44*(7), 1466–1477.

Nakagawa, H., Fukuda, H., Kawaida, M., Shiotani, A., & Kanzaki, J. (1998). Lubrication mechanism of the larynx during phonation: An experiment in excised canine larynges. *Folia Phoniatrica et Logopaedica, 50*(4), 183–194.

Novak, A., Dlouha, O., Capkova, B., & Vohradnik, M. (1991). Voice fatigue after theater performance in actors. *Folia Phoniatrica et Logopaedica, 43*(2), 74–78.

Ohlsson, A. C., Brink, O., & Lofqvist, A. (1989). A voice accumulator—validation and application. *Journal of Speech, Language, and Hearing Research, 32*(2), 451–457.

Ohlsson, A. C., Järvholm, B., & Löfqvist, A. (1987). Vocal symptoms and vocal behaviour in teachers. *Scandinavian Journal of Logopedics and Phoniatrics, 12*, 61–69.

O'Sullivan, P. B., Grahamslaw, K. M., Kendell, M., Lapenskie, S. C., Möller, N. E., & Richards, K. V. (2002). The effect of different standing and sitting postures on trunk muscle activity in a pain-free population. *Spine, 27*(11), 1238–1244.

Patovirta, R. L. (2005). *Teachers' health in moisture-damaged schools: A follow-up study.* Publication of the National Public Health Institute. Kuopio, Finland: National Public Health Institute.

Pekkarinen (Sala), E., Himberg, L., & Pentti, J. (1992). Prevalence of vocal symptoms among teachers compared with nurses: A questionnaire study. *Scandinavian Journal of Logopedics and Phoniatrics, 17*(2), 113–117.

Pekkarinen (Sala), E., & Viljancn, V. (1991). Acoustic conditions for speech communication in classrooms. *Scandinavian Audiology, 20*(4), 257–263.

Pellegrin-Garcha, D. (2011). *The role of classroom acoustics on vocal intensity regulation and speakers' comfort* (Doctoral thesis). Lyngby, Denmark: Technical University of Denmark.

Pinard, L. (2006). *Prevalence of otitis media and hearing loss and effects of sound-field FM amplification among First Nations elementary school children* (Master's thesis). Halifax, Nova Scotia, Canada: Dalhousie University.

Rantala, L. M., Hakala, S. J., Holmqvist, S., & Sala, E. (2012). Connections between voice ergonomic risk factors and voice symptoms, voice handicap, and respiratory tract diseases. *Journal of Voice, 26*(6), 819.e13–819.e20.

Rantala, L. M., Hakala, S., Holmqvist, S., & Sala, E. (2013). Connections between voice ergonomic risk factors in classrooms and teachers' voice production. *Folia Phoniatrica et Logopaedica, 64*(6), 278–282.

Rantala, L. M., Hakala, S., Holmqvist, S., & Sala, E. (2015a). Classroom noise and teachers' voice production. *Journal of Speech, Language, and Hearing Research, 58*(5), 1397–1406.

Rantala, L. M., Hakala, S., Holmqvist, S., & Sala, E. (2015b). Associations between voice ergonomic risk factors and acoustic features of the voice. *Logopedics Phoniatrics Vocology, 40*(3), 99–105.

Rantala, L., Vilkman, E., & Bloigu, R. (2002). Voice changes during work: Subjective complaints and objective measurements for female primary and secondary schoolteachers. *Journal of Voice, 16*(3), 344–355.

Rosenberg, G., Blake-Rahter, P., Allen, L., & Redmond, B. (1994). Improving classroom acoustics: A multi-distinct pilot study on FM classroom amplification. *American Academy of Audiology Annual Convention, 2*, 24–29.

Roto, P., & Sala, E. (1996). Occupational laryngitis caused by formaldehyde: A case report. *American Journal of Industrial Medicine, 29*(3), 275–277.

Roy, N., Merrill, R. M., Thibeault, S., Parsa, R. A., Gray, S. D., & Smith, E. M. (2004). Prevalence of voice disorders in teachers and the general population. *Journal of Speech, Language, and Hearing Research, 47*(2), 281–293.

Rubin, J. S., Blake, E., & Mathieson, L. (2007). Musculoskeletal patterns in patients with voice disorders. *Journal of Voice, 21*(4), 477–484.

Russell, A., Oates, J., & Greenwood, K. (1998). Prevalence of voice problems in teachers. *Journal of Voice, 12*(4), 467–479.

Sala, E., Airo, E., Olkinuora, P., Simberg, S., Ström, U., Laine, A., . . . Suonpää, J. (2002). Vocal loading among day care center teachers. *Logopedics Phoniatrics Vocology, 27*(1), 21–28.

Sala, E., Hellgren, U-M., Ketola, R., Laine, A., Olkinuora, P., Rantala, L., & Sihvo, M. (2009). *Ääniergonomian kartoitusopas työpaikalla tehtävää ääniergonomista kartoitusta varten. (Handboork and checklist for voice ergonomic assessment in work environment).* Helsinki, Finland: Työterveyslaitos (Institute of Occupational Health).

Sala, E., Hytönen, M., Tupasela, O., & Estlander, T. (1996). Occupational laryngitis with immediate allergic or immediate type specific chemical hypersensitivity. *Clinical Otolaryngology and Allied Sciences, 21*(1), 42–48.

Sala, E., Laine, A., Simberg, S., Pentti, J., & Suonpää, J. (2001). The prevalence of voice disorders among day care center teachers compared with nurses: A questionnaire and clinical study. *Journal of Voice, 15*(3), 413–423.

Sala, E., & Rantala, L. (2016). Acoustics and activity noise in school classrooms in Finland. *Applied Acoustics, 114*, 252–259.

Sala, E., Sihvo, M., & Laine, A. (2005). *Röstergonomi—Rösten- ett fungerande arbetsredskap. Institutet för arbetshygien och Arbetarskyddscentralen.* (Voice ergonomics—A functional voice as a working tool). Helsinki, Finland: Työterveyslaitos ja Työturvallisuuskeskus (Institute of Occupational Health and Centre for Occupational Safety).

Sala, E., Sihvo, M., & Laine, A. (2011). *Ääniergonomia—Toimiva ääni työvälineenä.* (Voice ergonomics—A functional voice as a working tool) (2nd ed.). Helsinki, Finland: Työterveyslaitos & Työturvallisuuskeskus (Institute of Occupational Health and Centre for Occupational Safety).

Sala, E., Viljanen, V., & Honka, J. (1995). Improvement of acoustic conditions for speech communication in classrooms. *Applied Acoustics, 45*, 81–91.

Sato, H., & Bradley, J. S. (2008). Evaluation of acoustical conditions for speech communication in working elementary school classrooms. *Journal of the Acoustical Society of America, 123*(4), 2064–2077.

Shield, B., Conetta, R., Dockrell, J., Connolly, D., Cox, T., & Mydlarz, C. (2015). A survey of acoustic conditions and noise levels in secondary school classrooms in England. *Journal of the Acoustical Society of America, 137*(1), 177–188.

Shield, B., & Dockrell, J. E. (2004). External and internal noise surveys of London primary schools. *Journal of the Acoustical Society of America, 115*(2), 730–738.

Shield, B., Greenland, E., & Dockrell, J. (2010). Noise in open plan classrooms in primary schools: A review. *Noise Health, 12*, 225–234. Retrieved from http://www.noiseandhealth.org/text.asp?2010/12/49/225/70501

Simberg, S., Sala, E., Tuomainen, J., & Rönnemaa, A. M. (2009). Vocal symptoms and allergy—a pilot study. *Journal of Voice, 23*(1), 136–139.

Simoni, M., Annesi-Maesano, I., Sigsgaard, T., Norback, D., Wieslander, G., Nystad, W., . . . Viegi, G. (2010). School air quality related to dry cough, rhinitis and nasal patency in children. *European Respiratory Journal, 35*(4), 742–749.

Simpson, S. A., & Cooke, M. (2005). Consonant identification in N-talker babble is a nonmonotonic function of N. *Journal of the Acoustical Society of America, 118*(5), 2775–2778.

Smith, E., Gray, S., Dove, H., Kirchner, L., & Heras, H. (1997). Frequency and effects of teachers' voice problems. *Journal of Voice, 11*(1), 81–87.

Södersten, M., Granqvist, S., Hammarberg, B., & Szabo, A. (2002). Vocal behavior and vocal loading factors for pre-school teachers at work studied with binaural DAT recordings. *Journal of Voice, 16*(3), 356–371.

Södersten, M., & Lindhe, C. (2011). *Kunskapsöversikt—Yrkestelaterade röststörningar och röstergonomi* (Scientific review—Occupation related voice disorders and voice ergonomics). Rapport (report) 6. Stockholm: Arbetsmiljöverket (Swedish Work Environment Authority). Retrived from https://www.av.se/en/search/?qry=S%C3%B6dersten+Lindhe

Stowe, L. M., & Golob, E. J. (2013). Evidence that the Lombard effect is frequency-specific in humans. *Journal of the Acoustical Society of America, 134*(1), 640–647.

Szeto, G. P., & Lee, R. (2002). An ergonomic evaluation comparing desktop, notebook, and subnotebook computers. *Archives of Physical Medicine and Rehabilitation, 83*(4), 527–532.

Van den Heuvel, S. G., de Looze, M. P., Hildebrandt, V. H., & Thé, K. H. (2003). Effects of software programs stimulating regular breaks and exercises on work-related neck and upper-limb disorders. *Scandinavian Journal of Work, Environment and Health, 29*(2), 106–116.

Van Heusden, E., Plomp, R., & Pols, L. C. W. (1979). Effect of ambient noise on the vocal output and the preferred listening level of conversational speech. *Applied Acoustics, 12*(1), 31–43.

Van Summers, W., Pisoni, D. B., Bernacki, R. H., Pedlow, R. I., & Stokes, M. A. (1988). Effects of noise on speech production: Acoustic and perceptual analyses. *Journal of the Acoustical Society of America, 84*(3), 917–928.

Vilkman, E., Lauri, E. R., Alku, P., Sala, E., & Sihvo, M. (1997). Loading changes in time-based parameters of glottal flow waveforms in different ergonomic conditions. *Folia Phoniatrica et Logopaedica, 49*(5), 247–263.

Vilkman, E., & Manninen, O. (1986). Changes in prosodic features of speech due to environmental factors. *Speech Communication, 5*(3–4), 331–345.

Vilkman, E., Sonninen, A., Hurme, P., & Körkkö, P. (1996). External laryngeal frame function in voice production revisited: A review. *Journal of Voice, 10*(1), 78–92.

Vintturi, J., Alku, P., Lauri, E. R., Sala, E., Sihvo, M., & Vilkman, E. (2001a). The effects of post-loading rest on acoustic parameters with special reference to gender and ergonomic factors. *Folia phoniatrica et Logopaedica, 53*(6), 338–350.

Vintturi, J., Alku, P., Lauri, E-R., Sala, E., Sihvo, M., & Vilkman, E. (2001b). Objective analysis of vocal warm-up with special reference to ergonomic factors. *Journal of Voice, 15*(1), 36–53.

Wålinder, R., Gunnarsson, K., Runeson, R., & Smedje, G. (2007). Physiological and psychological stress reactions in relation to classroom noise. *Scandinavian Journal of Work, Environment and Health, 33*(4), 260–266.

Walsh, D. P. (1975). Noise levels and annoyance in open plan educational facilities. *Journal of Architectural Research, 4*(2), 5–16.

Wilson, J. R. (2000). Fundamentals of ergonomics in theory and practice. *Applied Ergonomics, 31*(6), 557–567.

Witt, R. E., Taylor, L. N., Regner, M. F., & Jiang, J. J. (2011). Effects of surface dehydration on mucosal wave amplitude and frequency in excised canine larynges. *Otolaryngology-Head and Neck Surgery, 144*(1), 108–113.

Yip, C. H. T., Chiu, T. T. W., & Poon, A. T. K. (2008). The relationship between head posture and severity and disability of patients with neck pain. *Manual Therapy, 13*(2), 148–154.

CHAPTER 2

Test-Theory-Training-Transfer: Voice Training in Future Radio Presenters

Bernadette Timmermans and Marc De Bodt

Radio Landscape

Short Radio History

In Flanders one can listen to a public radio station from VRT (Vlaamse Radio en Televisie—Flemish Radio and Television, http://www.vrt.be) or to a commercial radio station from Medialaan ("Media avenue," http://www.medialaan.be). Next to these media houses, a lot of smaller radio stations operate as well (e.g., Radio Nostalgie or BRUZZ).

The Flemish Radio and Television (VRT) is the public broadcasting network of the Flemish Community. The mission and its stipulations are laid down in the media decree as well as in the management contract with the Flemish government. The management contract between the Flemish Community and the VRT regulates the special rules and conditions for granting the financial envelope—EUR 277 million in 2016 for radio and television—needed for the execution of its mission. The VRT submits an annual report on the degree to which the objectives and performance criteria laid down in the management contract have been met. In addition to the financial support of the Flemish government, advertisement is a source of income. The turnover of 2015 was EUR 441.2 million, the EBITDA (earnings before interest, taxes, depreciation, and amortization, December 2015) was EUR 4.8 million. Medialaan is a joint venture of two media groups (i.e., Persgroep and Roularta Media Group) and earns its income from advertisement only. The turnover of 2015 is EUR 442.6 million, the EBITDA amounted to EUR 41.8 million (December 2015).

On March 28, 1914, a pilot channel in Laeken (Brussels) transmits the first radio broadcast in Belgium. In 1930, the National Institute for Radio Broadcasting (NIR/INR) is granted a national monopoly, and in 1931 the NIR broadcasts its programs in Dutch (INR broadcasts in French). In 1947 the first regional channel Radio 2 (family radio) is launched, and in 1960 NIR becomes BRT and RTB (Belgian Radio and Television—Radio Télévision Belge). The radio stations from VRT in 2016 are Radio 1 (culture radio with news and sports), Radio 2 (family radio), MNM (hit radio), Klara (classical music), and Studio Brussel (radio for the youth). The core staff of the radio stations amounts to 262 individuals, 92 of whom are presenters and 37 journalists announce news reports (permanent or freelance personnel). Medialaan was founded in 2000, and in November 2001 Radio 4FM was launched. In 2009 4FM became "Q-music" with the slogan: "Q is good for you." In April 2009 "Joe" started with the slogan "your greatest hits." The core staff of the radio stations included 94 individuals, 14 of whom are announcers and 11 journalists make the news reports (permanent or freelance personnel).

Radio Training Program and Demographics

Most universities (bachelor or master degree) offer relevant courses in broadcasting, media, and communication, but a specific and unique education to become a radio maker is the artistic-oriented schooling "Bachelor or Master of Arts in Audiovisual Communication" of the Royal Institute of Theatre, Cinema, and Sound (RITCS). The RITCS in Brussels delivers polyvalent radio makers. This program has four basic components: radio documentary, sound art, radio drama, and radio program/presentation.

The future radio makers are young men and women between 18 and 25 years, lately more women than men are attending this training. They all belong to the Flemish community of Belgium. Sometimes students from the Netherlands participate in the training as well. All students have a high school degree at the beginning of their study. Since the start of the bachelor/master structure of higher education in Belgium, there has been an increasing interest of candidates with a bachelor or master degree (linguistics, politics, and sociology) to attend the course of radio maker.

In 1985 the training program for radio students contained 1 specialization year, preceded by 2 years in a wide-ranging program for audiovisual communication. The radio program gradually grew into an independent department, and in 1994 a full 4-year training was set up. In that first year, five students graduated (https//radio.ritcs.be/). Meanwhile, the radio program was well known and the number of students attending the radio training increased to an average of 40. Each year 5 to 10 students graduate. Usually, 15 to 18 students start in the first year.

Every candidate must pass an admission test where writing and communication skills, and cultural, political, and topical background are verified. Next to this, speech skills and voice

Box 2–1

Case 1
Male, 20 years old, 1st Bachelor Radio
Complaint: dyslexia
Responsible for Web content

This student had a nice voice and quite good diction, but due to his dyslexia, it was difficult to read a text in a proper way. He hesitated, made mistakes, and repeated a lot of syllables. But this young man was very inventive in hiding his reading problem. When he needed to read a text or bulletin, he always used a tablet with an auto cue prompter. This software made it possible to alter the speed of the text, and sentence by sentence occurred, in this way he could read much better. He learned that preparation was of utmost importance. As this student was very creative, had profound technical insights, good presentation skills, and could improvise as well, we believed that this reading problem should be no problem to him becoming a radio maker. He currently works for a commercial radio station and is responsible for Web content.

quality are assessed as well. Candidates with poor diction and/or a deviant voice quality are not permitted to start this education. If, however, the candidate excels in other qualities, an exception can be made under strict conditions (e.g., surgery and/or voice therapy).

Tasks of a Radio Maker

In the RITCS future radio makers are not trained to present radio shows only. The radio maker needs to be polyvalent and must excel in various skills. The term *radio maker* refers to the fact that he or she "makes" or designs a format for a radio program. It is also possible that this radio maker presents his or her own program. Radio makers may function as editors, researchers, presenters/announcers, technicians, or producers. Sometimes these functions also spill over into each other as every radio station has its own interpretation of the different jobs. Next to this, a radio career is very variable as a producer may become a presenter or a researcher may become a producer, and different kinds of career switches are possible. Whatever the task of the radio maker might be, he or she is always a part of the radio station. It must be clear that they work for a media house: for Medialaan (commercial radio stations) or for VRT (public radio stations) or for other more regional stations. The different media houses have websites of their brands, mentioning their presenters, producers, or researchers. In Belgium "known" presenters just start to use social media (Facebook: Jan Demeulemeester [Medialaan] and Jan Balliauw [VRT]) or make their own websites (http://www.petervandeveire.be). Until recently, presenters were not allowed to use social media or websites in their own name.

As an editor the radio maker needs to manage one or more radio shows in accordance of the concept and the target audience. He or she needs to have an extensive network and understand the contribution of every colleague. An editor arranges day/week/month and annual plans and follows the current events and news bulletins closely. An editor needs excellent communication skills.

As a researcher the radio maker prepares interviews, documentaries, and parts of a radio show. He contacts guests, looks for the necessary information, and makes sure that the content and/or audio files are ready for broadcasting. A researcher is creative and proposes topics or delivers other perspectives as a contribution to the show.

As a presenter the radio maker needs to absorb all information and briefings and convert them into an understandable content for the listeners. The presenter embodies the program and quite often his or her name is assigned to the program (e.g., https://radio1.be/programma/hautekiet, referring to the morning program "Hautekiet" of Jan Hautekiet). As a consequence, the presenter submits concepts, ideas, and topics. He or she is a good communicator and team player. The presenter may also write and/or deliver sports, news, and weather reports. Radio presenters who work mainly with music are called disc jockeys (DJ's) (e.g., Q music [Medialaan—commercial radio] presents "Maarten Vancoillie and Dorothee Dauwe" http://qmusic.be/programmas/maarten-dorothee). At times they may comment on certain songs while taking requests from listeners, though DJ's do not typically select most of the songs that are played. The presenters may become radio *personalities*, they may be called on to either host or make an appearance at charitable events and other public functions. For example, due to his status as a "known personality," Peter Van de Veire (DJ of MNM, VRT) presents TV shows as well (e.g., https://songfestival.be/eurosong2016/peter-van-de-veire-eurosong-2016-gaat-van-scherm-spatten/).

As a technician the presenter understands the basics of studio and editing programs. He or she is able to work the control board and takes care of a well-timed transition between announcement and music. He is able to make jingles and promo spots and takes care of the "sound" of the station.

As a producer the radio maker creates the conditions within which the program can be realized and is therefore in charge for a smooth flow of the radio show. During broadcasting he or she is responsible for the communication between everybody involved in the show (presenter, guests, and technician). A director checks timing and scenario, and he or she also welcomes and briefs the guests. He or she composes the team and takes care of an efficient and viable division of tasks for every member in a way that each of them knows what the outlines of everyone's mission is. Deadlines, agendas, website, and briefings are clearly communicated. The producer also keeps an eye on the long-term evolution of the show.

Vocal Demands of the Radio Maker as a Presenter

It is clear that the radio maker needs outstanding reading, writing, and communication skills. What about the vocal capabilities, and what are the tasks of a radio voice (Figure 2–1)? The radio voice must be able to present, to announce, to deliver radio promo spots or advertising, or function as a voice-over in documentaries. A presenter often works ad lib, an announcer "tells" the news while reading and in the role as a voice in spots or advertisements, interpretation skills are necessary. Whatever the function of the voice might be, the voice needs to sound pleasant, warm, mature, and attractive. The diction must be perfect without influences of a dialect, hesitations, or needless repetitions with an immediate intelligibility as a result. A natural and intelligent intonation is indispensable when news or sport bulletins are delivered. The presenter understands when loudness needs to be adapted: excited and thus louder to deliver sports and restrained and quieter in voice-over. The presenter comprehends the sound of every station, and knows exactly when the voice requires a low or high pitch. He or she is sensitive to breaks and pauses and uses them at the right moments without interrupting the flow of the program, and he or she varies in speed when necessary. According to the culture of the Northern part of Europe the quality of the voice needs to be clear, whereas in the more Southern part of Europe harsh voices are accepted. This "Mediterranean voice quality" seems to be peculiar to the southern temperament (Timmermans, 2003, 2008, 2013). This difference implies that the audience in Belgium is more sensitive to an outstanding quality of a voice.

In order to fully understand the impact of several parameters of the voice, we examined the influence of time on the pitch of women and men announcing news bulletins. Research revealed that the voices of women lowered significantly over the last 20 years (Niclaes, 2013). The changed position of the woman in our society may be responsible for this change. Next to this we also concluded that a presenter is allowed to talk quite fast, as long as he or she pauses long enough. The listener needs "cognitive pauses" to be able to fully understand the presenter (Coekaerts & Wuyts, 2014).

The Importance of Vocal Hygiene

Table 2–1 presents the parameters "duration, intensity, frequency, and quality" of voice use in relation to "dependency on the voice" in the function of the job. Research revealed that the parameter "time" is the most detrimental factor for the voice. Thus, the longer the voice use, the higher the risk on vocal pathology. The second factor should be frequency, followed by intensity (De Bodt et al., 2015).

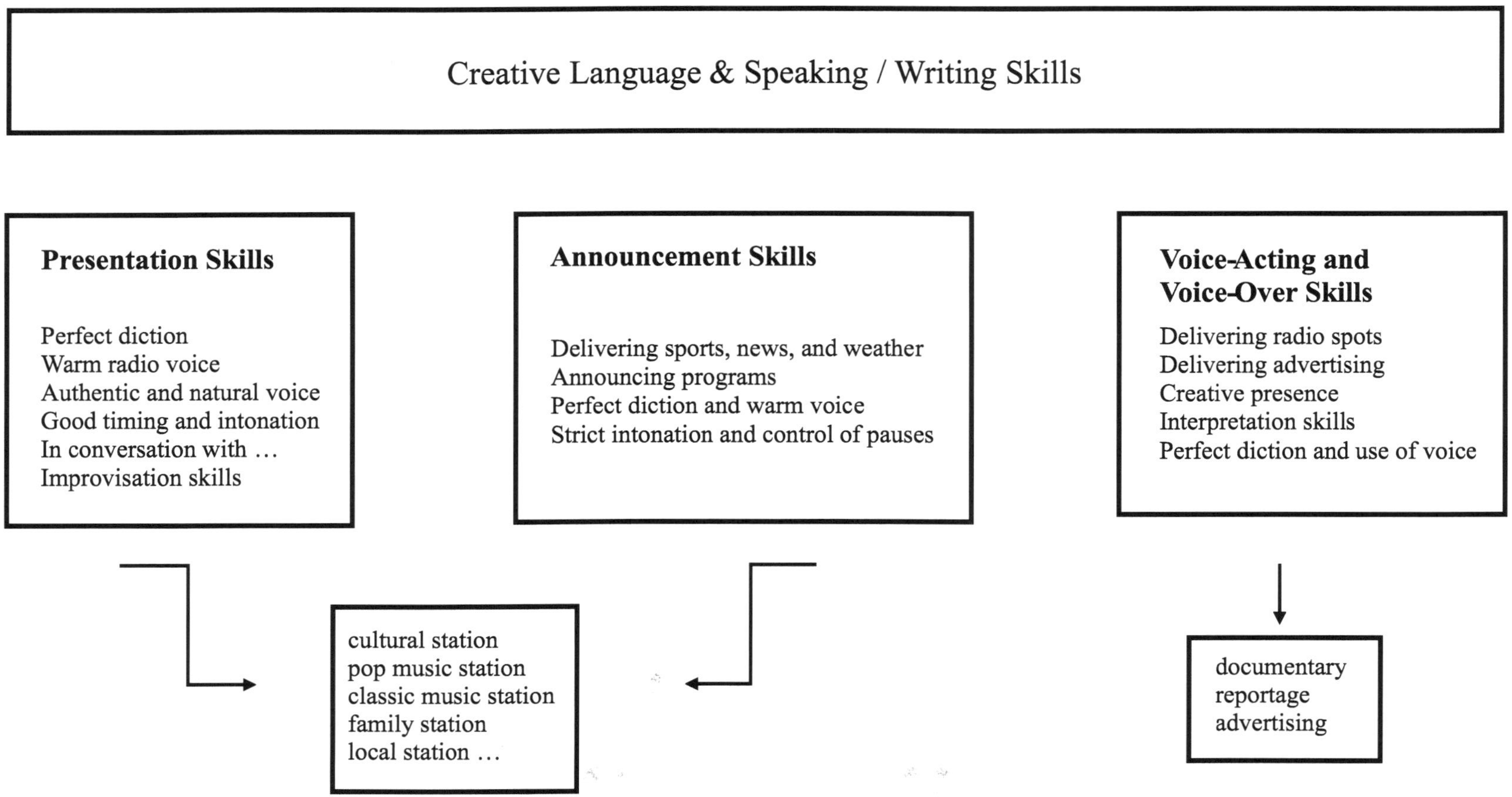

Figure 2–1. *Vocal capabilities and tasks of a radio presenter.*

Table 2–1. *The Parameters ofVoice Use in Function of the Job*

		Parameters			
		Duration Long	**Intensity Loud**	**Frequency Correct F_0**	**Quality High**
Voice-dependent job	Teachers	+++	++	++	Preferably
	Singers	++	++	++	Preferably
	Actors	++	++	++	Preferably
	Call-center personnel	+++	+	++	Preferably
	Sellers	++	–	++	Preferably
	Politicians	++	++	++	Preferably
	Presenters (radio and TV)	+	–	+++	Necessity
	Workers	–	–	–	–
	Professional drivers	–	–	–	–
	Office personnel	–	–	–	–

The radio presenter does not have to use the voice the whole day and since he or she uses a microphone he or she should not speak loudly all day, whereas the teacher uses the voice throughout the day and should speak rather loudly. The voice of a radio presenter must sound warm and appealing to listen to. It would be satisfying if the teacher has a pleasing voice as well, but that is not a necessary condition. This prerequisite asks for good vocal hygiene to guarantee superb voice quality.

In contrast to our expectations, research in future radio presenters/makers revealed that in spite of the awareness that they are absolutely dependent on their voices, they forget to take the appropriate precautions for voice care. Research by Timmermans et al. (2005) showed that in this population (n = 23) that received an intensive training in vocal hygiene, the smoking prevalence persisted (48%), 13% remained vocally abusive, and 26% ate late three times a week. Raphael (1991) states that smoking is always a problem in proper voice care and seems to be popular in the artistic and media environment. Seventy-three percent indicated that stress is an important factor affecting their voice. There is no plausible declaration for the neglected vocal hygiene, and the results of studies on vocal hygiene education are not unambiguous. Some studies are in favor of vocal hygiene (Chan, 1994; Roy et al., 2002; Yiu, 2002), while Timmermans et al. (2005) and Broaddus-Lawrence, Treole, McCabe, Allen, and Toppin (2000) found a relatively small impact of vocal hygiene education in "artistic" professional voice users. In a previous study Timmermans et al. (2003) questioned the vocal care of radio students (mean age = 22) and radio professionals (mean age = 41). It could be expected that age, maturity, and professional duties turn the vocal hygiene habits in favor. It is not shown that vocal hygiene in radio professionals is better than in radio students. These conclusions are surprising as one could expect that professional voice users are conscious about the voice and therefore take more care of the voice than any other individual would do.

Box 2–2

Case 2
Male, 20 years old, 2nd Bachelor Radio
Complaint: severe hoarseness and sore throat

This student had a warm voice at the end of the first bachelor. We refer to a warm voice when that voice sounds rather low, loud enough, and enriched with resonance. We also use the term *radiophonic* voice. Why this sudden change in voice quality? What happened during holidays? We decided to discuss the vocal hygiene questionnaire (Appendix 2–1) together and advised him to visit a laryngologist as well. The vocal hygiene questionnaire revealed an excessive intake of soft drinks (3 liters of an acidic soda). After 3 weeks of acidic soda barring, his voice was substantially better. Another 4 weeks later his voice turned to normal again. The laryngologist confirmed gastroesophageal reflux disease (GERD), and acid-blocking medication was prescribed. Afterward the student explained his change in vocal hygiene. During summer holidays he was diagnosed with diabetes, and as he was afraid of hypoglycemia, he decided to drink more soft drinks—this was absolutely not a good idea, neither for his voice nor for his diabetes.

Review of Literature

An overview of relevant research on artistic occupational voices (mainly actors and radio voices) is listed in Table 2–2. The population size of the studies varies between single cases and 165 subjects. The research focuses on specific vocal characteristics, such as vocal fatigue, speaker's formant, accent distribution, or on effects of specific voice training programs. There is no methodological uniformity among the studies, which makes comparison difficult. The majority of studies are restricted to acoustic measurements only, while a well-balanced approach implies optimally laryngeal imaging, case history taking, perceptual assessment, aerodynamic and acoustic measurements, and evaluation of quality of life. Outcomes after training are reported by Timmermans et al. (2004b; further reported in this chapter) and Walzak et al. (2008). In contrast with Timmermans, Walzak et al. found limited or negative changes for some measures, which indicates that further research is necessary to explore the benefits of voice training programs.

The Voice Training Program

The voice training program covers four necessary aspects in the process of voice training: test (baseline), theoretical background, training, and transfer (TTTT-approach; Table 2–3).

The Test

As we prepare the students for a future presentation job also, we first need to investigate several capabilities. The requirements to present for a radio station of VRT (Vlaamse Radio en Televisie, Flemish Radio and Television) are very strict and subject to obtaining the "voice certificate." The VRT standards for a good presenter are a warm and pretty voice to listen to, a "Standard Dutch" diction—free

Table 2–2. *Overview of Studies on "Artistic" Occupational Voice Users*

Authors	Year	Population	Subject of Study	Methods
Raphael & Scherer	1987	8 actors	Voice modifications	Acoustic analysis: spectral comparisons
Koufman & Blalock	1988	67 professionals	Vocal fatigue, dysphonia	Endurance test, voice assessment
Harvey, Fuedo, & Aronson	1989	84 actors	Objective analysis	Acoustic analysis, aerodynamics
Novak, Dlouha, Capkova, & Vohradnik	1991	45 actors	Vocal fatigue	Acoustic analysis, LTAS
Fuedo, Harvey, & Aronson	1992	44 actors	Comparative development	Acoustic analysis, aerodynamics
Novák & Vokrál	1995	165 professionals	Acoustic parameters	Acoustic analysis: LTAS, 3D-PAN
Leino & Rajamaki	1996	64 radio speakers	Spectral characteristics	Acoustic analysis: LTAS
Nawka, Anders, Cebulla, & Zurakowski	1997	15 different voices	The speaker's formant	Acoustic analysis: LTAS, 3D-PAN
Roy, Ryker, & Bless	2000	27 actors	Vocal violence	Acoustic analysis
Decoster & Debruyne	2000	20 male reporters (broadcasting)	Differences between identical passages with interval of 30 years	Acoustic analysis (speaking fundamental frequency [SFF], the standard deviation of the SFF [SFFsd], and the voice onset time [VOT])
Timmermans et al.	2003	27 radio students and 53 radio professionals	Vocal hygiene in radio students nd radio professionals	Specific questionnaire
Timmermans et al.	2004a	94 students audiovisual communication	Vocal quality changes after 9 months of training	Perceptual scale, videolaryngostroboscopy, maximum phonation time (MPT), jitter, lowest intensity (IL), highest frequency (F0H), Dysphonia Severity Index (DSI), and Voice Handicap Index (VHI)

Table 2–2. *continued*

Authors	Year	Population	Subject of Study	Methods
Timmermans et al.	2004b	23 trained and 23 untrained students	Outcome after 18 months of voice training	Stroboscopic, perceptual, acoustic and aerodynamic analysis, Voice Handicap Index, and specific questionnaire
Borrego et al.	2006	25 students of a radio announcing course	Effects of a training program	Perceptual and acoustic analysis
Walzak, McCabe, Madill, & Sheard	2008	18 student actors	Changes after 12 months of training	Acoustic measurements (cepstrum, energy ratio, noise-to-harmonic ratio, and soft phonation index)
Varosanec-Skarić	2008	45 acting students and 45 other students	Acoustic characteristics of voice and vocal care	Voice history data and acoustic analysis
Leino, Laukkanen, & Radolf	2011	1 male actor	Formation of the actor's formant	LTAS
Swerts & Marsi	2012	2 Flemish news readers	Accent distributions in spoken news bulletins	Perception study on real and synthesized samples
Guzman, Malebrán, Zavala, Saldívar, & Muñoz	2013a	8 radio broadcasters	Vocal fatigue in radio broadcasters	Acoustic analysis
Guzman, Correa, Muñoz, & Mayerhoff	2013b	37 actors	Influence of spectral energy distribution of emotional expression	Acoustic analysis
Warhurst, McCabe, Yiu, Heard, & Madill	2013	4 commercial and 11 public broadcasters	Acoustic characteristics of male broadcast voices	LTAS and CPP
Warhurst et al.	2016	9 radio educators and radio employers	Perceptions of radio employers and educators	Semistructured interviews

Table 2–3. *TTTT Approach*

	Test: Baseline	Theory: Lectures	Training: Workshops	Transfer: Coaching
1st Bachelor	1 hour (each student)	30 hours	30 hours	30 hours
2nd Bachelor			30 hours	30 hours
3rd Bachelor			30 hours	30 hours
Master			30 hours	

from every dialect—and an intelligent intonation. Therefore, the voice, the diction, and the intonation of every student are recorded and analyzed. It is important to set a baseline and to re-evaluate each student in order to measure the student's progress. The guidelines of the multidimensional voice assessment protocol as proposed by the European Laryngological Society (ELS; Dejonckere et al., 2001) are followed: a perceptual evaluation, a videolaryngostroboscopy, an aerodynamic measurement, acoustic analysis, and a self-assessment. A questionnaire on daily habits was presented in order to inspect vocal hygiene. Due to practical considerations it is impossible to perform a videolaryngostroboscopy for each student; only those students with a deviant voice quality are asked to visit an ear, nose, and throat (ENT) specialist.

An Overview of the Test Battery

The perceptual evaluation is performed using the GRBAS as designed by Hirano (1990), where the G stands for Grade of overall hoarseness, R for roughness, B for breathiness, A for asthenia, and S for strained. Each scale is rated as 0 (normal), 1 (slight), 2 (moderate), or 3 (severe).

The aerodynamic measurement is determined by the maximum phonation time (MPT/[s]). After a maximal inspiration, a vowel sound /a/ at habitual loudness and pitch is sustained. A stopwatch registers the length of time. The best trial out of three is the final MPT.

The acoustic analysis is performed using the Dysphonia Severity Index (DSI; Wuyts et al., 2000) and Acoustic Voice Quality Index (AVQI; Maryn, De Bodt, & Roy, 2010). The DSI is calculated to obtain an objective overall measure of voice quality. The DSI is based on the weighted combination of the following selected set of voice measurements: highest frequency (F0H, Hz), lowest intensity (IL, dB), maximum phonation time (MPT, s), and jitter (%). The DSI is the most optimal combination of independent variables that best reflects the degree of dysphonia as expressed by the G from the GRBAS. It is constructed as follows: $DSI = 0.13 \times MPT + 0.0053 \times F0H - 0.26 \times IL + 1.18 \times Jitter + 12.4$. The AVQI is an objective-acoustic measurement based on a combination of sustained vowel and connected speech. The AVQI is a multivariate construct based on linear regression analysis that combines several acoustic markers to yield a single score that correlates reasonably with the auditory-perceptual judgment of overall dysphonia severity (i.e., G from GRBAS).

A self-assessment is acquired using the Voice Handicap Index (VHI), as a validated Dutch translation is available (De Bodt et al., 2000; Jacobson et al., 1997). Using this index we have the opportunity to gain a better grasp on the perception of voice quality during several stages of the training. The VHI measures the psychosocial impact of the voice, as perceived by the subject. The questionnaire assesses the subject's perception of disability, handicap, and distress due to his or her voice difficulties. The VHI consists of three subscales with 10 questions each: the functional subscale, the emotional subscale, and the physical subscale. The functional subscale (VHI F) contains statements that describe the impact of a person's voice disorder or problem on the daily activities; the emotional subscale (VHI E) includes statements representing the affective responses to a voice disorder or problem, and the physical subscale (VHI P) reflects the self-perceptions of laryngeal discomfort and voice output characteristics (too low or too high pitched voice). Subjects self-rate the "severity" of their voice problem on a 0 to 3-point scale with "0" representing a self-perception of voice as normal: "1" representing mildly impaired voice and "3" representing self-perception of voice as severe impaired voice. Jacobson calculated a total score of the VHI of 33/120 as a function of a self-perceived mild voice problem, 44/120 as a moderate voice problem, and 61/120 as a severe voice problem.

A questionnaire on daily habits (Appendix 2–2) was administered to record "bad" habits such as smoking, late meals, vocal abuse, and stress affecting the voice. These topics were chosen as literature portrayed the artistic- and media-oriented population as vocally abusive, subject to stress and irregular working hours as a result of their professional duties (Raphael, 1991). Smoking was added to the topics because of its negative influence on vocal health and the supposition that a lot of these students smoked (Timmermans et al., 2002). Subjects indicated the number of late meals a week (ranging from 0 to 7); smoking, vocal abuse, and stress were reported by marking yes or no.

The Theory

In the lectures "Voice and Technique," the basic aspects of voice and speech training are expounded. Insights into the speech apparatus (anatomy and physiology of respiratory and articulatory system and larynx). The principles of vocal hygiene, the rules of pronunciation, and the use of the phonetic alphabet are explained. The several existing voice training programs as constructed by Grotowski, Linklater, Lessac, and Coblenzer are described as well (Coblenzer and Muhar, 2002; Grotowski, 1986; Lessac, 1997; Linklater, 1976). Vocal hygiene education is emphasized, and the consequences of tobacco smoke (vocal health), late meals (risk for GERD), vocal abuse (loud speaking and the use of too low or too high pitch), and stress affecting the voice are explained. Animation software is used to explain the functioning of the voice and the influence of bad vocal hygiene (http://www.bluetreepublishing.com). Students are recommended to change their lifestyle, and several assignments are given to encourage them herein. Students are asked to bring a bottle of water in every single lesson. If they forgot the bottle of water, they are obliged to get one immediately. The students learned about the FNAC diet, necessary for those who suffered from GERD. The abbreviation "FNAC" refers to fruit juice, alcohol, nicotine, coffee, caffeine drinks, and chocolate and are all nutrients with a possible negative influence on the stomach. The FNAC diet is an important issue as the students often work late for their radio station XLAIR (http://www.xlair.be). Furthermore, we can do no more than advise our students to take care of their voices as good as possible. Next to this, the students are tutored in auditory perception by the principles of the GRBAS of Hirano (1990). In these lectures a lot of pathologic and normal voices are presented, also known voices (singers, politicians, presenters) are described and analyzed by means of the GRBAS. It is necessary to learn to listen to the quality of voices in order to detect the parameters of roughness, breathiness, asthenia, and strain. Students are asked to search for good sounding voices in their own environment. With this task, students become more aware of their own voices. The rules of pronunciation are a central issue, they must be understood and properly used; for example, the influence of assimilation between consonants, and the exact and correct pronunciation of difficult words or words out of another language and names of cities worldwide. The basic aspects of the International Phonetic Alphabet (IPA) are important because students need to acquire a good understanding of the exact pronunciation of the vowels, diphthongs, and consonants. The lectures amount to 30 hours (see Tables 2–3 and 2–4) and take place in the first three months of the first bachelor. After 9 months, students are obliged to pass a theoretical exam on this material. This course is not repeated in the second bachelor. The theoretical background is presented in Klink Klaar (Timmermans, 2003, 2008, 2013) and unpublished course material.

The Training

In the training students skill themselves in the proper use of their voice, breathing, and speech. Workshops are given in groups of two to five individuals and from January, students receive individual training. The training amounts to 30 hours for each student. The exercises are presented in "Klink Klaar" with an accompanying website (http://www.klinkklaaronline.be) where a lot of exercises are provided (Timmermans et al., 2003, 2008, 2013). Speech and voice use are monitored by the tutor and several aids or devices (e.g., flow ball and cork—Figures 2–2 and 2–3) are provided to give an insight in proper articulation, breathing, and vocal technique.

Basic capabilities are taught in the first bachelor. In the first two months correct positioning of the body, relaxation, natural posture, and healthy breathing are trained. Next to this, the drilling of a vivid and active open articulation, proper vowel and consonant pronunciation, rules of correct diction, exercises on voice projection, extinction of vocal abuse (vocal attacks, backward voicing, and wrong use of the voice) are the issues throughout the rest of the year.

Breathing and good posture are trained in several stages. First, students have to detect their own breathing: How do they breathe? What happens in their bodies? What is a good position of the body while sitting, standing, and presenting? Students learn that the chin should not be held up too much while speaking, a good neutral posture is much better and prevents too much tension in the neck. In the second stage they explore the elasticity of the diaphragm while simple words or sentences are said. This implies that they have to feel the bulging of the abdomen with every inhalation and a flattening of the belly with every exhalation when they are speaking. In the beginning it is necessary to put a hand on their belly to feel this movement. A flowball (Thomann GmbH) is used to train the breath support (Figure 2–2). The white little ball keeps floating high in the air only when the breath support is strong enough. When singing a simple melody, the movement of the little white ball will show the strength of the subglottal pressure. The proper rhythm of breathing is trained using poems for children, and later text, journals, and voice-over text are used to train correct breathing. In the final phase, students learn to adjust their breathing to the text by using proper breathing pauses. Indeed, it is very important that the breathing pauses are taken at the correct moment, between the text arches and not within them.

Table 2–4. *Different Stages of the Voice Training Program for Radio Students of the RITCS*

Lessons	**Phases**								
1st Bachelor	**October**	**November**	**December**	**January**	**February**	**March**	**April**	**May**	**June**
Lectures	Vocal hygiene education								
Workshop	Posture/breathing		Drilling of vivid articulation and pronunciation + voice projection						
Coaching					Vocal coaching in projects				
2nd Bachelor	**October**	**November**	**December**	**January**	**February**	**March**	**April**	**May**	**June**
Workshop	Loudness, pitch, resonance, intonation of news, sports, weather								
Coaching					Vocal coaching in projects				
3rd Bachelor	**October**	**November**	**December**	**January**	**February**	**March**	**April**	**May**	**June**
Workshop	Announcing traffic and voice-over								
Coaching					Vocal coaching in projects				
Master	**October**	**November**	**December**	**January**	**February**	**March**	**April**	**May**	**June**
Workshop					Voice certificate				

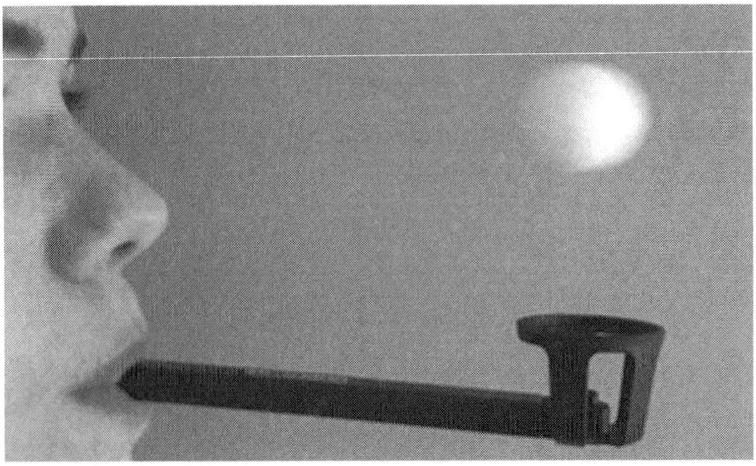

Figure 2–2. *Flow ball.*

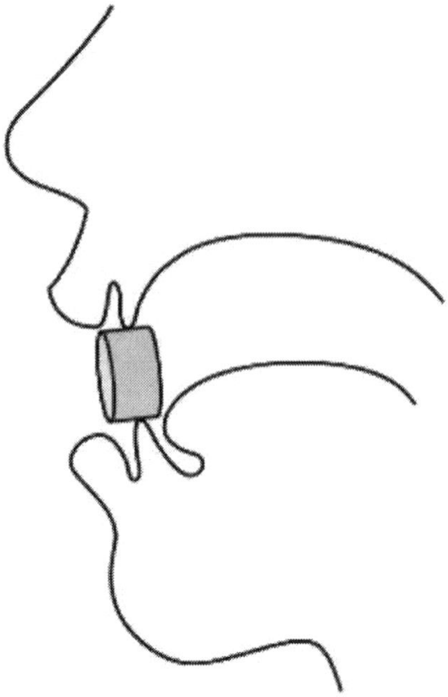

Figure 2–3. *The cork exercise.*

There are two basic exercises for the training of a vivid and open articulation that should be performed at least four times a week: the cork exercise and the pithiness exercise. A cork with a diameter of 20 mm is kept in interdental position (upper and lower teeth) while reading a list of polysyllabic words during 2 minutes (see Figure 2–3). Immediately after this task, students are invited to remove the cork while reading the rest of the polysyllabic words. Research indicated that the cork exercise is effective as the speech intelligibility of the students is significantly higher after the task (Ysenbaert, De Bodt, & Timmermans, 2004). The use of resistance tasks like the cork exercise relies on old traditions in drama education and eloquence. It is assumed that an increased jaw opening improves the distinctive features between phonemes, with more intelligible speech as a consequence. This kind of exercise is designed to improve jaw opening and to strengthen muscle activity. The cork exercise generates an adaptation effect and as a result students become more aware of their speech.

A pithiness exercise is an articulatory drill in which complex words have to be repeated quickly and be repetitive. The tongue tip strength and the resilience of the lips are trained in this way.

At the beginning of each year, students receive a weekly schedule on which they indi-

Box 2–3

An example of a pithiness exercise is as follows:

tippetappe tippetappe tiptaptop

tippetip tippetip tippetiptiptip

tippetiptiptip tappetaptaptap toppetoptoptop

tippetippetiptip tappetappetaptap toppetoppetoptop

pikkepakkepokke pikkepakkepokke pikkepakkepok

van rikkerde tikkerde tikkerde tik van rikkerde tikkerde tik

kipperde kopperde kap kap kipperde kopperde kap

pamperdepimperdepomperdepamp

piederie piedera piederoesasa

tanatanta tenetente tinitinti tonotonto

pamapampa pemepempe pimipimpi pomopompo

tammeramtamtam tommeromtomtom temmeremtemtem tummerumtumtum

danneranneranden dennerennerenden donneronnerondon dunnerunnerundun

cate which exercises they will perform and also when they will do so (Appendix 2–3).

Apart from these two fundamental exercises, the parameters of the vowels, diphthongs, and consonants are explained and trained. The parameters of the (Dutch) vowels and the diphthongs are jaw opening, rounding of the lips, tongue positioning, and length of the vowels. The dialect of every student is interpreted and compared to the standard in order to acquire a perfect diction. The parameters of the consonants are tongue positioning, voiced versus voiceless consonants, and length of the consonants. The influence of the microphone is important because the microphone may amplify every single "disturbing" detail. Therefore, students learn to keep the consonants short and vivid in order to avoid every annoying noise of, for example, "a wet T or a whistling S" (a wet T is a T with too much air in it, the consonant S may not have an accompanying whistling sound). The website http://www.klinkklaaronline.be guides the students in their exercises. For each vowel, diphthong, or consonant there are several exercises that have to be repeated by the student in order to anchor them. The exercises are expanded to reading lots of radio texts and spontaneous speech. Next to this they are trained to avoid swallowing sounds or the sound of sticky lips.

Proper breathing and vivid and open articulation are the base of a strong voice technique. These skills are essential in order to prevent the tension that may occur at the level of the vocal cords.

The second bachelor includes the training of the voice parameters loudness, pitch, and resonance and is taught in the first five months. What is the best mouth to microphone distance? Proper voice warmup is explained and trained (Van Lierde et al., 2001). Due to new insights new techniques are added in the training program, for example, Lax Vox (Mailänder, Mühre, & Barsties, 2016), semi-occluded vocal tract (Titze, 2006). Basic resonance exercises are given and students learn to adapt their pitch. It is clear that a warm voice is supported by a good resonance. An example of a resonance exercise is presented in Box 2–4.

Box 2–4

- Say [m] on a well-placed pitch and alter volume. Please note, only volume and not pitch.

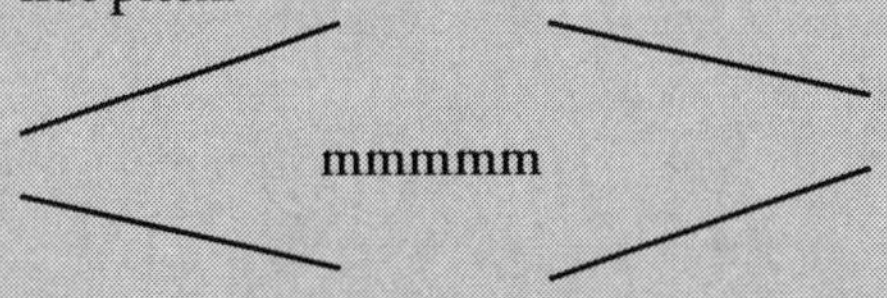

- Say [m] on well-placed pitch and play now with pitch, going from low to high, and vice versa. Please note, only pitch and not by volume.

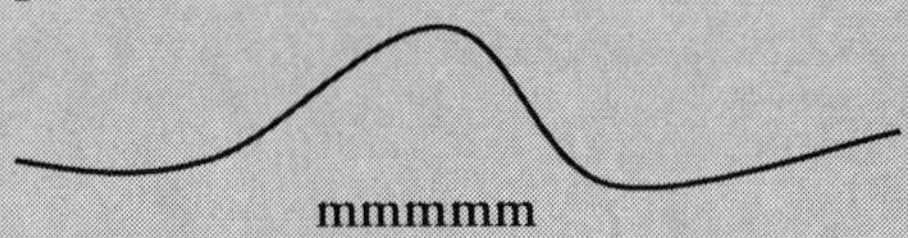

- Form a relaxed easy tone with a [m] and place a round vowel in-between.

mmom mmom mmom mmom

mmoem mmoem mmoem mmoem

mmuum mmuum mmuum mmuum

mmeum mmeum mmeum mmeum

mmom mmom mmom mmom

mmum mmum mmum mmum

Pitch and loudness are important as well. Natural pitch was measured at the beginning of their training and they understand that they have to stick to this pitch. Pitch can be controlled with the right "mind-set"—a calm attitude and a voice that can be associated with this. Just before they start to announce they evoke the right mind-set and start counting to three. The moment they feel that the pitch is right, they will start to speak. The pitch can alter a bit according to the style of the radio station: classic radio requires a calm and a rather low pitch, pop radio needs an enthusiastic and hence higher tone. A proper breathing is learned to control loudness, it is clear that an announcer does not have to talk loud as the microphone amplifies the voice. Nevertheless, loudness exercises are given to ensure that the voice is used correctly.

The rules of natural intonation and the intonation of news or sports announcements are explained. A news item is usually divided into three parts: (a) the fact and the reference to the source (e.g., a newspaper or a politician), (b) the explanation of that fact (= the body of the text), and (c) a conclusion (Table 2–5). Each part of a news item is read with a specific intonation by using a dynamic (loudness-louder), melodic (low pitch or high pitch), or tempo accent (a stop before a significant word).

It is important to use just only one type of accent because a combination of different accents can result in a too strong accent. Too strong accents are not favorable when a microphone is used since the news item can be misunderstood. The fact of a news item is always stressed with a loudness accent, the body of the text (where the fact is explained) a pitch accent (lower or higher pitch) is used, and the conclusion is served with a time accent or a lower pitch accent. The use of pitch accents and the speed of reading reflect the style of the radio station. A lot of high-pitched accents and fast reading are used in commercial and pop music stations, more low-pitched accents and a leisurely pace are used in cultural or classic music stations. Sometimes a high pitch is used in part A (fact) to express astonishment. Next to this, it is essential to learn to stress

Table 2–5. *The ABC-Structure of a News Item*

	Fact (A)	Body (B)	Conclusion (C)
Dynamic accent	↗		
	or		
Melodic accent	↗	↘ or ↗	↘
			or
Tempo accent			↘

the significant words to make sure that the message is correctly understood. There are no rules in choosing which words need to be stressed, common sense and a good text analysis are indispensable. The following guidelines are given: never stress old news, do not stress single words only but choose the right parts of a sentence, do not stress the last word of every sentence but try to "tell" the news and make it sound like a story, because that is just what it is. Sport announcements are read louder and faster to express the excitement, weather reports are important to the listeners and therefore the important words are firmly stressed. As the intonation of news, sports, and weather reports is quite specific and not easy to learn, a lot of exercises are given in the classroom but also in a radio studio. The last lessons are given in the radio studio (Figure 2–4). Mouth-to-microphone distance (20–30 cm max) is discussed (Figure 2–5), and the advantages of an upright position are stressed (e.g., better breathing and dynamic presenting).

In the third bachelor, the lessons are mostly given in a radio studio or in a read-in studio. Next to news, sports, and weather reports, traffic reports are also discussed and trained. Traffic reports are difficult because speech rate is quite high; thus a vivid articulation and a proper control of respiration are indispensable. Moreover, announcing traffic reports is often their first assignment as a sidekick in a radio show. From now on students come one by one to discuss their recorded exercises of news, sports, and weather reports or their own shows on XLair. Next to this, a "good voice-over technique" is another important skill. It is remarkable that radio presenters are often asked to lend their voices to read or to comment a documentary because of their attractive voices and excellent control of their intonation. The intonation of a voice-over is completely different because the voice is subordinate to the image. Therefore, the voice must sound subdued and soft. The dynamic, melodic, and tempo accents need to be emotive, and new characters are introduced by an inflection in their voice. In fact, students should therefore speak and sound totally different, more sensitive and more vivid. In the third bachelor a lot of exercises are given.

In the master, students can choose to follow the master class "radio program," and if they do so, they are coached to get the "voice certificate" of the public radio and television (VRT, Vlaamse Radio en Televisie/Flemmish Radio and Television). The voice certificate is an indispensable document that gives permission to present for one of the radio stations of the VRT. Students need to pass an exam to acquire this document. The exam is very strict, so students—once they get this certificate—can present in fact everywhere. Lessons are always in the radio studio, and a lot of exercises are given to spot the last small mistakes.

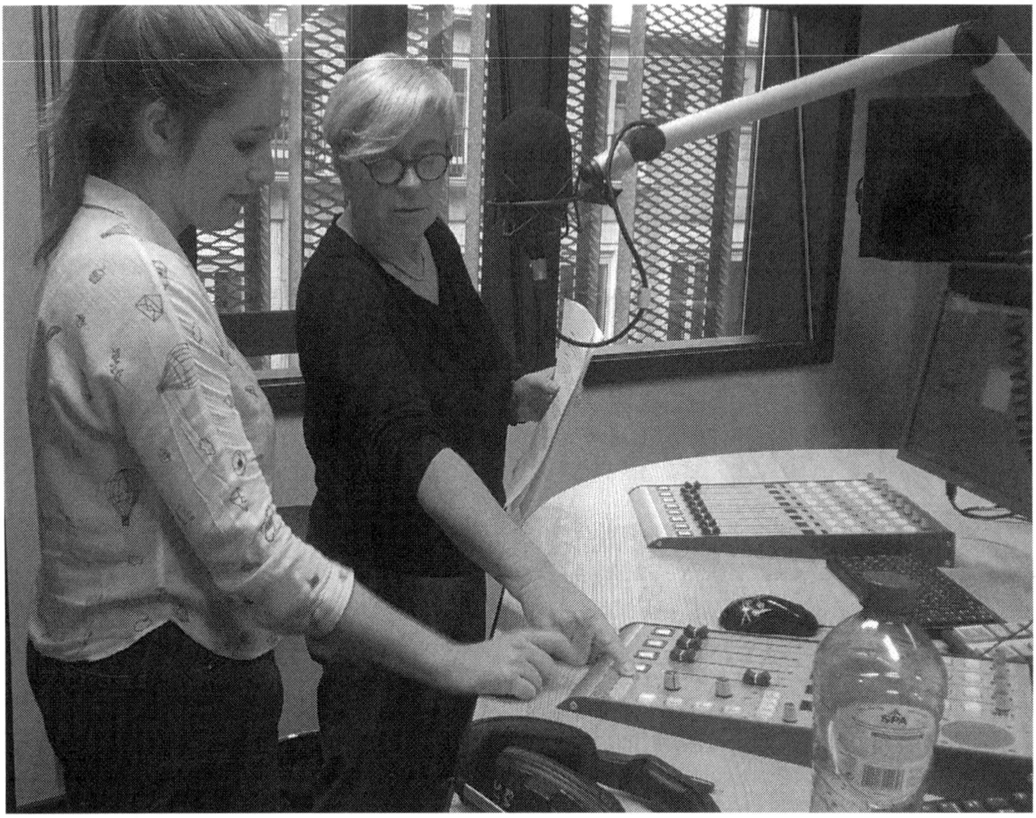

Figure 2–4. *Learning to use the control board.*

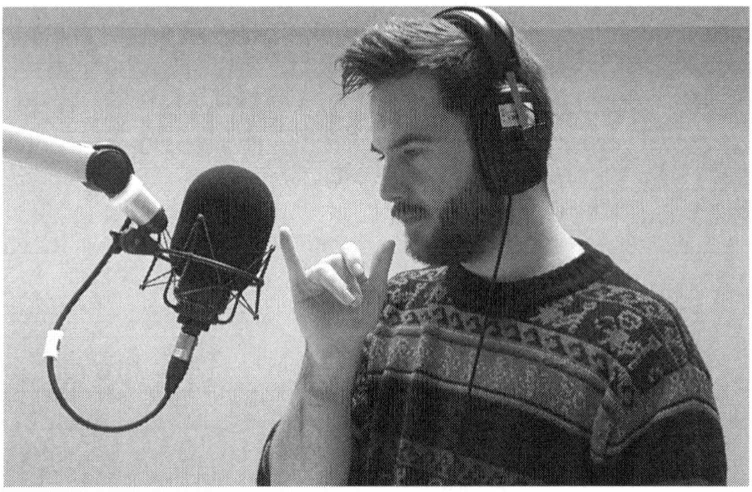

Figure 2–5. *Mouth-to-microphone distance.*

At the end of every school year students must pass an oral exam with specific demands for each level in order to move on to the next year. In the first bachelor the breathing technique, voice quality, and pronunciation of the vowels and diphthongs are evaluated. Students must be able to read an unprepared and an impromptu radio text. If the sounds are well anchored there will be almost no difference in the pronunciation of the vowels and diphthongs between the two texts. Next to this, their breathing and voice quality are evaluated as well. In case of voice problems, the student will be assessed just as in the beginning of the school year. In case the student fails, he or she gets another chance after summer. In the second and third bachelors, a jury of specialists of several public and commercial radio stations is asked to assist in the evaluation of the students. In the second bachelor the exam is attended by a radio colleague. Students read a prepared radio bulletin and an unprepared radio text. Both pronunciation and intonation are evaluated. The pronunciation has to be free of any dialect and the consonants must be vivid. The news bulletin should be read with correct accents and in a pertinent style. In the third bachelor three to five specialists of VRT, Medialaan, and BRUZZ (radio station in the center of Brussels, http://www.BRUZZ.be) are invited. First the jury listens to a recorded news, sports, and weather report, a voice over, and immediately after this the student presents a prepared topic for the jury. A joint evaluation is set up for pronunciation, voice quality, and intonation. It is of utmost

Box 2–5

Case 3

Female, 22 years old, Master

Complaint: quiet, sharp and high voice, intermittent and a nonfluent articulation in front of the microphone

Present job: Announcer

In the first bachelor no problem occurred when she presented her first bulletins, but in the second bachelor she becomes very uncertain as she enters the radio studio. Once she starts to talk her voice becomes quiet, very high and sharp, she is not able to talk without hesitation, and she cannot breathe properly. We advised her to consult the school psychologist, and after a month the student acknowledged that she suffered from performance anxiety. We tried to control this anxiety step by step and by giving her small tasks in the studio, in the beginning without presenting. At that stage it is important that she feels at ease in the environment of the studio, at first she is responsible for technical support in the studio. As she gains security and confidence, she starts to announce colleagues. In the third bachelor her voice was stronger, she spoke quite calm but the breathing was very irregular. She has more control of her voice, speech, and breathing before the microphone at the end of the third bachelor. Finally, she decided to make her master thesis—a radio drama—on this anxiety and her voice. The master thesis was a combination of recordings of fragments of our voice lessons, her own "little" voice, and the thoughts and feelings that went with it. At the end she was able to "crown" her work by presenting the outcome of the lottery at the national radio station Radio 1 (VRT). This was her first little victory in her struggle to become an announcer.

importance that the student is able to present bulletin in a natural and narrative way.

In order to ensure that the learned behavior is transferred to daily life, the *transfer*, the last phase, is organized. These coachings, take 30 hours a year. Students are evaluated by means of performance tasks such as radio programs presented on XLAir, and presentations of self-chosen topics. Sometimes a speech-language pathologist, together with a professional radio maker tutor the ateliers (i.e., lessons in radio presenting). The colleague radio maker supervises the proper form and flow of the program (e.g., a warm welcome to the listener at the beginning of the show, but also after a certain time a welcome is necessary for those who just turned on their radio). The SLP supervises the use of the microphone, the proper upright position, the use of correct language and/or pronunciation, and controlled breathing. Next to the coaching in the lessons, we also listen to the recorded programs they made and presented. In February every radio colleague listens to the students on XLAir, the necessary feedback is provided by means of a short note on any subject: the composition of the show, the way they address the listeners, the timing of the music, and so on.

The Outcome of the Training Program

The outcome of this program was first analyzed and evaluated in 2005 (Timmermans et al., 2005). An evaluation of the long-term effect (after 15 years) of this program is running at present and will be reported later on. Twenty-three professional voice users (13 males and 10 females) received voice training during 2 years (18 months) and vocal hygiene education during 1 year (9 months). Subjects are between 19 and 25 years old and students of the RITCS. This group, hereafter called the trained group, consists of future actors or radio makers/presenters. The study started with subjects beginning their schooling in 1998. The training was given as described in the beginning of this chapter.

A comparative analysis of the results of the three assessment moments—at study onset (Time 1), after 9 months (Time 2), and after 18 months (Time 3)—is performed in order to determine the impact of each training phase. Comparing results over time can reveal useful information about effectiveness, optimal duration of training, and the effect of vocal hygiene.

Data collection was based on multidimensional voice assessment protocol as proposed by the European Laryngological Society (ELS; Dejonckere et al., 2001). The following set of data was collected for each subject: perceptual evaluation (GRBAS; Hirano, 1990) by the investigator, acoustic parameters (DSI; Wuyts et al., 2000), an aerodynamic parameter (MPT/s), and self-assessment by the subject (VHI; De Bodt et al., 2000; Jacobson et al., 1997). Videolaryngostroboscopy was carried out at Time 1. A questionnaire (Appendix 2–2) on daily habits was administered to register habits such as smoking, eating, vocal abuse, and stress.

Data were analyzed with SPSS V11. The main purpose of the investigation was to evaluate the effect of the voice training program over time. The results of the variables DSI, jitter, lowest intensity (IL) and highest frequency (FoH), maximum phonation time (MPT), the VHI, and its subscales were investigated with a repeated measures ANOVA test. The post hoc Tukey multiple comparison test was used to study the effect of the training in and between the different training periods. The Kolmogorov-Smirnov test was used to investigate the normal distribution of the variables. The G score and the variables of the daily habits questionnaire (the presence of smoking, stress, vocal abuse, and the amount of late meals a week) were analyzed by the Friedman test that was used to calculate significant differences over time in each training period.

Table 2–6 presents the mean and standard error (SE) of the DSI, the VHI, and the subscores in Times 1, 2, and 3. The DSI score improves from 2 to 3.7 in Time 2 and to 4.6 in Time 3 (Figure 2–6). This is a remarkable improvement after 9 months of voice training. The results of the VHI improve but remain relatively high. The VHI/T scores changed from 18.4/120 in Time 1 to 19/120 in Time 2 and resulted in 14.4/120 in Time 3; the differences are not significant (Figure 2–7). The mean scores of the VHI/P and VHI/F show little or no improvement. The mean VHI/E score, on the contrary, is the only subscore that improves significantly (p = .003) after 18 months.

Table 2–6. *Results of the DSI, the VHI T, and Subscores from T1 to T3*

	Trained Group (n = 23)					
	T1	**T2**	**T3**	**T1/T2**	**T2/T3**	**T1/T3**
	Mean ± SE	Mean ± SE	Mean ± SE	p-value	p-value	p-value
DSI	2.0 ± 0.7	3.7 ± 0.7	4.6 ± 0.7	$p = .005$	$p = .2$	$p < .001$
VHI T	18.4 ± 0.7	19.0 ± 1.7	14.4 ± 1.7	$p = .9$	$p = .1$	$p = .2$
VHI P	8.0 ± 0.6	8.7 ± 0.6	8.3 ± 0.6	$p = .6$	$p = .8$	$p = .9$
VHI E	6.0 ± 0.9	5.4 ± 0.9	3.0 ± 0.9	$p = .9$	$p = .09$	$p = .03$
VHI F	4.3 ± 0.5	4.6 ± 0.5	3.3 ± 0.5	$p = .9$	$p = 1.20$	$p = .3$

Note. SE = standard error = SD/$\sqrt{n}$.

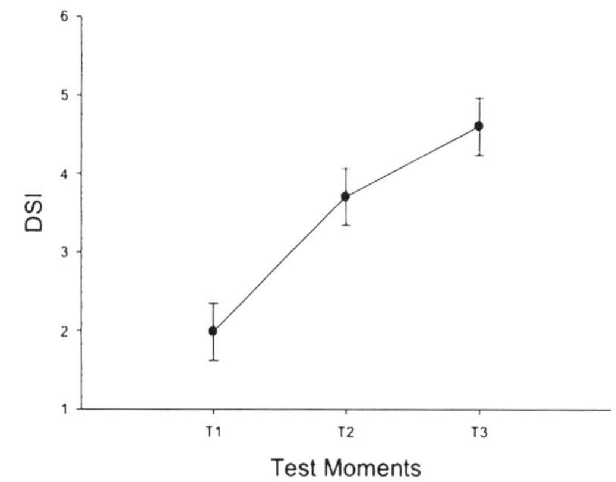

Figure 2–6. *The DSI scores from T1 to T2 and T3.*

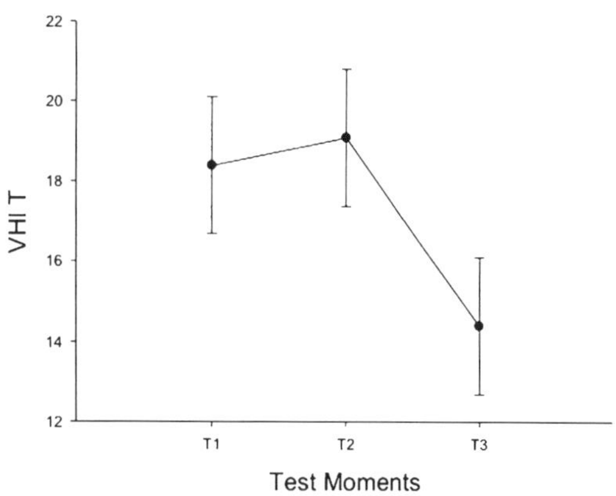

Figure 2–7. *The VHI scores from T1 to T2 and T3.*

The videolaryngostroboscopy was performed at Time 1 and only subjects with lesions were re-examined at the end of the study. The strobe rater detected four subjects with an incomplete glottal closure and three subjects with a disturbed mucosal wave. The perceptual evaluation of the four subjects with a lesion changed to G1 and the DSI score ameliorated in three subjects. The lesions of two subjects disappeared, one subject could not be examined, and one subjects' vocal folds status remained the same (erythema and edema). The G score confirms the improved calculated voice quality after 18 months, as G2 scores no longer occur. The perceptual evaluation changed significantly after 18 months (p = .04). The results demonstrate that perceived voice quality change is scored after 18 months only, illustrating that the categorical severity rating does not permit the scoring of minimal changes in voice quality.

In spite of the awareness that they are absolutely dependent on their voices, they do not take the necessary precautions for the care of their voices. Table 2–7 presents the three subsequent results (Times 1, 2, and 3) of smoking prevalence, vocal abuse, stress, and late meals. The smoking prevalence remains high after 9 and 18 months (from 39 to 48%): 13% is still vocally abusive, and 26% of the subjects instead of the 8% at the beginning of the study eat late. Stress affecting the voice increases dramatically and significantly ($p < .001$) from 17 to 43 to 73%. This could mean that the lectures have no effect on the daily habits.

In conclusion, it seems that the first training period is the most productive period; however, in the second training period the voice quality of 15 subjects (65%) still improves. It is important to note, however, that the presented results are the mean values of the 23 subjects, which does not reflect the individuals with better or worse scores. In spite of the improvement of their voice quality, vocal hygiene has not changed at all, meaning that their behavior is not modified as such by this program. Another concept should be formulated to modify lifestyle and daily habits.

Table 2–7. *Number and Percentage of Persons Who Smoke, Who Report Stress, Vocal Abuse, and Late Meals in T1, T2, and T3*

	Trained Group (n = 23)		
	T1	T2	T3
	n (%)	*n* (%)	*n* (%)
Smoke	9 (39%)	9 (39%)	11 (48%)
Stress	4 (17%)	10 (43%)	17 (73%)
Abuse	3 (13%)	5 (21%)	3 (13%)
Late meals	2 (8%)	9 (39%)	6 (26%)

References

Borrego, M. C., Gasparini, G., & Behlau, M. (2006). The effects of a specific speech and language training program on students of a radio announcing course. *Journal of Voice, 21*(4), 426–432.

Broaddus-Lawrence, P., Treole, K., McCabe, R., Allen, R., & Toppin, L. (2000). The effects of preventive vocal hygiene education on the vocal hygiene habits and perceptual vocal characteristics of training singers. *Journal of Voice, 14*(1), 58–71.

Chan, R. (1994). Does the voice improve with the vocal hygiene education? A study of some instrumental voice measures in a group of kindergarten teachers. *Journal of Voice, 8*(3), 297–291.

Coblenzer, H., & Muhar, F. (2002). *Atem und Stimme. Anleitung zum guten sprechten.* Wien, Austria: Öbv&Hpt.

Coekaerts, R., & Wuyts, C. (2014). Een vergelijking van de spreeksnelheid bij journaallezers van 1993 tot en met 2013. Master thesis, University of Ghent, Belgium.

De Bodt, M. S., Heylen, L., Mertens, F., Vanderwegen, J., & Van de Heyning, P. H. (2015). *Stemstoornissen. Handboek voor de klinische praktijk.* Antwerpen-Apeldoorn: Garant.

De Bodt, M. S., Jacobson, B., Musschoot, S., Zaman, S., Heylen, L., Mertens, F., Van de Heyning, P. H., & Wuyts, F. L. (2000). De Voice Handicap Index. Een instrument voor het kwantificeren van de psychosociale consequenties van stemstoornissen. *Logopedie, 13*, 29–33.

Decoster, W., & Debruyne, F. (2000). Longitudinal voice changes: Facts and interpretation. *Journal of Voice, 14*(2), 184–193.

Dejonckere, P. H., Bradley, P., Clemente, P., Cornut, G., Crevier-Buchman, L., Friedrich, G., Van de Heyning, P. H., Remacle, G., & Woisard, V. (2001). A basic protocol for functional assessment of voice pathology, especially for investigating the efficacy of (phonosurgical) treatments and evaluating new assessment techniques. *European Archives of Otorhinolaryngology, 258*, 77–82.

Fuedo, P., Harvey, P. L., & Aronson, D. B. (1992). Objective analysis of actors' voices: Comparative development across training. *Journal of Voice, 6*(3), 267–270.

Grotowski, J. (1986). *Naar een Sober theater.* Amsterdam, Netherlands: International Theatre Bookshop.

Guzman, M., Correa, S., Muñoz, D., & Mayerhoff, R. (2013b). Influence on spectral energy distribution of emotional expression. *Journal of Voice, 27*(1), 129.e1–129.e10.

Guzman, M., Malebrán, M. C., Zavala, P., Saldívar, P., & Muñoz, D. (2013a). Acoustic changes of the voice as signs of vocal fatigue in radio broadcasters: Preliminary findings. *Acta Otorrinolaringologica Espanola, 64*(3), 176–183.

Harvey, P. L., Feudo, P., & Aronson, D. B. (1989). Objective analysis of actors' voices: An initial report. *Journal of Voice, 3*, 143–147.

Hirano, M. (1990). Clinical application of voice tests. In National Institute on Deafness and Other Communication Disorders (Ed.), *Assessment of speech and voice production* (pp. 196–203). Bethesda, MD: National Institutes of Health.

Jacobson, B. H., Johnson, A., Grywalski, C., Silbergleit, A., Jacobson, G., Benniger, M. S., & Newman, C. W. (1997). The Voice Handicap Index (VHI): Development and validation. *American Journal of Speech-Language Pathology, 6*, 66–67.

Koufman, J. A., & Blalock, P. D. (1988). Vocal fatigue and dysphonia in the professional voice user: Bogart-Bacall syndrome. *Laryngoscope, 98*(5), 493–498.

Leino, T., Laukkanen, A. M., & Radolf, V. (2011). Formation of the actor's/speaker's formant: A study applying spectrum analysis and computer modeling. *Journal of Voice, 25*(2), 150–158.

Leino, T., & Rajamaki, T. (1996). *Voices on the air.* Scandinavian Voice Research: open symposium in honor ot Aatto Sonninen, Helsinki, Finland. September 14–15.

Lessac, A. (1997). *The use and training of the human voice. A biodynamic approach to vocal life.* Mountain View, CA: Mayfield.

Linklater, K. (1976). *Freeing the natural voice.* New York, NY: Drama Publishers.

Mailänder, E., Mühre, L., & Barsties, B. (2016). Lax Vox as a voice training program for teachers: A pilot study. *Journal of Voice*. Advance online publication. doi:10.1016/j.jvoice.2016.04.011

Maryn, Y., De Bodt, M., & Roy, N. (2010). The Acoustic Voice Quality Index: Toward improved treatment outcomes assessment in voice disorders. *Journal of Communication Disorders, 43*, 161–174.

Nawka, T., Anders, L. C., Cebulla, M., & Zurakowski, D. (1997). The speaker's formant in male voices. *Journal of Voice, 11*(4), 422–428.

Niclaes, L. (2013). *Spreektoonhoogte van radionieuwslezers door de Jaren heen*. Brussels, Belgium: Free University of Brussels – VUB, Master thesis.

Novak, A., Dlouha, O., Capkova, B., & Vohradnik, M. (1991). Voice fatigue after theatre performance in actors. *Folia Phoniatrica, 43*(2), 74–78.

Novák, A., & Vokrál, J. (1995). Acoustic parameters for the evaluation of voice of future voice professionals. *Folia Phoniatrica et Logopaedica, 47*, 279–285.

Raphael, B. (1991). Special considerations relating to members of the acting profession. In R. Sataloff (Ed.), *Professional voice. The science and art of clinical care* (pp. 85–89). New York, NY: Raven Press.

Raphael, B. N., & Scherer, R. C. (1987). Voice modifications of stage actors: Acoustic analyses. *Journal of Voice, 1*(1), 83–87.

Roy, N., Ryker, K. S., & Bless D. M. (2000). Vocal violence in actors; an investigation into its acoustic consequences and the effects of hygienic laryngeal release training. *Journal of Voice, 14*, 215–230.

Roy, N., Weinrich, B., Gray, S., Tanner, K., Toledo, S., Dove, H., . . . Stemple, J. (2002). Voice amplification versus vocal hygiene instruction for teachers with voice disorders: A treatment outcome study. *Journal of Speech, Language, and Hearing Research, 45*(4), 625–638.

Swerts, M., & Marsi, E. (2012). Prosodic evaluation of accent distributions in spoken news bulletins of Flemish newsreaders. *Journal of the Acoustical Society of America, 132*(4), 2616–2624.

Timmermans, B. (2003, 2008, 2013). *Klink Klaar. De eerste uitspraak- en intonatiegids voor het Nederlands*. Leuven, Netherlands: Davidsfonds.

Timmermans, B., De Bodt, M. S., Wuyts, F. L, & Van de Heyning, P. H. (2003). Vocal hygiene in future professional voice users and in professional voice users. *Logopedics, Phoniatrics, Vocology, 28*(3), 127–132.

Timmermans, B., De Bodt, M. S., Wuyts, F. L., & Van de Heyning, P. H. (2004a). Voice quality change in future professional voice users after 9 months of training. *European Archives of Otorhinolaryngology, 261*(1), 1–5.

Timmermans, B., De Bodt, M. S., Wuyts, F. L., & Van de Heyning, P. H. (2004b). Training outcome in future professional voice users after 18 months of voice training. *Folia Phoniatrica et Logopaedica, 56*(2), 120–129.

Timmermans, B., De Bodt, M. S., Wuyts, F. L., & Van De Heyning, P. H. (2005). Analysis of a voice training program in future voice professionals. *Journal of Voice, 19*(2), 102–110.

Titze, I. R. (2006). Voice training and therapy with a semi-occluded vocal tract: Rationale and scientific underpinnings. *Journal of Speech, Language, and Hearing Research, 49*(2), 448–459.

Van Lierde, K., D'haeseleer, E., Baudonck, N., Claeys, S., De Bodt, M. S., & Behlau, M. (2001). The impact of vocal warm-up exercises on the objective vocal quality in female students training to be speech language pathologists. *Journal of Voice, 25*(3), 115–121.

Varosanec-Skarić, G. (2008). Acoustics characteristics of voice and vocal care in acting and other students. *Clinical Linguistics and Phonetics, 22*, 10–11.

Walzak, P., McCabe, P., Madill, C., & Sheard, C. (2008). Acoustic changes in student actors' voices after 12 months of training. *Journal of Voice, 22*(3), 300–313.

Warhurst, S., Madill, C., McCabe, P., Ternström, S., Yiu, E., & Heard, R. (2016). Perceptual and acoustic analyses of good voice quality in male radio performers. *Journal of Voice*. Advance online publication. doi:10.1016/j.jvoice.2016.05.016

Warhurst, S., McCabe, P., Yiu, E., Heard, R., & Madill, C. (2013). Acoustic characteristics of male commercial and public radio broadcast voices. *Journal of Voice, 27*(5), 655.e1–655.e7.

Wuyts, F. L., De Bodt, M. S., Molenberghs, G., Remacle, M., Heylen, L., Millet, B. . . . Van de

Heyning, P. H. (2000). The Dysphonia Severity Index: An objective measure of vocal quality based on a multiparameter approach. *Journal of Speech, Language, and Hearing Research, 43*, 796–809.

Yiu, E. (2002). Impact and prevention of voice problems in the teaching profession: Embracing the consumers' view. *Journal of Voice, 16*(2), 215–228.

Ysenbaert, F., De Bodt, M. S., & Timmermans, B. (2004). De effectiviteit van de kurkoefening op de articulatorische precisie en de spraakverstaanbaarheid bij professionele stemgebruikers. *Logopedie, 28*(1), 27–31.

APPENDIX 2–1

Vocal Hygiene Questionnaire

General Information		
Year of birth:		
Sex:		
Amount of hours of radio presentation a week:		
Amount of years of radio presentation:		
Risk Factors		
	HOW MUCH	
Smoking	amount . . . /day	
Alcohol	drinks . . . /day	
Coffee	cups . . . /day	
Peppermint	amount . . . /day	
Soft drinks	amount . . . /day	
Late meals (<2 hours before going to bed)	amount . . . /week	
Voice-Related Factors		
Are you allergic?	YES/NO	If yes, please specify.
Do you have an acid-like taste in your mouth in the morning?	YES/NO	If yes, how often?
Do you abuse your voice? (screaming, shouting)	YES/NO	
Does your voice often sound hoarse?	YES/NO	If yes, how often?
Do you sing professionally?	YES/NO	
Is stress affecting your voice?	YES/NO	
Is fatigue affecting your voice?	YES/NO	

APPENDIX 2–2

Test Intake

QUESTIONNAIRE 1

Name: Age: Sex:

Classification:
- ☐ Elite vocal performer
- ☐ Professional voice user
- ☐ Nonvocal professional
- ☐ Nonvocal nonprofessional

- -

Please complete the list below and indicate the number of units of consumption of the listed products a day. For example, the number of cigarettes, the number of pints, and cups of coffee. Next to this, please indicate how many days a week you eat a meal less than 2 hours before going to bed.

Risk Factors: Units a day

- Alcohol ______ pints a day
- Coffee ______ cups a day
- Soft drinks ______ a day
- Peppermint ______ a day
- Late meals ______ days a week

Risk Factors: Voice use

- Vocal abuse yes ☐ no ☐
- Smoker yes ☐ no ☐

Medication:

Please write down the amount and kind of medication you take (sleeping pills, puffs for asthma, medication for the stomach, do not forget to mention the antacids)

____

____

Medical History:

Please mention surgical treatments for the stomach or throat.

APPENDIX 2–3

Weekly Schedule

1 Bach Radio	Monday	Tuesday	Wednesday	Thursday	Friday	Saturday	Sunday
Cork	x		x		x		x
Pithiness	x	x		x			x
Vowels/diphthongs			x		x		
Consonants		x			x		x
Assimilation		x			x		
Breath support	x		x				x

2 Bach Radio	Monday	Tuesday	Wednesday	Thursday	Friday	Saturday	Sunday
Cork							
Pithiness							
Articulation							
Voice exercises							
Intonation							

continues

Appendix 2–3. *continued*

3 Bach Radio	Monday	Tuesday	Wednesday	Thursday	Friday	Saturday	Sunday
Pithiness/cork							
Articulation							
Resonance							
Journals							
Voice-Over							

SECTION II

Practices and Outcomes of an Expert From Africa

CHAPTER 3

Developing an In-Class Voice Education and Training Program for Prospective Speech-Language Pathologists

Aliaa Khidr, Meredith Roper, and Michael Hull

Speech-Language Pathology Industry

U.S. News & World Report ranked speech-language pathology as 28th of the best 100 jobs and 19th of the best health care jobs (*U.S. News & World Report*, 2016a, 2016b), with 28,900 projected jobs, $71,550 median salary, and 0.9% unemployment rate.

The U.S. Bureau of Labor Statistics predicts 160,100 people will be employed as speech-language pathologists (SLPs) by 2022. Employment of SLPs is projected to grow 21% from 2014 to 2024, much faster than the average growth for all other occupations (7%) and for similar health occupations (17%) (Bureau of Labor Statistics [BLS], 2015).

Of the 134,100 American SLPs employed in 2012, about two out of every five worked in schools. Most of them worked full time: 48% in elementary and secondary schools; 19% in offices of physical, occupational, and speech therapists and audiologists; 13% in hospitals; 5% in nursing homes; and 4% in social assistance (BLS, 2015).

According to the American Speech-Language-Hearing Association (ASHA), 97% of the 2,544 school-based SLPs who responded to the ASHA 2010 Schools Survey were female. Their most common facility was elementary schools; 80% were clinical service providers, 80% worked full time, 48% worked in a suburban area, and 1% held a Ph.D. degree (ASHA, 2010). Similar results were found in the 2,539 school-based SLPs who responded to the ASHA 2012 Schools Survey. SLPs averaged 15 years of experience in the profession, and their most common facility was elementary schools. Ninety-one percent were clinical service providers, 79% worked full time, 50% worked in a suburban area, and 1% held a Ph.D. degree (ASHA, 2012).

Graduate SLP Clinical Training

To practice as a SLP in the United States, a master's degree from one of the 277 graduate programs accredited by the Council on Academic Accreditation is required. Graduate course work is expected to include an effective balance between traditional parameters of communication (articulation, phonology, voice, fluency, language, and hearing) and additional recognized and emerging areas of practice (e.g., swallowing, upper aerodigestive functions, etc.). Graduate programs are also required to provide supervised clinical experience sufficient in depth and breadth to achieve the targeted knowledge and skills. Finally, to earn a certification in speech-language pathology, students must complete a minimum of 400 hours of supervised clinical experience. Twenty-five hours must be spent in clinical observation, and 375 hours must be spent in direct client contact (ASHA, 2016).

Graduate SLP Voice Competencies

Despite the heavy clinical training component of SLP graduate programs, the training is not equal across all areas of practice. The reality is that there are far fewer opportunities for clinical hours in voice disorders, and it is one area in which many practicing clinicians reportedly feel a lack of competency. Many SLP graduate programs offer only limited course work and limited or no clinical practica in voice disorders prior to degree completion (Ruddy & Sapienza, 2004).

Tillard, Lawson, and Emmerson (2011) confirm this observation and relate the challenges with training graduate students in the evaluation and treatment of voice disorders to the low incidence of this clinical population. They also report that recent graduates and their employers perceive voice disorders as an area of preparation weakness. They explain that the difficulty of locating patients with voice disorders is not the only obstacle. The lack of funding for specialized equipment, hands-on practice, dedicated space for equipment, and expert faculty that can provide proper training all contribute to the challenges of graduate-level training in voice disorders.

Ruddy and Sapienza (2004) reported that many school-based SLPs have expressed apprehension in treating children with voice disorders because of their minimal education regarding voice evaluation and treatment and limited or nonexistent clinical exposure to voice disorders. The authors emphasize that the newly minted SLPs' lack of confidence in treating this population is probably the main cause of nonidentification and nontreatment of these disorders in the school.

Teten, DeVeney, and Friehe (2013, 2016a) developed a checklist for assessing graduate students' competencies in the area of voice disorders. The checklist contains 25 competencies across the prevention, assessment, and treatment of voice disorders. The authors recommend utilizing this checklist as a pre- and post-test measure to assess graduate students' preparation in the area of voice disorders. They used a five-level Likert scale rating to assess competency (1 = minimally competent; 2 = somewhat competent; 3 = moderately competent; 4 = very competent; 5 = extremely competent). Each checklist item is intended to measure and represent a discrete skill that aligns with competencies from ASHA's Graduate Curriculum on Voice and Voice Disorders (ASHA, 2009). They suggest that students ready to matriculate into an entry-level position should report competency levels of at least three or higher on the majority of the items in the checklist (Teten et al., 2013, 2016a).

Teten, DeVeney, and Friehe (2016b) used their checklist to study the self-perceived competence levels for the area of voice disorders in school-based SLPs in Nebraska. All of the surveyed SLPs reported feeling not particularly competent in their ability to assess or treat students with voice disorders. A score of 3 (i.e., moderate competence) is used to indicate minimum expected competence on each checklist item. Of the 25 surveyed items to which 153 SLPs responded, only one response

Box 3–1

Selected items from Teten et al.'s (2013) checklist for assessing graduate students' competencies in the area of voice disorders include the following:

Item #2. Develops preventative strategies for maintenance of vocal wellness and hygiene.

Item #4. Performs auditory-perceptual evaluations of voice quality using parameters of roughness, breathiness, strain, pitch, loudness, and overall severity of the voice.

Item #5. Considers environmental variables (e.g., emotional reactions, social pressures) that may impact the severity of the voice disorder.

Item #13. Plans and implements a treatment program to address the individual needs of the client and communication styles of family members based on the results of comprehensive assessment and client and/or family consultation.

Item #15. Demonstrates various therapeutic strategies for facilitating the restoration of normal balance between respiration, phonation, and resonance to achieve balanced voice production.

mean was above 3: "Develops preventative strategies for maintenance of vocal wellness." All other item means were at or below 3. Findings did not indicate a significant correlation between academic course work in voice disorders during the SLP's graduate program and the SLP's overall self-perceived competence in voice. The authors attribute the low self-perception of preparation to evaluate to the low incidence of voice disorders (Teten et al., 2016b).

Interestingly, the study also showed no correlation between graduate-level clinical practica with voice clients and self-perceived competence in working with voice disorders. Furthermore, there was a slight negative correlation between experience with adult clients with voice disorders during clinical practicum and feeling competent treating people with voice disorders (Teten et al., 2016b). In this scenario, having a new voice patient may be a reminder of their incompetence rather than an opportunity to build them up. These data support the notion that regular classwork and patient-targeted competence alone, without SLP self-targeted competence, are not enough to develop the needed competencies in voice.

But SLPs in this population reportedly felt more competent, though still below the score of 3, if they had been pursuing academic continuing education (CE) in the general area of voice within the last 5 years. This is a good indication of the need for more practical CE opportunities targeting the perceptual and performance voice skills necessary for caring for both self and others.

Graduate SLP Voice Challenges

Voice Challenges as Prospective Professional Voice Users

Speech-language pathologists work with communication and swallowing disorders in individuals of all ages. Verbal communication is the basis of almost all of their evaluations and accompanies all of their physical examinations.

Verbal communication, speech, language, and voice modeling, as well as verbal instructions and verbal feedback, are central to all treatment sessions. Most of these verbal interactions need to be carried out through clear, lively, animated, modulated, and appealing voices that can successfully engage and stimulate their communicatively impaired clients. Vocal demands increase with children, group therapy settings, hearing impaired populations, and elderly patients. Some techniques, such as the Lee Silverman Voice Treatment for patients with Parkinson's disease, involve modeling loud phonation throughout the session (Sapir, Ramig, & Fox, 2011). In addition to their vocal use with patients, SLPs use verbal communication to provide counseling, training, and education to family members, caregivers, team members, and professionals across disciplines.

Simberg, Sala, and Rönnemaa (2004) reported that students studying to become teachers have a greater number of frequently occurring vocal symptoms than do other university students. SLPs, especially school-based SLPs, have similar vocal profiles to teachers. They both place heavy demands on their voice, often instructing for many hours in acoustically challenging environments without much time for the voice to rest (Roy, Merrill, Thibeault, Gray, & Smith, 2004). SLPs also share similar risk factors for voice problems among teachers: female gender (Roy et al., 2004), number of years teaching (Roy et al., 2004; Russell, Oates, & Greenwood, 2005), and poor classroom environment (Simberg, Sala, Vehmas, & Laine, 2005; de Medeiros, Barreto, & Assunção, 2008).

Gottliebson, Lee, Weinrich, and Sanders (2007) studied voice problems in 104 first-year graduate SLP students at two universities. All students participated in voice screenings. Fourteen percent (n = 15) of the participants failed the voice screening by demonstrating two or more abnormal voice characteristics, including persistent glottal fry (present in all who failed); low habitual pitch; juvenile resonance; hoarse, breathy, or strained phonation; abnormally low pitch on sustained vowels; and voice breaks. Twelve percent (n = 12) failed both the screening and follow-up questionnaire regarding voice disorders. Responses included self-reported dysphonia, medical history with voice-related side effects, difficulty with excessive voice use, and voice problems occurring daily or weekly. Their results suggest that voice problems among future SLPs are more common than the 3 to 9% reported in the general population (Verdolini & Ramig, 2001) and similar to the 11% reported for teachers (Roy et al., 2004).

Voice Challenges as College Students

Graduate and undergraduate SLP students share the same demographic, social, and student work profile as their college peers. Therefore, it is expected that they share similar challenges related to the vocal demands of college life. Hartley, Breen, and Thibeault (2016) conducted a comprehensive investigation describing the prevalence of vocal health concerns in 652 college students, predominately aged 18 to 25 years. Lifetime prevalence of a voice disorder was 34%, and 46% reported voice problems or difficulties within the past 12 months. They tended to use their voice more during social or extracurricular activities than during class or work, particularly for more vocally demanding activities, such as shouting, yelling, cheering, or singing. For employed students, however, substantial voice-related requirements were present, with more than 90% talking often or all the time and 45% reporting a frequent need to talk loudly. Student perceptions of vocal health concerns largely mirrored activity patterns, with the majority of students identifying social or extracurricular activities as the likely source of voice difficulties (Hartley et al., 2016).

SLPs' Beliefs Regarding Their Own Voice

Over the last two decades, there has been increased awareness regarding the effect of voice disorders on the social, psychological, and occupational aspects of teachers' lives. This research started with the growing recognition and affirmation of teachers as "vocal athletes" and professional voice users. Such an appreciation does not exist yet for SLPs. Throughout the past 5 years, graduate SLP students attending the voice disorders class at the University of Virginia (UVA) have participated in surveys approved by the institutional review board (IRB). These surveys were designed to increase students' awareness of their own vocal load, demands, and challenges and necessary voice training and care as future professional voice users. They were completed throughout the semester, and their results were discussed to reiterate the point of vocal awareness. They targeted concepts such as students' goals for the class, their perceptions regarding their own and others' vocal behaviors, their understanding of professional voice use, and their beliefs regarding implications of vocal changes in self and others.

A study by Gillingham, Brenner, and Khidr (2012) compared the perceptual skills of 26 students (24 females, 2 males) attending the graduate voice disorders course at UVA in the fall of 2012 to that of three voice experts, including the first author. All students were tested regarding their auditory-perceptual skills and were found to be competent. Students were then asked to rate the percentage of time in which vocal fry was used during a recording of continuous speech (0%, 25%, 50%, 75%, or 100% of the time). Students rated three recordings: their own, a classmate's, and Sabrina Farhi, a former announcer for National Public Radio (NPR). The study showed that students consistently reported less vocal fry in their own voice and that of their classmate. Their ratings for vocal fry in the unfamiliar voice of Sabrina Farhi were consistent with the scoring of the expert raters. The study highlighted a surprising disparity regarding the graduate students' evaluation of possible health, occupational impact, and need for voice care for the professional voice user who used habitual vocal fry 50 to 75% of the time. Almost all students reported that the habitual use of vocal fry by the radio announcer might affect the longevity of her voice and her career, and voice therapy was recommended. On the other hand, students reported that similar habitual vocal fry behavior would not have an affect on their own future career or that of their classmate (Gillingham et al., 2012). Both findings suggest that graduate SLP students may be less sensitive to changes in their own voice or that of someone close to them, such as their classmates, and more sensitive to similar changes in unfamiliar voices of potential clients. This may affect their decision regarding if and when to seek clinical care for their own voice problems.

A more recent study by Khidr (2015) surveyed 24 female students ages 23 to 35 years at the University of Virginia on the first day of their voice disorders class in order to understand their vocal awareness baseline. It should be noted that graduate SLP students at UVA take the voice disorders class in the fall semester of the second year. By that time they all have been in the program for three semesters. For Track I students who have an undergraduate degree in communication disorders, it is the last semester before leaving for their internship. For Track II students who have an undergraduate degree in something other than communication disorders, they still have one semester of course work ahead of them. In both cases, students have already had two (Track II) or three (Track I) semesters of clinical practicum.

Students were asked about their goals for the class. Most of the students reported generic goals, including learning about voice therapy, voice diagnosis, voice knowledge, voice disorders, anatomy, counseling, and teamwork. A smaller number of students reported more specific goals directly related to personal voice education and training, including perceptual analysis of voice, self-care of voice, preventive voice care, advocating for professional voice users, promoting vocal hygiene, and confidence in vocal exercises. It is important to note that most students at this stage in the graduate program do not feel the need to learn how to care for or train their voice.

Although 15 of the 24 students identified themselves as professional voice users, these same students had not previously educated themselves about how to care for their voice, paid attention to negative feelings in their throat, sought educational material, or planned vocal rest or therapy.

When asked for examples of professional voice users, one quarter of the students (6/24) did not name SLPs. Sixty-one percent (14/24) of students reported not knowing or having access to voice resources. The 39% (9/24) who reported knowing voice resources listed the instructor of the course, the speech clinic at UVA, and the course textbook as their resources. This realization confirms the need for students to become aware of the vocal nature of their profession and be comfortable in identifying and using online, literature, clinical, and coaching resources (Khidr, 2015). There is a clear need to establish a voice care program for self and others.

Thirty-nine percent (9/24) reported experiencing voice problems in the past year (during their graduate program), but none sought clinical help. While 79% (19/24) experienced "notable throat sensations" related to talking, 90% (17/19) of those students ignored the sensation, and only 10% (2/19) planned periods of vocal rest. Seventeen percent (4/24) of the students were assigned voice clients and had been treating voice problems before starting the course (Khidr, 2015). This realization confirms the need for students to become aware of how their throat feels and voice sounds when talking, and how and when to seek clinical help.

The Field of Phoniatrics

Hermann Gutzmann (1865–1922) is known as the father of phoniatrics in Europe. He argued that medical students were not informed about communication disorders during their medical studies and advocated for adding a new medical specialty that addressed this void in medical education and clinical services. His 1905 lecture, "Speech Disorders as a Topic of Clinical Education," is considered the birth of phoniatrics. The incorporation of his newly established clinic into the Clinic of Otolaryngology of the Charite Hospital in Berlin solidified the field (Kuczkowski, Cieszyńska, Plichta, Tretiakow, & Stodulski, 2015). This physical and collaborative relationship became the model for future phoniatrics and otolaryngology practices around the world.

On the other side of the Mediterranean, Dr. Nasser Kotby, professor at Ain Shams University, is considered the father of phoniatrics in the Middle East. He established the specialty of Phoniatrics and Logopedics (medical and nonmedical speech-language pathology) at Ain Shams University in Egypt in 1974 and chaired the department until 1998. (Kotby, 2006). He is currently president of the Egyptian Society of Phoniatrics and Logopedics (ESPL).

By 2010, the field of Phoniatrics in Egypt grew from one phoniatrician (medical SLP) and two logopedists (nonmedical SLP) to approximately 125 phoniatricians and 250 logopedists. This team established phoniatrics education and services in all state university hospitals in Egypt, as well as in major public and private hospitals over all the Middle East.

In addition, several resettled and resumed practicing phoniatrics and logopedics in Europe, the United States, and Canada (Kotby, El-Sady, & Hegazi, 2010; Kotby, 2014).

Dr. Kotby served on the board of the International Association of Logopedics and Phoniatrics (IALP) from 1983 to 2007. He was IALP treasurer for two terms in the 1980s and 1990s and president in 1995. His previous roles with IALP, along with his current role as an honored member, have developed strong ties between the growing ESPL professional community and their large international family. This manifested in the participation of many European colleagues in the education and training of new professionals in Egypt and ongoing collaborations toward advancing the field (Kotby, 1980, 2014).

Graduate Training in Phoniatrics

The Union of the European Phoniatricians (UEP) and the European Union of Medical Specialists (UEMS) collaborated to develop a program for phoniatric training. The graduate medical student enters the specialist training program after passing the basic training period, typically in the Phoniatric Department of a University Hospital. The training program includes supervised clinical work and theoretical studies covering nine major sections with special emphasis on the voice disorders section. The different stages of experience and independent competence for each section are evaluated as (a) acquired basic knowledge and skills, (b) requires supervision, or (c) independent (UEP & UEMS, 2010).

The phoniatrician's voice training includes competencies in the areas of voice diagnosis, voice prevention, voice rehabilitation, voice medical treatment, and laryngeal surgery. Specific examples of these competencies include auditory-perceptual evaluation of voice, assessment of voice ergonomics, care of professional speakers, providing and supervising voice therapy, understanding influences of drug treatments on voice, and performing laryngeal surgical techniques.

The Egyptian Educational Program for Master's Degree in Phoniatrics (Fadly & Kotby, 1978) includes similar guidelines, which requires competency in vocal self-training as a prerequisite to voice rehabilitation and training others on voice care. It states that the trainee is required to "practice the 'Accent Method' for voice therapy in order to be able to participate in giving therapy for patients with selected types of dysphonia" (Fadly & Kotby, 1978).

Phoniatricians trained in Ain Shams Medical School, including the first author, have experienced first-hand the value of practicing voice therapy exercises to take care of their own voices before attempting to care for voices of their patients. The Phoniatrics program of Ain Shams University invested generously in auditory-perceptual training, and weekly grand rounds were imperative to the training. Students were required to conduct a full evaluation (case history, subjective evaluations, objective analysis, laryngeal examination, etc.) on a voice patient every week. They presented their findings and therapy plan to a panel of phoniatric voice experts who collectively re-examined the patient to confirm or dispute the students' findings. The final therapy plan was approved in that setting and student phoniatricians were given a set time to re-present their findings after their patient started voice therapy or underwent laryngeal surgery. Behavioral voice therapy was provided for each patient at least twice per week, with an average caseload of five patients per student phoniatrician, whether in individual or group therapy format. These prospective phoniatricians did not provide voice therapy until they received a full program of voice therapy by one of their senior colleagues or faculty and demonstrated the ability and confidence to perform the necessary skills. This heavy voice training is typical for most phoniatrics programs.

Voice Education and Training Programs

Students studying to become professional voice users should have access to voice care programs during their graduate education. It is too late to wait until they are already in the workforce to receive vocal care and training. Fortunately, there has been a gradual buildup of such programs for licensed teachers, both across the globe and in the United States. However, there are few programs that exist for student teachers and even fewer for SLPs prior to entering the workforce.

The programs that do exist for preservice teachers range from a 6-hour training program provided by Timmermans in Belgium (Timmermans et al., 2011), a weeklong in-class training provided by Morrissey in Iowa (2003), and a 14-week curriculum provided by Duffy and Hazlett in Ireland (2004). These programs cover a wide range of activities including lectures (Duffy & Hazlett, 2004; Morrissey, 2003; Timmermans et al., 2011), hands-on vocal and breathing exercises (Duffy & Hazlett, 2004; Morrissey, 2003; Timmermans et al., 2011), homework assignments, and readings (Morrissey, 2003).

These published studies target student teachers preparing to enter the workforce as professional voice users. No studies to date target graduate SLP students entering a similar workforce. The voice education and training (VET) program described later in this chapter is the first reported program that targets graduate SLPs. It is administered for 9 weeks as an in-class program that consists of similar activities, including lectures, hands-on vocal and breathing exercises, homework assignments, and readings. In addition, it includes training perceptual voice and voice exercise skills and engaging graduate SLP students in activities that target voice well-being of self, familiar partners, and professional voice users.

Outcome Measures

The most commonly reported outcome measures of voice education and training programs are objective acoustic voice measures, subjective voice qualities, and self-rated vocal functions and dysfunctions. Timmermans et al. (2011) reported on objective acoustic measures of pitch and pitch deviation, phonatory measurement (maximum phonation time), and the dysphonia severity index, which includes measures of highest frequency, lowest intensity, maximum phonation time, and jitter. They also reported on subjective auditory-perceptual analysis of voice performed by the clinicians using the GRBAS (grade, roughness, breathiness, asthenia, strain) scale. Duffy and Hazlett (2004) used a combination of objective and subjective measures. For objective acoustic measures, they reported on the dysphonia severity index; for subjective outcomes they reported on the frequency of occurrence of 18 vocal symptoms on the Vocology Screening Profile and the scores of the Vocal Handicap Index to quantify the self-perceived impact of voice disorders.

The VET program described later in this chapter is the only one that reports on students' perception of changes in their (a) vocal awareness, (b) implementation of vocal behaviors, and (c) confidence in performing newly acquired auditory-perceptual and voice exercise skills as outcomes for a voice education and training program. These outcomes were scored along a five-level Likert scale (0 = not at all confident; 1 = not so confident; 2 = reasonably confident; 3 = very confident; 4 = extremely confident) for their confidence in practicing Smith Accent voice exercise skills. Outcomes were also dichotomously scored (0, 1) for awareness and implementation of vocal hygiene strategies.

Graduate SLP Voice Education and Training (VET) Program

VET Program Development

The first author's medical phoniatric training with an intensive focus on voice and her passion for preventive voice education and training were key in developing this program. Soon after accepting a faculty position at the Communication Disorders program at UVA in 1998, the first author reached out to the otolaryngology department and offered her services in developing a voice lab that could serve her voice education and training vision. The head of the otolaryngology department put her in charge of this project (Khidr, 2003). In a few months, the newly developed voice lab moved to a bigger space, and in few years it moved to a new building. During this time, the first author headed two reputable institutional projects (Noordzij et al., 2001, 2002), earned the lab a grant to participate in a follow-up multicenter research project (Carrau et al., 2004, 2005), and provided multiple opportunities for the graduate SLP students to intern with her. These graduate students received one-on-one clinical education and training in auditory-perceptual evaluation, laryngeal examination, and voice therapy. Interns first observed and slowly eased into helping with assessments and therapy before conducting supervised assessments and therapy.

In addition, the first author, in conjunction with Kate Burke in the drama department, started providing comprehensive voice evaluations for each incoming class of drama students. This provided opportunities for graduate SLP students to interview, analyze, and examine the larynx and provide comprehensive feedback for a professional voice user. However, this meaningful, early training benefited only a limited number of highly engaged graduate SLP students. In order to make voice education and training available to all graduate SLP students, the first author lobbied for the addition of a voice care course to the SLP curriculum. Realizing that this option was not feasible at the time, she started providing optional voice therapy workshops at the end of each semester to students in the SLP program, the local chapter of National Student Speech-Language-Hearing Association (NSSLHA), and interested clinicians through regional, national, and international venues (Khidr, 2003a, 2003b, 2004, 2005a, 2005b; Khidr & Samlan, 2003).

By the end of the last decade, a shift in the vocal behavior of college students became evident. A clear voice quality was no longer the norm, and a dysphonic voice was no longer a cause for worry or reason to seek help. It was then that the first author decided to make voice education and training part of the graduate and undergraduate curriculum at UVA so that all students attending the SLP program would benefit. She designed a three-unit voice education and training program for the graduate class, which was included in their voice disorders course, and a one-unit program for the undergraduate class, which was included in their anatomy and physiology course. Both programs involved a semester-long, student-led, IRB-approved research project that collected data from surveys describing the students' vocal profile, impressions regarding different vocal qualities, and attitudes toward seeking voice therapy. The results of each of these surveys were shared in class with the students, and the implications of their responses were discussed and presented by the first author, as well as her graduate and undergraduate students, in local, national, and international conferences (Khidr, 2014a, 2014b, 2014c; 2015; Ligon, Rank, & Khidr, 2013; Ligon, Rank, Khidr, & Hull, 2016a, 2016b; Maddox, Khidr, & Hull, 2016; Roper

& Khidr, 2015a, 2015b, 2015c; Khidr, Roper, & Hull, 2017). The targeted competencies and outcomes of this voice education and training program have evolved throughout the years to meet the growing personal and professional needs of the graduate SLP students.

Targeted Competencies and Outcomes

The foundational focus of the phoniatrics program model is to train the voice of the clinicians before expecting them to provide voice therapy to their patients. This element is missing from most graduate speech pathology programs, which usually recommend, but do not require, that students treating a voice client should be currently enrolled in or have completed a voice class. Those few students who have voice clients usually observe voice therapy for the first time as their clinical supervisor administers it to their client. Students are expected to provide voice therapy on their own after just a few sessions. This may work well for speech or language clients because the graduate students already possess necessary underlying articulation and language skills. However, this is not true in the case of voice. The underlying skills needed to administer voice therapy involve far more than simply having a clear voice.

SLP students need to acquire the following basic competencies in order to care for their own voices and therefore provide adequate care for clients with voice disorders: (a) acquire voice awareness, (b) implement healthy vocal behaviors, (c) perform basic auditory-perceptual analysis, and (d) perform selected voice therapy techniques with appropriate confidence (Figure 3–1).

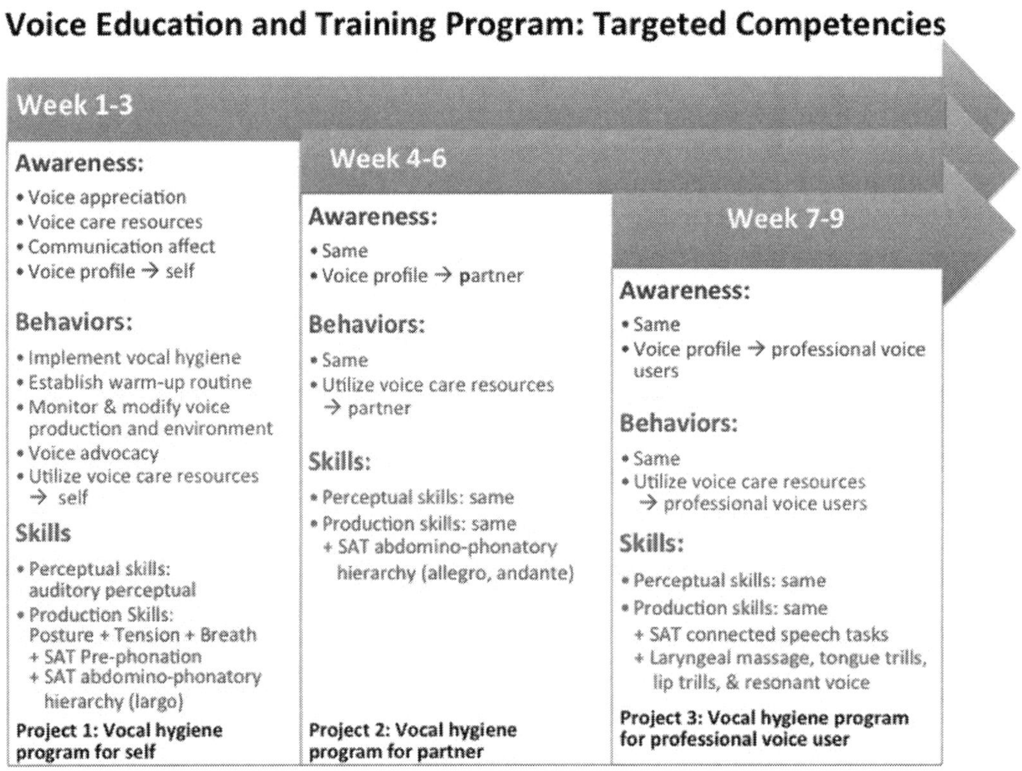

Figure 3–1. *Voice Education and Training Program: Targeted Competencies.*

The first author used the phoniatrics model as the foundation for the SLP voice education and training program. She provided students with multiple opportunities to (a) reflect on the value of the human voice in general, as well as the value and challenges of the professional voice; (b) realize that they are pursuing the career of a professional voice user; (c) notice how their voice sounds and feels and how their posture, muscle tension, and breathing feel when voicing; (d) design vocal hygiene programs for self and others; (e) record their daily vocal habits; (f) perform auditory-perceptual analysis on familiar and unfamiliar voice samples; (g) schedule one-on-one sessions with their instructor to get feedback (Figure 3–2); and (h) practice selected voice exercises in and out of class to habituate the new routine. Additionally, students were provided an opportunity to (i) participate in fun voice awareness activities on campus (Figure 3–3); (j) research a selected professional

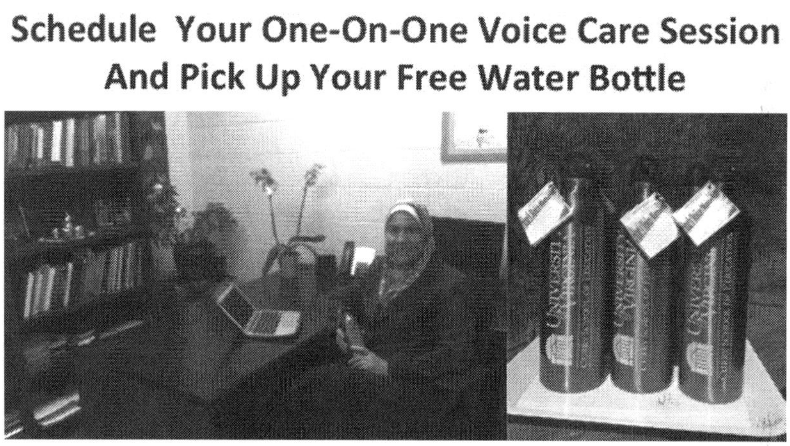

Figure 3–2. *Scheduling one-on-one voice care sessions with the instructor.*

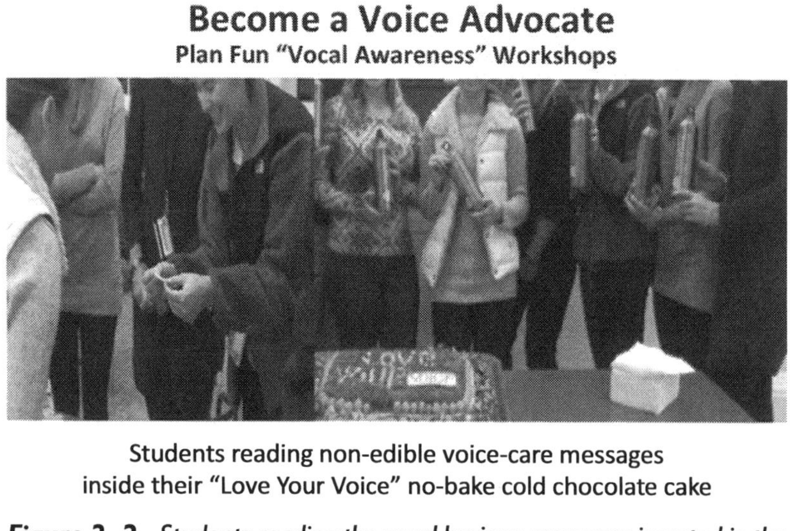
Become a Voice Advocate
Plan Fun "Vocal Awareness" Workshops
Students reading non-edible voice-care messages
inside their "Love Your Voice" no-bake cold chocolate cake

Figure 3–3. *Students reading the vocal hygiene messages inserted in the "Love Your Voice" cake.*

voice using population; (k) share in research addressing their own vocal profile and challenges; (l) present their research in local, regional and national meetings (Figure 3–4); and (m) design and deliver a community service activity aiming to teach their selected population how to care for their voice (Figures 3–5 and 3–6). Targeted professional voice users served by this class included other graduate and undergraduate SLP students, graduate education students, university professors, university singers, university athletes, university tour guides, local schoolteachers as well as staff and customers of a local brewery.

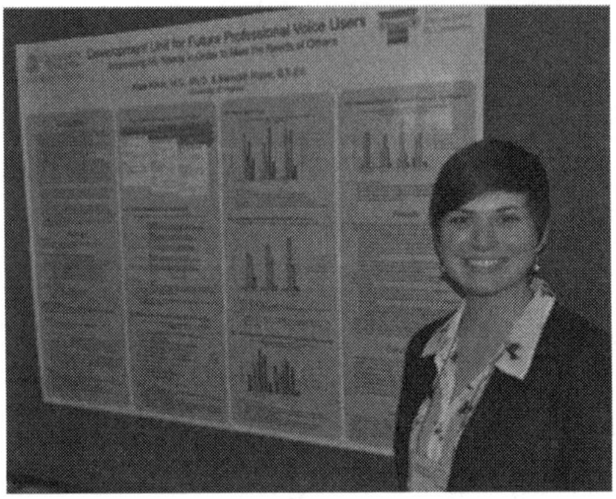

Figure 3–4. *Student poster presentation in SHAV, March 2015.*

Vocal Awareness

Voice Appreciation. Students were given assignments that build awareness of the value of the human voice, which is fundamental for appreciating the unique cultural aesthetics of the abundant vocal traditions and performances across the globe. They were also given assignments to reflect on the implications of considering professional voice users as vocal athletes. This helps them understand the unique psychological, social, and occupational impact of preserving and treating their own voice, as well as the voices of other professional

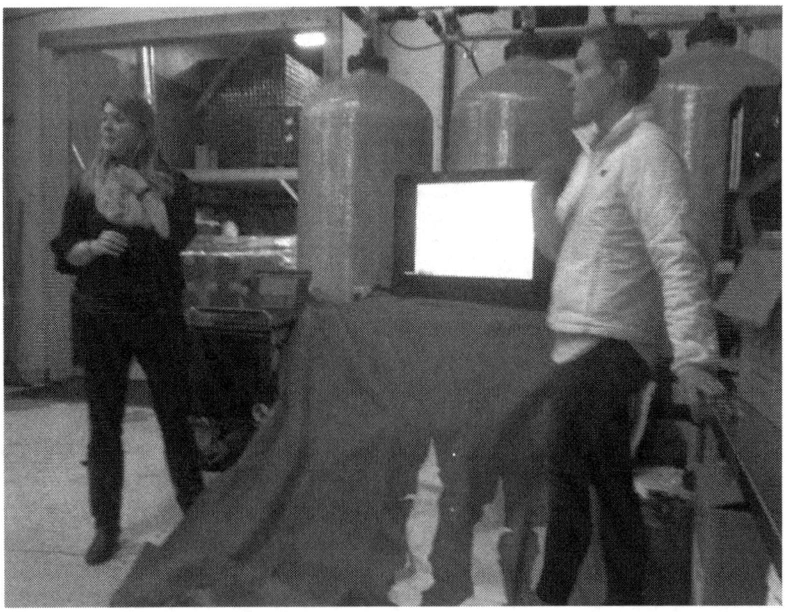

Figure 3–5. *Students presenting in a community vocal awareness activity.*

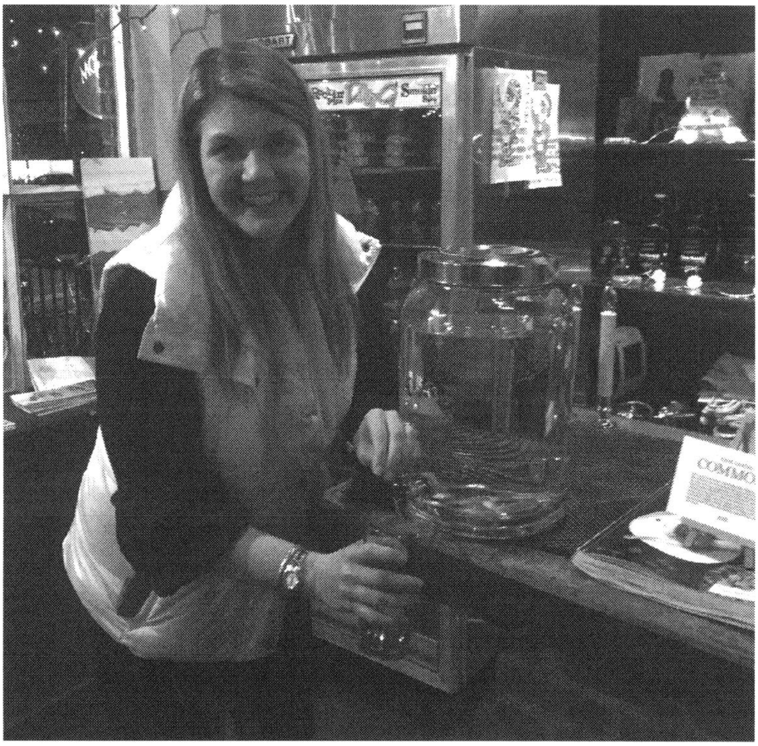

Figure 3–6. *Student advocating for hydration in a community vocal awareness activity.*

voice users. In order to cultivate this vocal awareness students were asked to respond to an online forum regarding a vocal performance that has special meaning, describing what the human voice means to them, and commenting on classmates' posts to appreciate their point of view.

Communication Effect. Students completed surveys and engaged in class discussions to raise awareness of the effect of voice on communication. Most students do not take time to think about how others perceive them through their voice. Students were asked to review relevant literature covering this topic and participate in related class activities.

Ligon, Rank, Khidr, and Hull (2016a) asked 23 graduate SLP students attending the voice disorders class of 2013 to describe listeners' possible perceptions of the communication affect (attitude, mood, emotion, etc.) of female speakers. Students were then asked to evaluate the desirability of the 25 adjectives on a 3-point scale (1 = undesirable; 2 = neither desirable nor undesirable; 3 = desirable). Ten adjectives were rated as desirable (confident, mature, engaged, lively, sophisticated, relaxed/chill, cool, sweet, feminine, sexy), two were rated as in between (nonaggressive and flirtatious), and 13 were rated as undesirable (apathetic/disinterested, aggressive, sleepy, vain, bored/unengaged, manly, insecure/hesitant, uneducated, unhealthy/sick, tense/stressed, depressed, painful, obnoxious). Later on, students were asked to use these 25 adjectives to describe eight vocal qualities: rough, breathy, strained, loud, soft/weak, high pitch, low pitch, and vocal fry. This class described vocal fry as vain (56%), apathetic/disinterested (48%), sleepy (38%), relaxed/chill (38%), and bored/ unengaged (36%). Students discussed their impressions as listeners of different vocal qualities and how that may affect social and professional interactions, reiterating the effect of voice on communication.

Voice Care Resources. Students explored online resources such as the University of Iowa "Voice Academy" interactive program (University of Iowa, 2016), as well as relevant literature and book chapters (Colton, Casper, & Leonard, 2006; Khidr, 2010, 2012; Kotby, 1995; LeBorgne & Rosenberg, 2014; Stemple & Fry, 2010). In order to easily receive or recommend voice therapy services, students were also made aware of the physical location of local facilities that provide voice services, including the speech clinic at UVA, drama program, university hospital, and private practitioners.

Voice Profile. Voice profile refers to how one's voice sounds and feels during or after talking; unhealthy vocal behaviors one engages in; vocal hygiene behaviors one observes; vocal demands one has in their social, professional, and academic life; challenges one has that may affect their ability to continue talking with ease and clarity throughout the day; environments one regularly talks in; and stressors one has on a daily basis.

Students were expected to become aware of their own vocal profile, that of a classmate, and that of a selected professional voice user by conducting formal interviews, following a standardized voice protocol, and completing the Vocal Handicap Index. These hands-on activities served to solidify the students' appreciation of the effect of one's personal vocal profile on their voice outcome.

Vocal Behaviors

Implementing Vocal Hygiene. In order to help students acquire healthy vocal habits, they were asked record their daily vocal practices using the Vocal Hygiene Weekly Log (Appendix 3–1) three times each week. This helped them monitor their vocal habits and habituate implementation of healthy vocal behaviors.

Students also filled out the Unit Feedback Survey (Appendix 3–2) at the end of each 3-week unit. The Unit Feedback Survey used a 5-point rating scale to describe students' confidence. Engaging the students in recording their own responses was intended not only to help them take care of their own voices but also to help them connect with their future clients and share their own experiences regarding strategies that may have worked for them.

Implementing a Warm-Up Routine. The Smith Accent (SA) Technique is considered one of the most holistic voice therapy techniques used by phoniatricians and logopedists in Europe, Africa, and Asia. Its popularity is due to its physiological basis, logical hierarchy of skills, holistic nature in addressing body posture, muscle tension, body movements, and relaxed breathing, and the coordination of breathing with phonation (abdomino-phonatory control). The habituation of this control is achieved through a hierarchy of tasks that gradually increase in speed, length, phonatory complexity (nonvoiced and voiced fricatives, vowels), linguistic complexity (single syllables, multiple syllables, words, sentences), communicative complexity (reading, monologues, discussing prepared topics, discussing novel topics), and conversational turn-taking (Khidr, 2010; Kotby, 1995; Thyme-Frøkjær & Frøkjær-Jensen, 2001).

Originally, relaxation and stretching exercises were not used in the SA Technique because breathing exercises resulted in relaxation. As a holistic method, it trains not only alternating tension and relaxation of the respiratory, phonatory, and articulatory muscles, but also the coordination and balance between breathing muscles and all muscles used for movement and posture. However, Thyme-Frøkjær and Frøkjær-Jensen (2001) introduced a set of relaxation and stretching exercises to be completed before the SA exercises in order to combat the increased stress observed in today's modern life. They reported that many people have increased tension in the neck and shoulders, causing discomfort, pain, and headaches. This tension influences the muscles of the larynx and therefore the vocal functions.

These exercises include stretching and relaxing the shoulders, neck, and articulatory muscles. In the SLP vocal education and training program, the combination of the stretching exercises, basic abdomino-diaphragmatic breathing exercises, pre-phonatory SA exercises, and the vowel play of the phonatory phase using the largo rhythm were collectively named "Vocal Warm-Ups." The first author led the students in these vocal warm-ups (Figure 3–7) for 10 minutes at the beginning of each class. She demonstrated the exercises and provided individual feedback to the students, similar to group therapy format. Students were asked to perform these vocal warm-ups twice a day, 3 days a week, and report completion on the Vocal Hygiene Weekly Log.

Voice Advocacy. Students were asked to advocate for vocal health by designing voice awareness brochures or vocal hygiene activities. Students reviewed and commented on the submissions of their classmates. They were encouraged to share their products on social media or in other classes to advocate for vocal health.

Utilizing Voice Care Resources. By the end of each 3-week unit, students were asked to submit a voice care project, which involved identifying and utilizing relevant voice care literature and online resources to design an

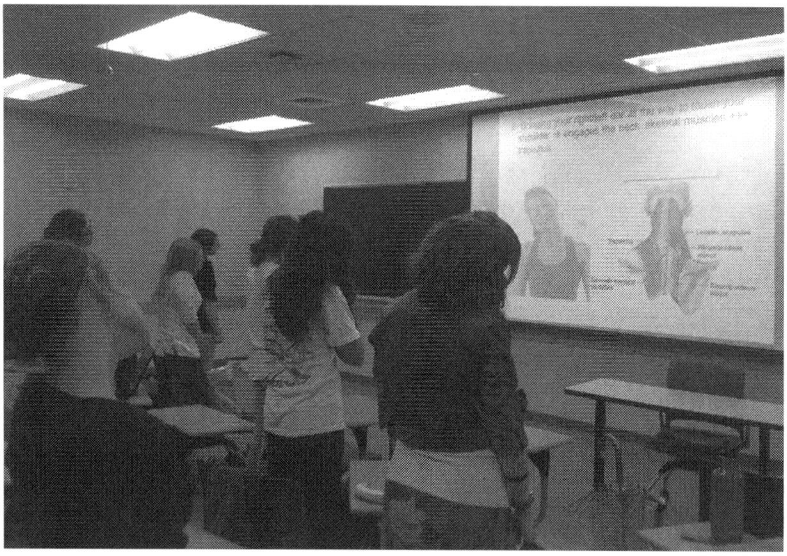

***Figure 3–7.** In-class neck stretches.*

individualized vocal hygiene plan for themselves, a classmate, and a selected professional voice user that addressed their unique vocal profile and challenges.

Vocal Skills

Voice Perception Skills. Basic voice perception skills entail (a) the ability to perform visual observations and analysis of body posture, muscle tension (mouth, face, neck, shoulders, etc.), breathing patterns, and abdomino-phonatory control used during voice production; (b) the ability to palpate the neck and identify areas of tension in the extrinsic laryngeal and neck muscles; and (c) the ability to perform auditory-perceptual analysis on one's own voice, familiar voices, and unfamiliar voices.

Auditory-perceptual analysis of voice is the most fundamental skill that needs to be developed first. A solid appreciation of the product (voice) is needed for the clinician to appreciate the physiological ingredients (posture, muscle tension, breath support, etc.) that contribute to it. In order to acquire new auditory-perceptual skills, students were asked to self-monitor and correct suboptimal vocal behaviors. As a precursor to acquiring perceptual analysis skills, students were asked to study the physiological correlates of auditory-perceptual voice characteristics and describe normal and dysphonic voices. To assess their readiness to acquire basic auditory-perceptual skills, students studied the GRBAS and CAPE-V (Consensus Auditory-Perceptual Evaluation of Voice) scales (Nemr et al., 2012) and completed an auditory-perceptual quiz. Then, students were asked to listen to online voice case simulations from the University of Wisconsin-Madison (2008) and voice case simulations from La Trobe University, Melbourne, Australia (Oates & Russell, 2003). Students read the experts' auditory-perceptual evaluations included in both resources after listening to each case.

In the first unit (Weeks 1–3) of the voice education and training program, students were asked to record the Rainbow Passage using any free application of their choice, such as Praat (Boersma & Weenink, 2016), listen to their recordings, and describe their voice using the auditory-perceptual parameters of voicing, resonance, register, pitch, and loudness, and the voice quality parameters describing grade of dysphonia, roughness, breathiness, asthenia, and strain. In the second (Weeks 4–6) and third (Weeks 7–9) units, students recorded and analyzed the Rainbow Passage read by a classmate. Gillingham et al. (2012) tested the auditory-perceptual skills of 26 graduate SLP students before and after attending the voice education and training program. Students' perceptual ratings of audio recordings of 10 unfamiliar voices were used to calculate the score. The researchers observed that the students' auditory-perceptual analysis scores were significantly improved after completion of the auditory-perceptual analysis listening and rating activities of the program.

Voice Production Skills. Once the basic warm-up routine was established, the students were taught the higher levels of the SA abdomino-phonatory hierarchy (Khidr, 2010; Kotby, 1995; Thyme-Frøkjær & Frøkjær-Jensen, 2001), in addition to manual laryngeal massage, tongue trills, lip trills, and resonant voice. Manual laryngeal massage involves kneading the laryngeal muscles and joints to alleviate excessive tension in those areas. This helps the larynx to descend, allowing for easier and clearer voice production. Tongue trills involve quickly rolling the tongue against the roof of the mouth while slowly and steadily exhaling. This helps relax the tongue and avoid unnecessary muscle tension in the larynx. Lip trills, similar to tongue trills, involve trilling the lips together while slowly and steadily exhaling. This helps release lip tension, avoid unnecessary tension in the larynx, and focus on breath control, which makes the voice more efficient. Finally, resonant voice involves humming and focusing on vibrations in the facial bones during voice production, which releases tension in the vocal folds, allowing the vocal folds to vibrate more freely (Colton, Casper, & Leonard, 2006). Students were asked to practice the exercises performed in class three times a week, commenting on its ease and on their confidence in the practice.

Program Outcome Measures

Basic competencies needed by graduate SLP students to care for their own voices and provide adequate care for clients with voice disorders are used as outcome measures for the VET program. These include the students' ability to (a) acquire voice awareness, (b) implement healthy vocal behaviors and voice warm-up exercises in their daily routine, and (c) perform basic auditory-perceptual analysis and selected voice therapy techniques with appropriate confidence (Figure 3–8). All these targeted competencies and outcome measures have been described earlier in the chapter.

Undergraduate SLP Voice Education and Training (VET) Program

The undergraduate course of "Anatomy and Physiology of the Speech and Hearing Mechanism" is one of the prerequisites for the graduate voice disorders course. This course has a

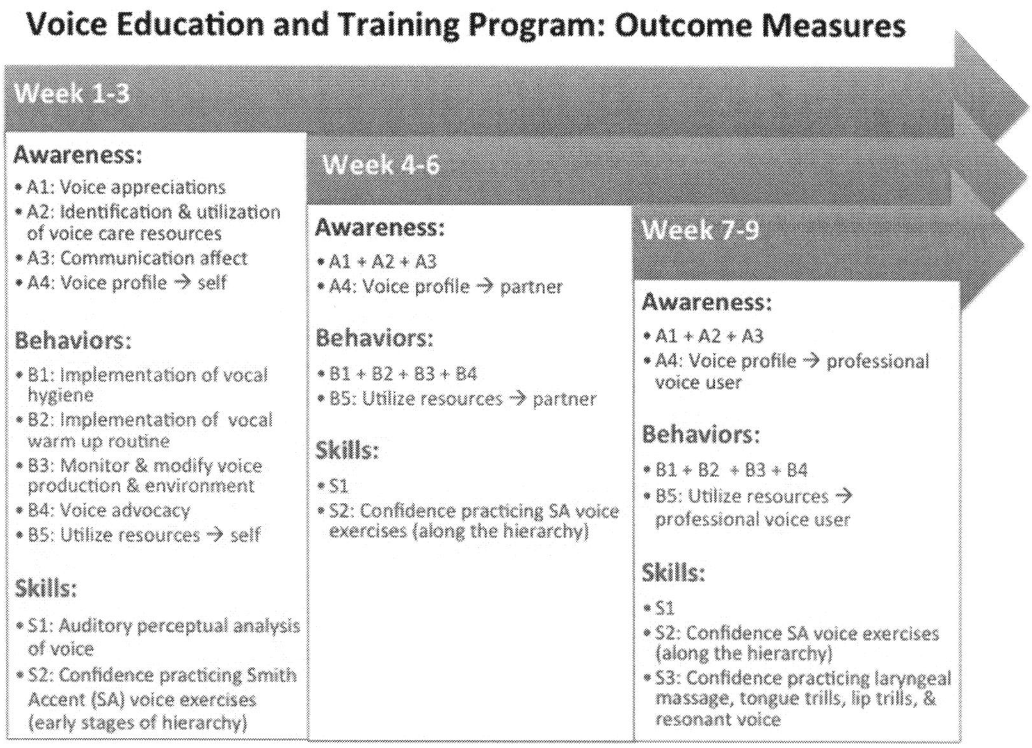

Figure 3–8. *Voice Education and Training Program: Outcome Measures.*

unit covering anatomy and physiology of phonation that spans over six one-hour classes, provided as three classes per week for 2 weeks. It is during this unit that undergraduate students receive their in-class VET Program. The undergraduate program is modeled after unit 1 of the graduate program. The graduate end-of-unit project of creating a vocal hygiene program for self is replaced by the undergraduates designing an engaging voice advocacy project. As the anatomy and physiology class is usually offered in the spring semester, students are asked to design an activity that can take place on campus to advocate for voice and celebrate World Voice Day on April 16.

Withers and Khidr (2017) studied 84 students attending the Anatomy and Physiology of the Ear and Voice Mechanism course at James Madison University (JMU). All received the undergraduate in-class VET program as part of their unit on anatomy and physiology of phonation. The program included one 60-minute presentation highlighting voice care and four 15-minute in-class vocal warm-ups. Students completed the Vocal Hygiene Weekly Log (see Appendix 3–1) three times per week for 4 weeks (extending beyond the in-class unit), completed the Unit Feedback Survey (see Appendix 3–2) at the end of the program, and created a voice care campaign for World Voice Day. It also included a pre- and post-program Vocal Appreciation Survey. The students were required to answer all surveys as part of their homework; however, a consent form gave them the option to remove their results from the study. All surveys were approved by JMU's Institutional Review Board of Social and Behavioral Sciences.

Withers and Khidr (2017) found that 82% of the undergraduate SLP class had never received information regarding potential vocal challenges as future SLPs, 89% were not aware of voice care services available to them at JMU, and 96% had never had a vocal evaluation before. Researchers reported a 31% improvement in the amount of water students were drinking (from 1 to 3 cups per day to 4 to 6 cups per day), 75% increase in their confidence in monitoring their own voice, and 63% increase in their confidence in using the stretching exercises as well as the SA technique for pre-phonatory and basic (largo rhythm) abdomino-phonatory exercises.

The undergraduate students designed and shared posters and activities that advocated for voice care on the 2016 World Voice Day. They also posted voice-care messages on their social media networks and provided examples of the feedback they received. The researchers concluded that the implementation of a 2-week in-class VET program in the required undergraduate anatomy course resulted in substantial improvement in the voice care behaviors of undergraduate SLP students. Engaging undergraduate SLP students in advocating for voice care among their peers on campus served as an additional way for students to educate themselves about the importance of their voice while serving as voice advocates (Withers & Khidr, 2017).

Case Study

In 2014, 22 female students ages 23 to 35 received the voice education and training (VET) program described earlier in the chapter as part of their graduate voice class curriculum. The VET program and all the surveys used were approved by the University of Virginia's Institutional Review Board of Health and Science Research (IRB-SBS #2013-0451). Each student was assigned a randomized code to use when answering the surveys for the data to remain anonymous. Students had the option to ask for their data to be removed from the study through contacting the research assistant. No students asked for their data to be removed but a few did not complete their surveys as required (Khidr, Roper, & Hull, 2017, submitted).

The VET program contained three units. Each unit lasted 3 weeks and consisted of two 30-minute in-class activities per week, totaling 3 hours per unit (9 hours total). Students filled out the Vocal Hygiene Weekly Log (see Appendix 3–1) three times per week and the Unit Feedback Survey (see Appendix 3–2) at the end of each 3-week unit of the voice education and training (VET) program. They also completed individual and group assignments outside of class.

The Vocal Hygiene Weekly Log (see Appendix 3–1) monitored their vocal behaviors, vocal hygiene, and use of voice warm-up routines. The Unit Feedback Survey (see Appendix 3–2) assessed their (a) development of voice awareness, (b) implementation of vocal hygiene strategies and utilization of educational voice resources, and (c) confidence in newly developed skills of self-monitoring and correction of vocal behaviors and environments, perceptual voice analysis, and performing Smith Accent voice exercises and four other voice therapy exercises.

While completion of all questions on the Unit Feedback Survey was required, there is only complete data for 13 students for Units 1 and 2, and for 18 students for Unit 3. In addition, responses for some survey questions (Questions 6 through 8) were only collected after Unit 3.

Khidr, Roper, and Hull (2017, submitted) used responses on the Vocal Hygiene Weekly Log (see Appendix 3–1) to create a voice exercise variable by summing the scores for Question 1, a healthy consumption variable by summing the scores for Questions 2 through 6, a healthy behavior variable by summing the scores on Question 7, and a vocal hygiene strategy/modification use variable by summing the scores on Question 8. The scoring method for each question is detailed in Appendix 3–1. The researchers then used a repeated measures analysis of variance (ANOVA) to examine mean change across the weeks of data collection. None of the four ANOVA models, one for each variable described above, revealed significant mean differences.

As with the data from the Vocal Hygiene Weekly Log, Khidr, Roper, and Hull (2017, submitted) used responses on the Unit Feedback Survey (see Appendix 3–2) to create an awareness variable, an implementation variable, and a confidence in practicing Smith Accent (SA) exercise skills variable. The construction of these variables is described below the discussion of descriptive statistics from the Unit 3 feedback. Three repeated measures ANOVA models were used to evaluate mean differences in subject awareness, subject implementation, and subject confidence in practicing SA voice exercise skills. The results showed significant increases in mean scores for subject awareness, subject implementation, and subject confidence in practicing SA voice exercise skills. Moreover, omega squared indicated that 10% of the variation in subjects reported awareness, 28% in subject reported implementation, and 45% of the variance in subjects reported confidence in practicing SA voice exercise skills were attributable to the change in unit. These effect sizes—medium, very large, and extremely large, respectively—indicate that the material and activities provided in the units produced a significant practical increase in awareness, implementation, and confidence in practicing SA voice exercise skills after controlling for the sample size associated with the repeated measures statistical significance testing.

Descriptive statistics are used to discuss results from the Unit Feedback Survey after Unit 3 that are not reported elsewhere. Responses to Questions 1 through 5 on the Unit Feedback Survey (see Appendix 3–2) were used to create variables that represented subject awareness, implementation, and confidence in practicing Smith Accent (SA) voice exercise skills. The awareness variable was created by combining the responses to Questions 1 and 2 of the Unit Feedback Survey. Each question asks the respondent to select all that apply from a group of options, which were scored as either a zero (not endorsed) or a one (endorsed). The scores were then summed to create each subject's awareness score with a potential range from zero to nine. Table 3–1 displays the total, median, mean, and standard deviation for each option as well as for the combined awareness variable for Unit 3. Figure 3–9 displays a histogram of the awareness variable for Unit 3. As Table 3–1 shows,

Table 3–1. *Descriptive Statistics for "Voice Care Awareness" After Unit Three*

	Total[a]	Mdn	M	SD
A. How my voice sounds	18	1	1	0
B. How my voice feels	15	1	0.83	0.38
C. My daily vocal demands and challenges	15	1	0.83	0.38
D. My vocal environment (noise, distance, groups, etc.)	15	1	0.83	0.38
E. My unhealthy vocal behaviors (throat clearing, hard coughing, hard glottal attacks, etc.)	17	1	0.94	0.24
F. How others' voices sound	18	1	1	0
G. Others' daily vocal demands and challenges	16	1	0.89	0.32
H. Others' vocal environments (noise, distance, groups, etc.)	16	1	0.89	0.32
I. Others' unhealthy vocal behaviors (throat clearing, hard coughing, hard glottal attacks, etc.)	17	1	0.94	0.24
Total	147	9	8.17	1.86

[a]Total endorsements for A through I had a potential range from 0 to 18 and Total Awareness for all subjects had a potential range from 0 to 162. (For each subject the potential range was from 0 to 9.)

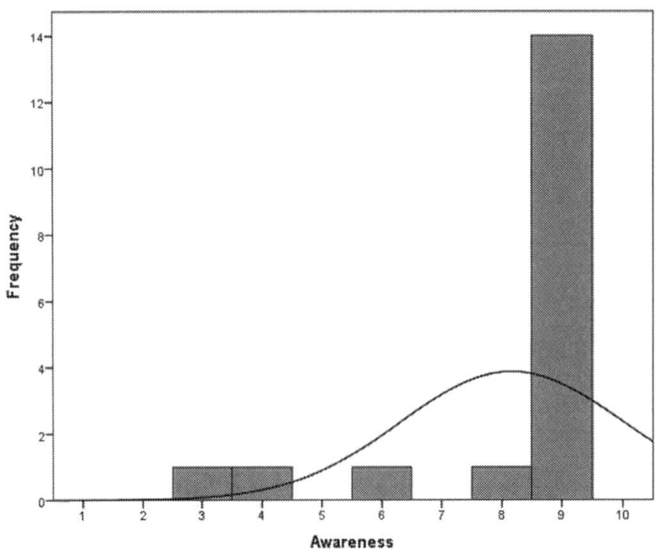

Figure 3–9. *Histogram with normal curve overlay displaying awareness scores for Unit 3.*

the subjects indicated high awareness across all options and, subsequently, on the total awareness variable. Additionally, Figure 3–9 shows that all but four subjects endorsed all of the awareness indicator responses and only three subjects endorsed less than eight of the nine options.

The implementation variable was created by combining responses to Questions 3 and 4 of the Unit Feedback Survey. As with the awareness variable, options were scored as either a zero (not endorsed) or a one (endorsed), which resulted in an implementation score with a potential range from zero to seventeen. Table 3–2 displays the total, median, mean, and standard deviation for each option as well as for the combined implementation variable for Unit 3. Figure 3–10 displays a histogram

Table 3–2. *Descriptive Statistics for "Implementation of New Behaviors" After Unit Three*

	Total[a]	Mdn	M	SD
A. Increase hydration	17	1	0.94	0.24
B. Decrease caffeine	6	0	0.33	0.49
C. Plan voice rest throughout my high-demand talking times of the day	16	1	0.89	0.32
D. Avoid sources of noise when talking	12	1	0.67	0.49
E. Modify talking environment to be less challenging	13	1	0.72	0.46
F. Monitor/decrease abusive vocal behaviors	13	1	0.72	0.46
G. Avoid talking in noisy environments (bars, concerts, gatherings)	11	1	0.61	0.50
H. Avoid/decrease talking on the phone in the car	7	1	0.39	0.50
I. Acknowledge and start working on stressors that I could identify	11	1	0.61	0.50
J. Seek support when I experience a negative mind-set	6	0	0.33	0.49
K. Vocal appreciation	12	1	0.67	0.49
L. Basic vocal knowledge (anatomy and physiology)	10	1	0.56	0.51
M. Vocal hygiene practices	15	1	0.83	0.38
N. Vocal challenges/disorders	14	1	0.78	0.43
O. Diagnosis of voice disorders	15	1	0.83	0.38
P. Management of voice disorders	11	1	0.61	0.50
Q. Voice research trends	4	0	0.22	0.43
Total	193	11	10.72	3.82

[a]Total endorsements for A through Q had a potential range from 0 to 18, and Total Implementation for all subjects had a potential range from 0 to 306. (For each subject the potential range was from 0 to 17.)

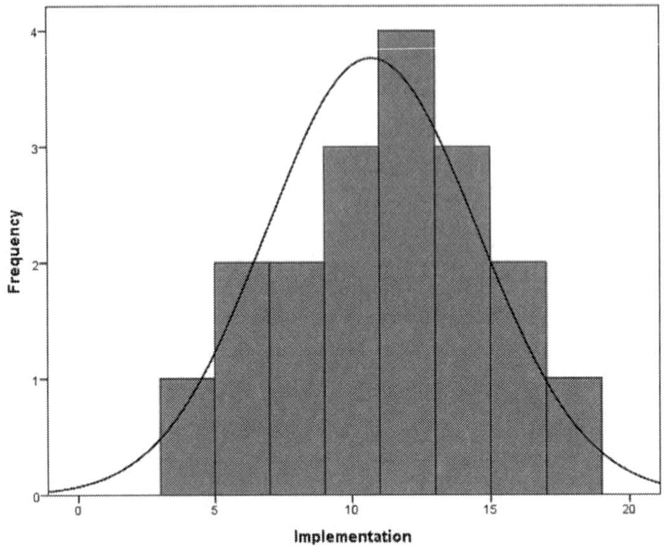

***Figure 3–10.** Histogram with normal curve overlay displaying implementation scores for Unit 3.*

of the implementation variable for Unit 3. As Table 3–2 shows, the mean value of the total implementation is only slightly greater than what would be expected by chance alone. Across all options, "Decrease caffeine" (6), "Avoid/decrease talking on the phone in the car" (7), "Seek support when I experience a negative mind-set" (6), and [utilize] "Voice research trends" (4) were the only options that were endorsed by less than half of the subjects. Figure 3–10 shows that the implementation variable is much more normally distributed than the awareness variable in Unit 3.

The confidence in practicing SA voice exercise skills was created from subject responses to Question 5 of the feedback survey. The subjects rated their confidence in applying each skill by using a five-level Likert scale ranging from "Not at all confident" (scored zero) to "Extremely confident" (scored four). The Likert scale scores were summed across the 13 voicing skills to create each subject's confidence in voicing skills score with a potential range from 0 to 52. Table 3–3 displays the total, median, mean, and standard deviation for each skill as well as for the combined confidence in practicing SA voice exercise skills variable for Unit 3. Figure 3–11 displays a histogram of the confidence in practicing SA voice exercise skills variable for Unit 3.

As Table 3–3 shows, the median for six of the SA skills was 3 (Very confident). Namely, in descending order, the subjects were "Very Confident" in SA skills B, A, C, F, and G (tied), and D.

For seven of the SA skills, the median value was at the scale midpoint of 2 (Reasonably confident). In descending order of confidence, these skills are E, H, I, J, K, and L and M (tied). Figure 3–11 shows that the confidence in practicing the Smith Accent exercise skills variable is reasonably normally distributed in Unit 3. Additionally, the mean of the confidence in practicing these seven Smith Accent exercise skills is only slightly greater than what would be expected by chance alone.

Table 3–3. *Descriptive Statistics for "Confidence in Practicing the Smith Accent Exercises" After Unit Three*

	Total[a]	Mdn	M	SD
A. Monitor/adjust posture	51	3	2.83	0.71
B. Monitor/control abdomino-diaphragmatic breathing	52	3	2.89	0.58
C. Monitor/adjust muscle tension in shoulders, head and neck, face, temporo-mandibular joint, and articulator muscles	50	3	2.78	0.65
D. Monitor/control volume, speed, rhythm, and intonation	44	3	2.44	0.78
E. Monitor/control timing of volitional expiration	43	2	2.39	0.61
F. Use proper breath support for nonvoiced sounds	45	3	2.50	0.62
G. Use proper breath support for voice sounds	45	3	2.50	0.62
H. Use proper breath support for vowel play	42	2	2.33	0.77
I. Use proper breath support for slow-speed syllables and speech	39	2	2.17	0.71
J. Use proper breath support for fast-speed syllables and speech	37	2	2.06	0.73
K. Use proper breath support during monologues	35	2	1.94	0.94
L. Use proper breath support during dialogues	34	2	1.89	0.90
M. Use proper breath support in group discussions	34	2	1.89	0.90
Total	551	31.50	30.61	5.92

[a]Total scores for A through M had a potential range from 0 to 72, and Total Confidence in Practicing the Smith Accent Exercise Skills for all subjects had a potential range from 0 to 936. (For each subject the possible range was from 0 to 52.)

Box 3–2

Smith Accent skills rated by students as "Very confident" in descending order:

B. Monitor/control abdomino-diaphragmatic breathing

A. Monitor/adjust posture

C. Monitor/adjust muscle tension in shoulders, head, and neck

F.* Use proper breath support for nonvoiced sounds

G.* Use proper breath support for voice sounds

D. Monitor/control volume, speed, rhythm, and intonation

(*) tie

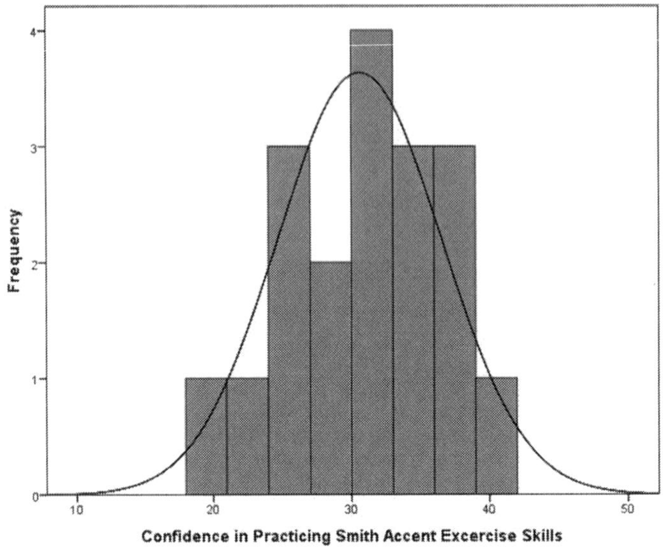

Figure 3–11. *Histogram with normal curve overlay displaying confidence in practicing Smith Accent voice exercise skills scores for Unit 3.*

Box 3–3

Smith Accent skills rated by students as "Reasonably confident" in descending order:

E. Monitor/control timing of volitional expiration

H. Use proper breath support for vowel play

I. Use proper breath support for slow-speed syllables and speech

J. Use proper breath support for fast-speed syllables and speech

K. Use proper breath support during monologues

L.* Use proper breath support during dialogues

M.* Use proper breath support in group discussions

(*) tie

Responses to Questions 6 through 8 on the Unit Feedback Survey were only gathered after completion of the VET program (end of Unit 3). Therefore, while Unit Feedback Questions 1 through 5 could be examined longitudinally (Khidr, Roper, & Hull, 2017, submitted), Questions 6 through 8 are limited to descriptive statistics. The behaviors within Questions 6 through 8 all use the same five-level Likert scale ranging from "Not at all confident" (scored zero) to "Extremely confident" (scored four). The Likert scale scores were summed across the behaviors within each question to create a total score for each subject on that question.

Question 6 asks whether Unit 3 helped the subjects develop confidence practicing four voice therapy exercises, namely, laryngeal massage, tongue trills, lip trills, and resonant voice. Confidence in practicing these four exercises had a total score with a potential range from 0 to 16. Table 3–4 shows the total score, median, mean, and standard deviation for each voice exercise as well as the combined confidence practicing voice exercises.

As Table 3–4 shows, the subjects as a group were slightly more confident in practicing lip and tongue trills, on average "Reasonably confident," than the manual laryngeal massage or resonant voice exercises, on average "Not so confident." Figure 3–12 displays the distribution of the total confidence in practicing these four voice therapy exercises.

Question 7 asks whether Unit 3 helped the subjects develop confidence in self-monitoring and self-correction. Confidence

Table 3–4. *Descriptive Statistics for "Confidence in Practicing Selected Voice Exercises" After Unit Three*

	Total[a]	Mdn	M	SD
A. Use manual laryngeal massage to decrease vocal hyperfunction	25	1.00	1.39	0.61
B. Use tongue trills to decrease vocal hyperfunction	38	2.00	2.11	0.90
C. Use lip trills to decrease vocal hyperfunction	41	2.00	2.28	0.75
D. Use resonant voice to decrease vocal hyperfunction	28	1.50	1.56	0.98
Total	132	8.00	7.33	2.54

[a]Totals for A through D had a potential range from 0 to 72, and Total Confidence in Practicing Selected Voice Exercises had a potential range from 0 to 288. (For each subject the possible range was from 0 to 16.)

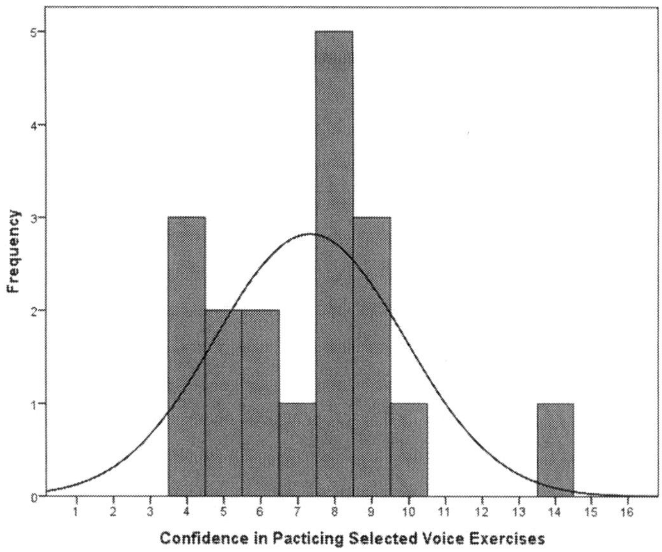

Figure 3–12. *Histogram with normal curve overlay displaying the total confidence in practicing selected voice exercises scores for Unit 3.*

in self-monitoring and self-correction was measured with three behaviors that had a total score with a potential range from 0 to 12. Table 3–5 shows the total score, median, mean, and standard deviation for confidence in each behavior as well as the combined confidence in self-monitoring and self-correction.

Table 3–5 shows that the subjects as a group were more confident in self-monitoring and self-correcting, on average "Very Confident," than they were in their confidence in practicing facilitating voice exercises. Figure 3–13 displays the distribution of the total confidence in self-monitoring and self-correction.

Question 8 asks whether Unit 3 helped the subjects develop confidence in their auditory-perceptual analysis skills. Confidence in auditory-perceptual analysis skills

Table 3–5. *Descriptive Statistics for "Confidence in Self-Monitoring and Self-Correction" After Unit Three*

	Total[a]	Mdn	M	SD
A. Use vocal hygiene log in monitoring vocal behavior.	56	3.00	3.11	0.68
B. Use vocal hygiene log in modifying vocal behavior.	55	3.00	3.06	0.73
C. Implement vocal hygiene measures.	55	3.00	3.06	0.64
Total	166	9.00	9.22	1.93

[a]Totals for A through C had a potential range from 0 to 72, and Total Confidence in Self-Monitoring and Self-Correction had a potential range from 0 to 216. (For each subject the possible range was from 0 to 12.)

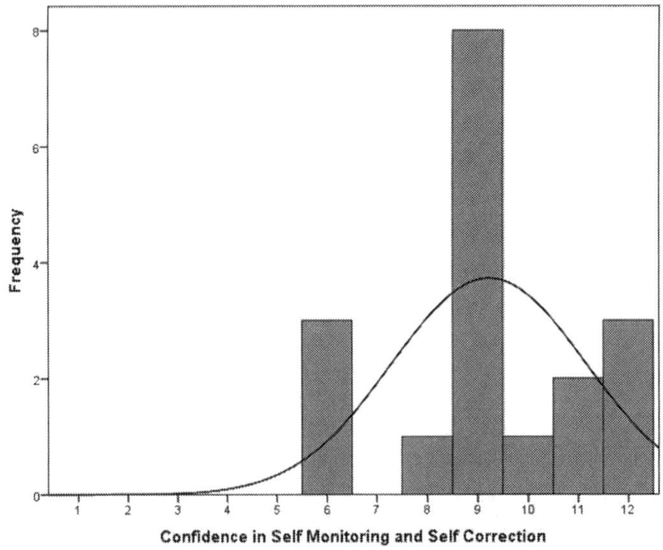

Figure 3–13. *Histogram with normal curve overlay displaying the confidence in self-monitoring and self-correction sores for Unit 3.*

was measured with three behaviors that had a total score with a potential range from 0 to 12. Table 3–6 shows the total score, median, mean, and standard deviation for confidence in each behavior as well as the combined confidence in auditory-perceptual analysis skills.

Table 3–6 shows that the subjects as a group were, on average, between "Reasonably confident" and "Very confident" in their auditory-perceptual analysis skills. Figure 3–14 displays the distribution of the total confidence in auditory-perceptual analysis skills.

Table 3–6. *Descriptive Statistics for "Confidence in Auditory Perceptual Analysis Skills" After Unit Three*

	Total[a]	Mdn	M	SD
A. Use of auditory perceptual skills in monitoring and analyzing my own voice	48	3.00	2.67	0.69
B. Use of auditory perceptual skills in monitoring and analyzing familiar (classmates) voices	44	2.00	2.44	0.51
C. Use of auditory perceptual skills in monitoring and analyzing unfamiliar/stranger (clients) voices	42	2.00	2.33	0.49
Total Confidence in Auditory Perceptual Analysis Skills	134	7.50	7.44	1.42

[a]Totals for A through C had a potential range from 0 to 72, and Total Confidence in Auditory Perceptual Analysis Skills had a potential range from 0 to 216. (For each subject the possible range was from 0 to 12.)

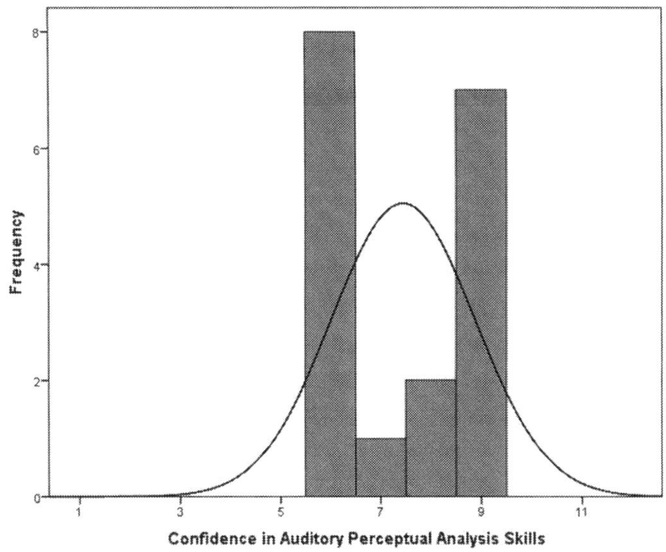

Figure 3–14. *Histogram with normal curve overlay displaying the total confidence in auditory perceptual analysis skills scores for Unit 3.*

Conclusion

The voice education and training (VET) program led to significant improvement (in mean scores) for graduate speech-language pathologists' (a) awareness regarding their own voices and the voices of others, (b) implementation of vocal hygiene and warm-up voice exercises in their daily routine, and (c) confidence in practicing the Smith Accent (SA) voice exercises. This baseline acquisition of vocal awareness, application of vocal hygiene behaviors, and confidence in SA voice exercises is fundamental for prospective speech-language pathologists as future professional voices.

By the end of the VET program, graduate SLP students were also (a) "Very confident" in self-monitoring and self-correcting vocal behaviors and vocal environments, (b) "Reasonably confident" or "Very confident" in their auditory-perceptual analysis skills, and (c) "Reasonably confident" in practicing lip and tongue trills. This was not the case for their confidence in practicing manual laryngeal massage or resonant voice exercises. Students reported they were "Not so confident" in practicing these two voice therapy exercises.

The graduate SLP VET program was able to achieve almost all of its targeted basic vocal competencies. The Smith Accent technique was the most practiced technique during the in-class training sessions and outside of the class with warm-up exercises. It was introduced at the beginning of Unit 1 and was practiced throughout the three units. Students, on average, showed a significant increase in their confidence in practicing the Smith Accent exercises introduced earlier along the hierarchy. The VET program also achieved its targeted competencies for easier voice therapy exercises, such as tongue and lip trills, which were not introduced until Unit 3. Voice therapy exercises that required more hands-on training, such as exercises in the later stages of the SA hierarchy, manual laryngeal massage, and resonant voice exercises, need additional time in student training to acquire the desired competencies.

Recommendations

Recommendations for Caring for Self

Graduate speech-language pathologists, just like other college students, are at high risk for developing voice problems during their college years. They also, like graduate teachers, are examples of future voice professionals who will depend on their voices to fulfill the requirements of their jobs. In spite of this reality, there are no published data describing voice care education and training by graduate SLP programs. In addition, almost none of the postgraduate professional development programs provided by the local and national associations, such as ASHA, address this crucial need.

Voice screenings and vocal health should be explicitly addressed in all university programs. Sufficient information about ergonomic factors in vocal behavior and factors that increase the risk for suffering from voice disorders should be part of every college student's compulsory course work. This practice has become routine at Turku University in Finland since 1988 (Simberg, Sala, Laine, & Rönnemaa, 2001).

In addition, graduate SLP programs should have a special focus on voice care for their students as a prerequisite for providing voice care and training to voice clients. The definition of voice disorder should be linked to the demands made on the voice; the voice disorders of SLP students and others preparing for occupations with high vocal demands should be cured before entering the workforce. Basic care should be expanded to include voice education, voice training, and voice screening.

Follow-up voice evaluations, medical examinations, and on-site resources for direct voice therapy should also be readily available.

Local and national professional institutions, school districts, and medical centers need to add voice care and training professional development programs to the year-round CE programs they provide to their members.

Recommendations for Caring for Others

Coursework and clinical practica targeting voice clients may not be the most efficient way to acquire necessary skills and build self-perceived competence in managing patients with voice disorders (Teten et al., 2016b). It is crucial to build these skills throughout the undergraduate and graduate programs by adding voice education and training programs to their requirements for clinical competence. A focus on caring for self as a precursor for managing others should be emphasized. The same need exists for those who are already in the workforce. There is a growing need for providing voice training professional development programs to licensed SLPs who do not feel confident enough to care for their own voice or provide therapy to patients with different voice disorders. ASHA needs to provide SLPs with more practical CE opportunities targeting voice perception and production skills needed to take care of their own voices as well as the voices of their clients.

Acknowledgment. To my students, the ever-growing members of our exciting family of voice advocates, researchers, teachers, and clinicians. Working with you all has always been the best part of my professional career. My co-authors reflect the genuine passion I have seen in all of you across my 20 years at UVA. Meredith started research in voice as an undergraduate student and Mike joined us as a PhD student. It is this genuine curiosity and love of science across disciplines that make our family of "Academia" a special family worth joining.

References

American Speech-Language-Hearing Association. (2009). Graduate curriculum on voice and voice disorders. *ASHA Special Interest Division 3, Voice and Voice Disorders.* Retrieved from http://www.asha.org/uploadedFiles/slp/clinical/VoiceGradCurric.pdf

American Speech-Language-Hearing Association. (2010). *2010 Schools survey report: Survey methodology, respondent demographics, and glossary.* Retrieved from http://www.asha.org/research

American Speech-Language-Hearing Association. (2012). *2012 Schools survey report: Survey methodology, respondent demographics, and glossary.* Retrieved from http://www.asha.org/research/memberdata/schoolssurvey/

American Speech-Language-Hearing Association. (2016). *2014 Standards and implementation procedures for the Certificate of Clinical Competence in Speech-Language Pathology.* Retrieved from http://www.asha.org/Certification/2014-Speech-Language Pathology-Certification-Standards/

Boersma, P., & Weenink, D. (2016). Praat: Doing phonetics by computer [Computer software]. Version 6.0.23. Retrieved from http://www.praat.org/

Bureau of Labor Statistics. (2015). Speech language pathologists. *Occupational Outlook Handbook.* U.S. Department of Labor. Retrieved from https://www.bls.gov/ooh/healthcare/speech-language-pathologists.htm

Carrau, R. L., Khidr, A. A., Crawley, J. A., Hillson, E. M., Davis, J. K., & Pashos, C. L. (2004). The Impact of laryngopharyngeal reflux on patient-reported quality of life. *Laryngoscope, 114*(4), 670–674. doi:10.1097/00005537-200404000-00014

Carrau, R. L., Khidr, A. A., Gold, K. F., Crawley, J. A., Hillson, E. M., Koufman, J. A., & Pashos, C. L. (2005). Validation of a quality-of-life instrument for laryngopharyngeal reflux.

Archives of Otolaryngology-Head and Neck Surgery, 131(4), 315.

Colton, R. H., Casper, J. K., & Leonard, R. (2006). Vocal rehabilitation. In *Understanding voice problems: A physiological perspective for diagnosis and treatment* (4th ed., pp. 313–359). Philadelphia, PA: Lippincott Williams & Wilkins.

De Medeiros, A. M., Barreto, S. M., & Assunção, A. Á. (2008). Voice disorders (dysphonia) in public school female teachers working in Belo Horizonte: Prevalence and associated factors. *Journal of Voice, 22*(6), 676–687. doi:10.1016/j.jvoice.2007.03.008

Duffy, O. M., & Hazlett, D. E. (2004). The impact of preventive voice care programs for training teachers: A longitudinal study. *Journal of Voice, 18*(1), 63–70. doi:10.1016/s0892-1997(03)00088-2

Fadly, M. D., & Kotby, M. N. (1978). Project for curriculum for the master degree in phoniatrics. Faculty of Medicine, Ain Shams University. In A. Sonnien (Ed.), *Proceedings of the 7th Congress of the European Union of Phoniatricians* (pp. 183), Jyvaskyla, Finland.

Gillingham, L., Brenner, H., & Khidr, A. A. (2012, March). *Raising self-awareness in future voice professionals.* Poster presented at the Speech-Language-Hearing Association of Virginia Conference, Tysons Corner, VA.

Gottliebson, R. O., Lee, L., Weinrich, B., & Sanders, J. (2007). Voice problems of future speech-language pathologists. *Journal of Voice, 21*(6), 699–704. doi:10.1016/j.jvoice.2006.07.003

Hartley, N. A., Breen, E., & Thibeault, S. L. (2016). Epidemiology of vocal health in young adults attending college in the United States. *Journal of Speech, Language and Hearing Research, 59*(5), 973–993. doi:10.1044/2016_jslhr-s-15-0214

Khidr, A. A. (2003a, March). *The Smith Accent Technique voice therapy.* Presented at the Speech-Language-Hearing Association of Virginia Conference, Fredericksburg, VA.

Khidr, A. A. (2003b, June). *Establishing a voice lab: Science and business.* Presented at the 27th Annual Fitz-Hugh Symposium, Charlottesville, VA.

Khidr, A. A. (2004, March). *Clinical applications of the Smith Accent technique.* Presented at the Speech-Language-Hearing Association of Virginia Conference, Fredericksburg, VA.

Khidr, A. A. (2005a, September). *The physiological basis, procedures and applications of a holistic voice therapy technique.* Presented at James Madison University, Harrisonburg, VA.

Khidr, A. A. (2005b, March). *The Smith Accent technique.* Presented at the Speech-Language-Hearing Association of Virginia Conference, Charlottesville, VA.

Khidr, A. A. (2010). Introduction to the Smith Accent technique. In J. C. Stemple & L. T. Fry (Eds.), *Voice therapy: Clinical case studies. Introduction to the Smith Accent Technique* (3rd ed., pp. 153–159. San Diego, CA: Plural.

Khidr, A. A. (2012). Functional voice disorders. In E. M. Abdel-Rahman & R. A. Balogun (Eds.), *Functional impairment: Management, types and challenges* (pp. 43–80). Hauppauge, NY: Nova Science.

Khidr, A. A. (2014a, November). *Vocal hygiene workshop.* Presented at Charlottesville High School, Charlottesville, VA.

Khidr, A. A. (2014b, November). *Vocal hygiene workshop.* Presented at the University of Virginia, Charlottesville, VA.

Khidr, A. A. (2014c, November). *Hoo's voice matters workshop.* Presented at the University of Virginia, Charlottesville, VA.

Khidr, A. A. (2015, April). *Students, teachers and professors as professional voice users.* Presented at University of Virginia's First Annual World Voice Day Celebration and Concert, Charlottesville, VA.

Khidr, A. A., Roper, M., & Hull, M. (2017, March). *Graduate voice education and training programs: Setting goals and evaluating outcomes.* Presented at the 7th Egyptian Society for Phoniatrics and Logopedics Congress, Cairo, Egypt.

Khidr, A. A., Roper, M., & Hull, M. (2017). *Preparing graduate speech language pathologists for a professional voice user career.* Submitted for publication.

Khidr, A. A., & Samlan, R. (2003, June). *An introduction to the Smith Accent technique of voice therapy.* Presented at The Voice Foundation in Philadelphia, PA.

Kotby, M. N. (1980). *Egypt.* Retrieved from Union of European Phoniatrics http://www.phoniatrics.eu/uep/downloads/h_egypt.pdf

Kotby, M. N. (1995). The Accent Method: Technical considerations. In *The Accent Method of voice therapy* (pp. 55–83). San Diego, CA: Singular.

Kotby, M. N. (2006). Egypt: Four decades of voice research and clinical application. *The ASHA Leader, 11*, 30–32. doi:10.1044/leader.WB3.11072006.30

Kotby, M. N. (2014, March). *The story of phoniatrics and logopedics in Egypt*. Presented at the 4th Egyptian Society for Phoniatrics and Logopedics Congress, Cairo, Egypt.

Kotby, M. N., El-Sady, S., & Hegazi, M. (2010). Thirty-five years of care of child language in Egypt. *Topics in Language Disorders, 30*(1), 84–91. doi:10.1097/tld.0b013e3181d08273

Kuczkowski, J., Cieszyńska, J., Plichta, Ł, Tretiakow, D., & Stodulski, D. (2015). Hermann Gutzmann (1865–1922): The father of phoniatrics, an independent specialty. *Journal of Voice, 29*(3), 263–264. doi:10.1016/j.jvoice.2014.09.001

LeBorgne, W. D., & Rosenberg, M. D. (2014). *The vocal athlete*. San Diego, CA: Plural.

Ligon, C., Rank, N., & Khidr, A. A. (2013, June). *Vocal fry in female college students*. Poster presented at the Voice Foundation, Philadelphia, PA.

Ligon, C., Rank, N., Khidr, A. A., & Hull, M. (2016a, June). *Perceived desirability of vocal fry among graduate female speech pathology students*. Presented at the Voice Foundation, Philadelphia, PA.

Ligon, C., Rank, N., Khidr, A. A., & Hull, M. (2016b, June). *Perceived influence of the media on the use of vocal fry in comparison with other vocal characters*. Presented at the Voice Foundation, Philadelphia, PA.

Maddox, M., Khidr, A. A., & Hull, M. (2016, June). *Laryngeal symptoms in weightlifting*. Presented at the Voice Foundation, Philadelphia, PA.

Milback, L., & Khidr, A. A. (2001, November). *The Accent method of voice therapy: A student clinician's perspective*. Presented to American Speech-Language-Hearing Association (ASHA), New Orleans, LA.

Morrissey, M. L. (2003). Vocal health in teacher training programs. *The Phenomenon of Singing, 4*, 111–117. Retrieved from http://journals.library.mun.ca/ojs/index.php/singing/article/view/568

Nemr, K., Simões-Zenari, M., Cordeiro, G. F., Tsuji, D., Ogawa, A. I., Ubrig, M. T., & Menezes, M. H. (2012). GRBAS and Cape-V scales: High reliability and consensus when applied at different times. *Journal of Voice, 26*(6), 812.e17–812.e22. doi:10.1016/j.jvoice.2012.03.005

Noordzij, J. P., Khidr, A. A., Evans, B. A., Desper, E., Mittal, R. K., Reibel, J. F., & Levine, P. A. (2001). Evaluation of omeprazole in the treatment of reflux laryngitis: A prospective, placebo-controlled, randomized, double-blind study. *Laryngoscope, 111*(12), 2147–2151. doi:10.1097/00005537-200112000-00013

Noordzij, J. P., Khidr, A. A., Desper, E., Meek, R. B., Reibel, J. F., & Levine P. A. (2002). Correlations of pH-probe measured laryngopharyngeal reflux with symptoms and signs of reflux laryngitis. *Laryngoscope, 112*, 2192–2195.

Oates, J. (2009). Auditory-perceptual evaluation of disordered voice quality: Pros, cons and future directions. *Folia Phoniatrica et Logopaedica, 61*(1), 49–56. doi:10.1159/000200768

Oates, J., & Russell, A. (1998). Learning voice analysis using an interactive multi-media package: Development and preliminary evaluation. *Journal of Voice, 12*(4), 500–512. doi:10.1016/s0892-1997(98)80059-3

Oates, J., & Russell, A. (2003). A sound judgment [Computer software]. Multimedia Production Unit. La Trobe University, Melbourne, Australia. http://trove.nla.gov.au/work/8793217?selectedversion=NBD25468646

Roper, M., & Khidr, A. A. (2015a, March). *Graduate SLP program focus: Care for others versus care for self.* Presented at Speech-Language-Hearing Association of Virginia Conference, Richmond, VA.

Roper, M., & Khidr, A. A. (2015b, March). *Development unit for future and current professional voice users.* Poster presented at Speech-Language-Hearing Association of Virginia Conference, Richmond, VA.

Roper, M., & Khidr, A. A. (2015c, March). *Development unit for future and current professional voice users.* Poster presented at Curry Research

Conference at University of Virginia, Charlottesville, VA.

Roy, N., Merrill, R., Thibeault, S., Parsa, R. A., Gray, S. D., & Smith, E. M. (2004). Prevalence of voice disorders in teachers and the general population. *Journal of Speech, Language and Hearing Research, 47*(2), 281–293. doi:10.1044/1092-4388(2004/023)

Ruddy, B. H., & Sapienza, C. M. (2004). Treating voice disorders in the school-based setting: Working within the framework of IDEA. *Language Speech and Hearing Services in Schools, 35*(4), 327–332. doi:10.1044/0161-1461(2004/032)

Russell, A., Oates, J., & Greenwood, K. (2005). Prevalence of self-reported voice problems in the general population in South Australia. *Advances in Speech Language Pathology, 7*(1), 24–30. doi:10.1080/14417040500055193

Sapir, S., Ramig, L. O., & Fox, C. M. (2011). Intensive voice treatment in Parkinson's disease: Lee Silverman Voice Treatment. *Expert Review of Neurotherapeutics, 11*(6), 815–830. doi:10.1586/ern.11.43

Simberg, S., Sala, E., Laine, A., & Rönnemaa, A. (2001). A fast and easy screening method for voice disorders among teacher students. *Logopedics Phoniatrics Vocology, 26*(1), 10–16. doi:10.1080/14015430119481

Simberg, S., Sala, E., & Rönnemaa, A. (2004). A comparison of the prevalence of vocal symptoms among teacher students and other university students. *Journal of Voice, 18*(3), 363–368. doi:10.1016/j.jvoice.2003.12.005

Simberg, S., Sala, E., Vehmas, K., & Laine, A. (2005). Changes in the prevalence of vocal symptoms among teachers during a twelve-year period. *Journal of Voice, 19*(1), 95–102. doi:10.1016/j.jvoice.2004.02.009

Stemple, J. C., & Fry, L. T. (2010). *Voice therapy: Clinical case studies* (3rd ed., pp. 153–159). San Diego, CA: Plural.

Teten, A., DeVeney, S., & Friehe, M. (2013). Checklist for assessing graduate student competencies in voice disorders. *Special Education and Communication Disorders Faculty Publications, paper 20.* doi:10.1044/vvd23.3.95

Teten, A., DeVeney, S., & Friehe, M. J. (2016a). Use of student perceptions to measure voice disorders course impact on learning. *Journal of Curriculum, Teaching, Learning and Leadership in Education, 1*(1), 84–93. Retrieved from http://digitalcommons.unomaha.edu/ctlle/vol1/iss1/10

Teten, A. F., DeVeney, S. L., & Friehe, M. J. (2016b). Voice disorder management competencies: A survey of school-based speech-language pathologists in Nebraska. *Special Education and Communication Disorders Faculty Publications.* doi:10.1044/2015_LSHSS-14-0098

Thyme-Frøkjær, K., & Frøkjær-Jensen, B. (2001). Teaching the Accent Method. In K. Thyme- Frøkjær & B. Frøkjær-Jensen (Eds.), *The Accent method: A rational voice therapy in theory and practice* (pp. 94–134). Bicester, UK: Speechmark.

Tillard, G., Lawson, K., & Emmerson, S. (2011). Perceptions of the clinical competence of new speech-language pathology graduates in New Zealand: A research note. *The Open Rehabilitation Journal, 4*(1), 23–27. doi:10.2174/1874943701104010023

Timmermans, B., Coveliers, Y., Meeus, W., Vandenabeele, F., Looy, L. V., & Wuyts, F. (2011). The effect of a short voice training program in future teachers. *Journal of Voice, 25*(4), e191–e198. doi:10.1016/j.jvoice.2010.04.005

Union of the European Phoniatricians and European Union of Medical Specialists. (2010). *Phoniatrics Training Programme and Logbook.* Retrieved from http://www.phoniatrics.eu/uep/education/logbook-phoniatrics-uems-2010/index.html

University of Iowa. (2016). Voice-academy [Computer software]. Retrieved from https://uiowa.edu/voice-academy/

University of Wisconsin-Madison. (2008). Voice disorders: Simulations and games [Computer software]. Retrieved from https://csd.wisc.edu/slpgames/sims.html

U.S. News & World Report. (2016a). The 100 best jobs of 2016. Retrieved from http://money.usnews.com/careers/best-jobs/rankings/the-100-best-jobs

U.S. News & World Report. (2016b). Best healthcare jobs. Retrieved from http://money.usnews.com/careers/best-jobs/rankings/best-healthcare-jobs

Verdolini, K., & Ramig, L. O. (2001). Review: Occupational risks for voice problems. *Logope-*

dics Phoniatrics Vocology, 26(1), 37–46. doi:10.1080/14015430119969

Withers, G., & Khidr, A. A. (2017, March). *In-class World Voice Day campaign: JMU's SLP undergraduate program.* Poster presented at Speech-Language Hearing Association of Virginia Conference, Richmond, VA.

APPENDIX 3–1

Vocal Hygiene Weekly Log

Scoring Method

Item 1 and 8: (yes, no)

Items 2 through 6: (zero, <1, 1–3, 4–6, 7–9, and >9)

Items 7 and 12: (none of the time, a little bit, some of the time, most of the time, a good bit, all of the time)

Item 11: (0% of the time, up to 25% of the time, 25–50% of the time, 50% of the time, 50–75% of the time, 75–100% of the time)

Scored Items

1. Select the warm-up exercises you completed today (check all that apply):
   - AM/PM stretching exercises
   - AM/PM breathing exercises
   - AM/PM vocalizing exercises
2. Indicate your consumption of water throughout the day (in cups)
3. Indicate your consumption of herbal teas and noncaffeinated drinks throughout the day (in cups)
4. Indicate your consumption of caffeinated drinks (coffee/tea/coke/etc.) (in cups)
5. Indicate your consumption of alcohol throughout the day (beer 12 oz, wine 5 oz, spirits 1.5 oz)
6. Indicate your consumption of cigarettes throughout the day.
7. Unhealthy vocal behaviors—Select the frequency of which you noticed the following behaviors today:
   - Throat clearing
   - Hard coughing
   - Shouting, yelling, screaming
   - Speaking loudly
   - Speaking over loud noise
   - Forcing voice out
   - Speaking in unnatural pitch (too high/low)
   - Speaking in unnatural voice quality (character voice)
   - Excessive talking
   - Talking while driving
   - Cheering/rooting with a crowd
8. Implemented vocal hygiene strategies/modifications today:
   - Plan voice rest throughout my high-demand talking times of the day
   - Take water breaks throughout the day
   - Consume a cup of water before or right after my caffeinated beverage
   - Avoid sources of noise when talking
   - Modify talking environment to be less challenging
   - Avoid talking in noisy environments
   - Avoid talking on the phone in the car
   - Acknowledge and start working on stressors I could identify
   - Seek support for any negative mind-sets

- Rearrange clinical setting so that I am closer to my client
- Rearrange clinical setting so that we are farther away from the source of noise in the room

9. Hours of voice USE today
10. Hours of voice REST today
11. Vocal experiences throughout the day—Select the percentage of time you noticed the following experiences:
    - Clear voice quality
    - Full breath support during voicing
    - Uncontrollable voice quality changes throughout the day
    - Voice fatigue after voicing
    - Voice fatigue during voicing
12. Emotional status today
    - Full of lot/lots of energy
    - Worn out/tired
    - Down/depressed
    - Calm/peaceful
    - Stressed from work-related issues
    - Stressed from family-related issues
    - Stressed from health-related issues
13. Select your vocal experience at the end of the day
    - Clear voice
    - Strong voice
    - Easy flowing voice
    - Voice changes
    - Voice fatigue
    - Strained voice
    - Voice loss

APPENDIX 3–2

Unit Feedback Survey

Scoring Method

Items 1–4: (yes, no)

Items 5–8: (0 = Not at all confident; 1= Not so confident; 2 = Reasonably confident; 3 = Very confident; 4 = Extremely confident)

Scored Items

1. This unit's vocal hygiene log helped me gain self-awareness regarding:
   - How my voice sounds
   - How my voice feels
   - My daily vocal demands and challenges (duration, volume, animation, individual versus group therapy, etc.)
   - My vocal environment (noise source, dryness, space size, distance to listener, etc.)
   - My unhealthy vocal behaviors (throat clearing, hard coughing, hard glottal attacks, etc.)
2. This unit's vocal hygiene log helped me gain awareness regarding:
   - How others' voices sound
   - Others' daily vocal demands and challenges (duration, volume, animation, individual versus group therapy, etc.)
   - Others' environment (noise source, dryness, space size, distance to listener, etc.)
   - Others' unhealthy vocal behaviors (throat clearing, hard coughing, hard glottal attacks, etc.)
3. This unit's vocal hygiene log helped me implement the following modifications:
   - Increase hydration
   - Decrease caffeine
   - Plan voice rest throughout my high-demand talking times of the day
   - Avoid sources of noise when talking
   - Modify talking environment to be less challenging
   - Monitor/decrease abusive vocal behaviors
   - Avoid talking in noisy environments (bars, concerts, gatherings)
   - Avoid/decrease talking on the phone in the car
   - Acknowledge and start working on stressors that I could identify
   - Seek support when I experience a negative mind-set
4. This unit's voice awareness material has helped me identify and utilize new resources that address the following areas:
   - Vocal appreciation
   - Basic vocal knowledge (anatomy and physiology)
   - Vocal hygiene practices
   - Vocal challenges/disorders
   - Diagnosis of voice disorders
   - Management of voice disorders
   - Voice research trends
5. This unit helped me develop confidence practicing the Smith Accent exercises:
   - Monitor/adjust posture
   - Monitor/control abdomino-diaphragmatic breathing
   - Monitor/adjust muscle tension in shoulders, head and neck, face,

temporomandibular joint, and articulator muscles
- Monitor/control volume, speed, rhythm, and intonation
- Monitor/control timing of volitional expiration
- Use proper breath support for nonvoiced sounds
- Use proper breath support for voice sounds
- Use proper breath support for vowel play
- Use proper breath support for slow speed syllables and speech
- Use proper breath support for fast speech syllables and speech
- Use proper breath support during monologues
- Use proper breath support during dialogues
- Use proper breath support in group discussions

6. This unit helped me develop confidence practicing these facilitating voice exercises:
   - Use manual laryngeal massage to decrease vocal hyperfunction
   - Use tongue trills to decrease vocal hyperfunction
   - Use lip trills to decrease vocal hyperfunction
   - Use resonant voice to decrease vocal hyperfunction

7. This unit helped me develop confidence in self-monitoring and self-correction:
   - Use vocal hygiene log in monitoring vocal behavior
   - Use vocal hygiene log in modifying vocal behavior
   - Implement vocal hygiene measures

8. This unit helped me develop confidence in my auditory-perceptual analysis skills:
   - Use of auditory-perceptual skills in monitoring and analyzing my own voice
   - Use of auditory-perceptual skills in monitoring and analyzing familiar (classmates) voices
   - Use of auditory-perceptual skills in monitoring and analyzing unfamiliar/stranger (clients) voices

SECTION III

Practices and Outcomes of an Expert From Australia

CHAPTER 4

Keeping the Voice Fit: Voice Education and Training for the Fitness Industry

Anna Rumbach

The Fitness Industry

Fitness professionals "direct, instruct and guide individuals and groups in the pursuit of physical fitness and well being" (Australian Bureau of Statistics [ABS], 2006). The demand for fitness industry services is growing rapidly as a result of population growth, changes in population age demographics, government investment in preventive health and infrastructure, and the evidence of health benefits of physical activity. There are over 30,000 registered fitness professionals within Australia, with group fitness instructors (GFIs) making up approximately 30% of the industry workforce (Fitness Australia, 2012). The gender mix of the industry is relatively balanced (56% female, 44% male), and almost two-thirds (62%) of fitness professionals are aged between 22 and 39 years (mean = 34 years; Fitness Australia, 2012). Data reporting employment type estimates 68% of fitness professionals are employed on a casual basis, 18% permanent full time, 12% part time, and 2% are working proprietors and partners (ABS, 2006).

Voice Problems in the Fitness Industry

In recent decades, the fitness industry has evolved, shifting away from the focus on looking good, to one that embraces feeling good and improving overall health and quality of life (Fitness Australia, 2012). With this shift, the industry has embraced a myriad of new service offerings that inspire the masses to exercise together. GFIs (also known as aerobics or group exercise instructors) instruct and demonstrate complete freestyle, prechoreographed or circuit-style exercise sessions to groups of exercise participants of varying ages and fitness levels with limited individual interaction (Fitness Australia, 2014). Despite acknowledging that the voice is a critical tool to ensure consumer engagement, motivation, and safety, up to 71% of GFIs reportedly suffer from voice difficulties at some point in their career (Fontan, Fraval, Michon, Dejean, & Welby-Gieusse, in press; Long, Williford, Olson, & Wolfe, 1998; Newman & Kersner, 1998; Rumbach, 2013a), with voice difficulties negatively influencing work performance, work efficiency, and personal identity (Long et al., 1998; Newman & Kersner, 1998; Rumbach, 2013b; Sapir, Atias, & Shahar, 1990; Sapir, Keidar, & Mathers-Schmidt, 1993).

Prevalence and Predictive Factors

Voice problems represent a significant occupational hazard for fitness professionals. Despite this, exploration of the prevalence and nature of the acute and chronic voice problems experienced by GFIs has been limited to small cohort studies conducted using self-report questionnaire designs (Heidel & Torgerson, 1993; Long et al., 1998; Newman & Kersner, 1998; Rumbach, 2013a). The prevalence of voice disorders in GFIs was first investigated by Heidel and Torgerson (1993). This study compared the vocal symptomatology of 50 female GFIs with 50 female group fitness consumers. The results found GFIs to be at significantly higher risk for voice problems than consumers; compared to only 4% of consumers (n = 2), 58% (n = 29) of GFIs reported hoarseness immediately following a class (Heidel & Torgerson, 1993). Subsequently, Long et al. (1998) surveyed 50 female and 4 male GFIs, aged between 20 and 54 years (M = 34.1) from various fitness settings within the United States, finding 42.6% (n = 23) experienced partial voice loss either during or immediately following instruction. Significant variables associated with voice problems included sore throat, hoarseness following instruction, and use of shouting while teaching. In the same year, Newman and Kersner (1998) surveyed 48 female GFIs in Britain, of which 52% (n = 25) reported experiencing voice problems. Instructing classes for more than 10 hours per week was significantly associated with the report of current voice difficulties. Instructors with more than 6 years' experience within the industry were more likely to report a history of voice difficulties than those who had been active within the industry for shorter periods.

A more recent study surveyed 280 frmale and 81 male GFIs (N = 361), aged between 18 and 67 years (M = 37.3, SD = 1.42) who were currently active in the Australian fitness industry (Rumbach, 2013a, 2013b). All participants indicated that they had no history of voice problems prior to entering the fitness industry. Chronic voice symptoms (sensory or perceptual) were prevalent in 71% (n = 256) of the cohort. A large proportion of the cohort (78.95%, n = 285) reported acute onset of voice difficulties during or immediately after periods of exercise instruction. The amount of vocal abuse encountered while teaching (e.g., screaming and no amplification, minimal or no consumption of water) and circumstances surrounding instructor health (e.g., illness, inadequate sleep, stress, voice overuse) were reported to be contributing factors. A formal diagnosis of a voice disorder was present in 10.53% of the total cohort (n = 38). Factors significantly associated with the report of chronic hoarseness included, with consideration of younger age and less years in the industry: partial voice loss during or after instructing, increased vocal volume above normal speaking level while instructing, teaching when sick, teaching with a sore throat, having a sore throat often, experiencing cold/flu often, and consistently using a microphone (Rumbach, Khan, Brown, Eloff, & Poetschke, 2015).

Small sample sizes, a strong gender bias toward females, and a natural bias for participation from those with voice concerns means that these results may not be extrapolated to the industry at large. However, overall similarities throughout the available group data suggest that voice problems are present in the profession globally.

Auditory-Perceptual and Sensory Symptoms

Self-report has been the primary measure used within the literature to report the presence of voice symptoms in this population. GFIs have reported both auditory-perceptual and sensory symptoms, with hoarseness, general throat discomfort, and a speaking voice lower in pitch among those most commonly experienced (Figure 4–1; Heidel & Torgerson, 1993; Long et al., 1998; Newman & Kersner, 1998; Rumbach, 2013a).

Voice Impairment and Associated Activity Limitation and Participation Restriction

The World Health Organization's International Classification of Functioning (WHO, 2001) can be useful in recognizing the impact a voice disorder can have on all aspects of an individual's life. In relation to voice disorders, "impairment" is defined as an abnormality in physical function (e.g., abnormal laryngeal function represented perceptually through hoarseness). "Activity limitation" refers to the limitation in performance caused by the impairment (e.g., inability to produce a voice with clear quality which means it cannot be easily heard), while "participation restriction" is defined as a loss of role function due to the impairment or disability (e.g., no longer able to perform the job as required). Voice impairments can create ongoing activity limitation and participation restriction, impacting not only the GFIs ability to fulfil their vocational role, but function across personal, social, and other professional settings. In a study examining the effect of diagnosed voice disorders on quality of life (QOL) in 38 GFIs with formal voice diagnoses, GFIs expressed frustration, sadness, and concern with regard to the longevity of their teaching career (Rumbach, 2013b). Inability to perform their regular vocational tasks due to voice difficulties resulted in GFIs ceasing or altering their work program (e.g., periods of absenteeism, reduction in teaching hours, discontinuing programs of exercise that placed added demands on the voice) and their instruction approach (e.g., increasing nonverbal cueing, decreasing music volume, and increasing microphone volume) to compensate for their impairment. The consequences of voice impairment were far reaching, with 50% (n = 19) noting that they had become increasingly withdrawn from social aspects of life due to the need for voice preservation for work and/or severity and nature of the voice problem. Voice impairments may also contribute to other occupational and economic problems as the majority of GFIs are casual employees, with their primary sources of income coming from vocations that require stable and well-controlled voices and the ability to speak for extended periods of time (e.g., primary, secondary, and tertiary educators, police officers, retail assistants, and managers; Rumbach, 2013b). A considerable body of evidence indicates that inability to communicate verbally as desired across all environments may lead to increased stress, frustration, and depression (Mathieson, 2001; Sapir et al., 1993; Smith, Taylor, Mendoza, Lemke, & Hoffman, 1998), which in themselves can be significant stressors contributing to participation restriction across social and occupational domains.

Management of Voice Disorders in the Fitness Industry

Considering the heavy vocal load associated with the profession and the high prevalence of self-reported voice difficulties, GFIs appear to be a large group of occupational voice users who are currently underserviced.

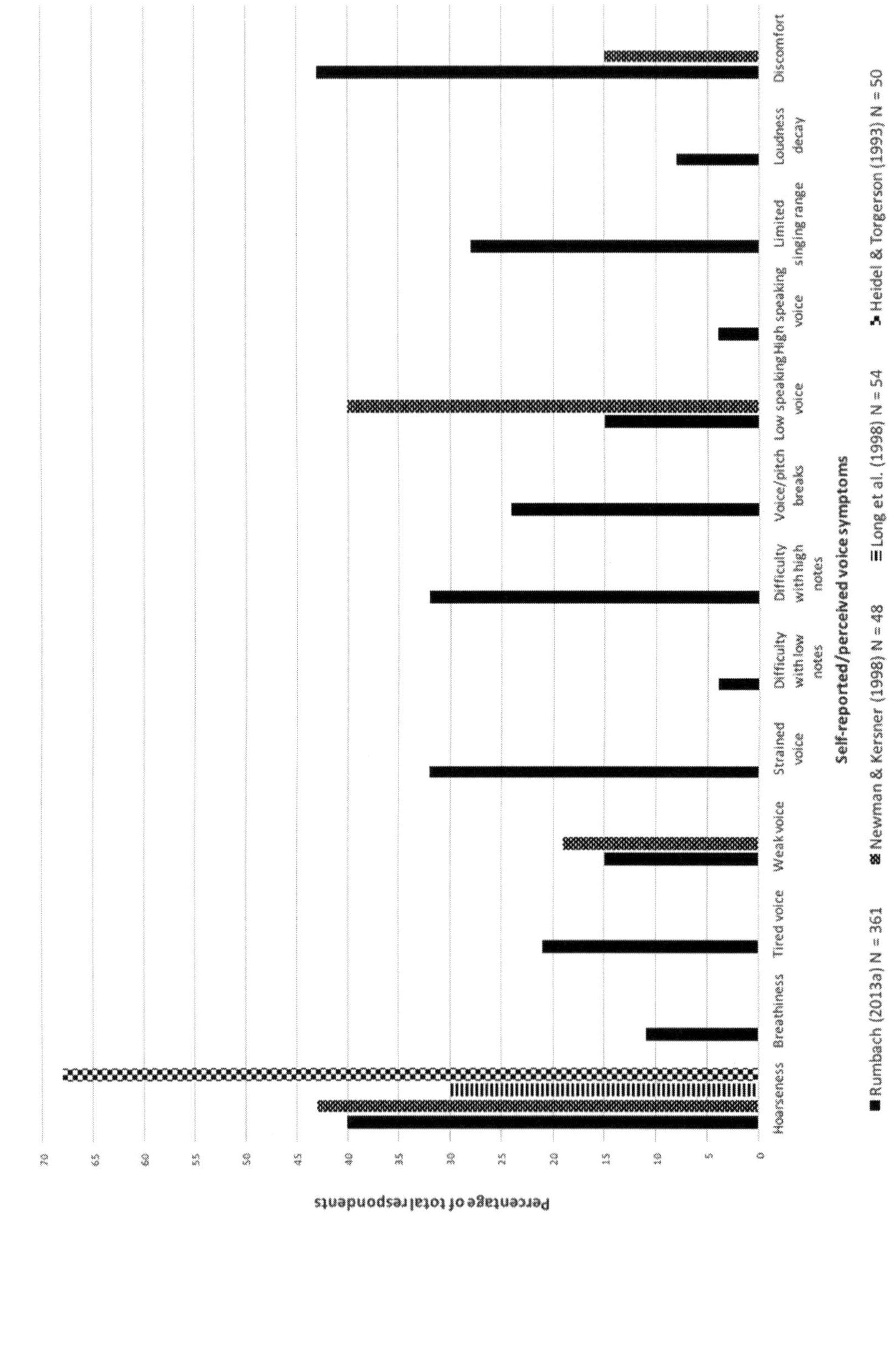

Figure 4–1. *Summary of self-reported auditory-perceptual and sensory voice symptoms experienced by GFIs.*

Approximately one in six to seven instructors who experience voice difficulties actually seek a medical opinion, despite seven out of ten GFIs reporting chronic voice symptoms (Rumbach, 2013a). Reasons for this may include the following:

- Vocational dysphonia and vocal attrition in this population seems to be an accepted consequence of the occupation (Rumbach, 2013b).
- GFIs are unaware of what constitutes a voice problem.
- GFIs are unaware of the benefits of voice therapy and the services available to them (Rumbach, 2013b).
- GFIs choose not to seek intervention for their voice problems because of the expense and time involved, as well as the reluctance for co-workers, management, and health insurance companies to lend support (Rumbach, 2013b).

Prevention and treatment of voice problems in the fitness industry require a systematic education and training approach tailored to the demands of the profession that targets all industry stakeholders.

Voice Education and Training

In Australia, there is no uniform approach to voice education and training in the fitness industry (Newman & Kersner, 1998; Rumbach, 2013a). Despite instructors reaching near unanimous agreement (98.06%) that voice care should be covered as part of industry training (Rumbach, 2013a), only 30% report formal exposure to voice education, with even fewer (2–10%) receiving any practical voice training (Newman & Kersner, 1998; Rumbach, 2013a). Voice education and training is not required by law, and vocational dysphonia is often considered an acceptable consequence of the occupation (Rumbach, 2013b). Thus for a proactive and systematic approach toward education and training to be implemented, multiple stakeholders—industry leaders, workplace management, health care professionals, and GFIs—must understand the potential benefits of taking a proactive and/or reactive stance.

In Australia, Safe Work Australia and Workplace Health and Safety (WHS) authorities in each state or territory have the responsibility of enforcing WHS/occupational health and safety legislation (acts and regulations). Employers must meet legislated WHS requirements or face penalties. The employer must provide information, instruction, and training on how employees can perform their job safely and employees must cooperate with health and safety arrangements. To ensure WHS legislation is upheld, workplace management in fitness facilities should implement a risk assessment framework, with potential hazards and risks to vocal health being identified and regularly reviewed to ensure that assumptions regarding levels of risk and the controls required remain adequate. A longitudinal multidimensional approach that incorporates ongoing risk assessment of work design, workplace design, and worker behavior should be utilized, in addition to designing, delivering, and reinforcing vocal health policies and models of voice education and training that are appropriate for the needs of GFIs instead of only selecting those models that are cheaper and easier to implement and manage.

To be successful, WHS intervention begins with all stakeholders understanding that favorable ergonomic conditions for voice use can reduce health risks to GFIs and improve exercise participant satisfaction and safety. Stakeholders need to have clearly defined roles and responsibilities to ensure favorable ergonomic conditions are established and maintained. The onus for education and training relies not only on the employer and industry at large, but the GFIs who must be responsible for following company WHS policies, acknowledging and investigating voice symptoms early and following any necessary treatment guidelines prescribed by health professionals. The overall goal of the GFI voice education and training programs is to increase fitness industry stakeholders' awareness of how caring for the voice contributes to overall health and well-being. Understanding normal phonatory behavior, the nature of voice difficulties that may arise as a result of the occupation, and strategies to make the occupational voice load safer may (a) reduce presenteeism and absenteeism rates, (b) promote longevity of a GFIs' career, and (c) facilitate a more positive and united attitude to voice care. Furthermore, it may encourage more instructors to seek help when faced with voice difficulties.

How Do We Get Involved?

As health professionals, we need to take both an indirect and direct approach to voice education. As the realms of the fitness industry are vast and varied, it is likely that voice education and training services for GFIs will not be readily available in a permanent or full-time capacity. In Australia, speech-language pathologists (SLPs) are usually employed in a casual capacity by industry leaders/management to deliver large-scale educational workshops, or by GFIs to deliver face-to-face individualized training. Currently there is no established systematic, longitudinal approach to voice education and training in the fitness industry. SLPs are encouraged to actively approach industry leaders and individual fitness facilities to form partnerships to develop and implement voice education and training to those entering the profession and those already entrenched in it. The vocal health programs presented in this chapter have been developed by an SLP who is a qualified and practicing fitness professional. However, absence of fitness qualifications does not preclude SLPs from successfully implementing these programs. SLPs are encouraged to seek support from a fitness industry mentor who may provide information regarding exercise physiology, technique for execution of physical exercise, and fitness teaching practices.

It is beneficial for SLPs to be cognizant of the demands of the profession and the exercise programs being taught so that education and training can be tailored accordingly. GFIs want to hear from someone who understands what they do on a day-to-day basis, and they prefer SLPs who recommend treatment that is logical as well as compatible and achievable within the restrictions of their professional lifestyle. If you have never stepped foot into a gym or participated in a group fitness class, running this type of education and training program may be challenging. Immerse yourself in the culture of the industry!

The remainder of this chapter outlines three versions of a voice education and training program, taking both proactive and reactive stances, which are derived from clinical experience with this population. Each program can be implemented in isolation; however, a blended approach that is implemented longitudinally will most likely provide better results and higher levels of GFI satisfaction.

Models of Service Delivery

Involving all stakeholders is likely to be the key to success to changing the culture surrounding voice education and training in the fitness industry. With this in mind, each stakeholder will have different needs and desired outcomes and thus different models of service delivery need to be considered. Small and large group seminars, workshops, and small group practical sessions as well as individualized education, and training are all feasible options. Table 4–1 provides a broad overview of each service delivery model presented here. Although it is beneficial for companies to promote and implement a phased, longitudinal approach incorporating all actions, many companies choose to adopt an isolated approach. The target audience for voice education and training includes (a) industry leaders and fitness facility managers, (b) instructors training to enter the profession, (c) established instructors without voice complaint, and (d) established instructors with voice complaint. Each approach is suitable for all stakeholders; however, industry leaders and fitness facility managers typically do not actively participate in small group practical sessions and are not involved in individualized education and training. However, they should remain informed of the findings of the vocoergonomic assessment, the education and training program being implemented, and the outcomes of such programs for GFI vocal health so that they can help establish and promote a vocally safe working environment.

Table 4–1. *Models of Service Delivery for Voice Education and Training*

	Group Seminar and Workshop Sessions	Small Group Practical Sessions	Individualized Education and Training
Intended audience	Industry leaders and fitness facility managers; instructors training to enter the profession; established instructors without voice complaint; established instructors with voice complaint	Instructors training to enter the profession; established instructors without voice complaint; established instructors with voice complaint	Established instructors without voice complaint; established instructors with voice complaint
Audience size	Small (<10 people) and large (>10 people) groups	Small groups (<10 people)	One-on-one
Session duration	2 hours	1–2 hours	30 minutes–1 hour
Frequency of intervention	Once-off session	Two to four sessions over a few weeks/months (desirable) *or* a longer once-off session	Approximately once a week, up to 6 weeks
Proposed venue	Group fitness room/studio. Venue size will vary depending on the facility.	Group fitness room/studio. Venue size will vary depending on the facility.	Small therapy room within clinical setting (assessment + intervention); group fitness room/studio (assessment + carryover of tasks)

Group Seminar and Workshop Sessions

Group seminar and workshop sessions promote vocal health awareness to all stakeholders. Sessions can be conducted as frequently as desired, with each session running for approximately 2 hours. However, shorter and longer sessions can be arranged to suit the needs of the consumer. It is recommended that a "refresher" session be conducted every 12 months. Content on vocal anatomy and physiology, vocal hygiene, microphone training and troubleshooting, and how and when to seek professional support to promote vocal health is delivered via multimedia presentation. GFIs are also oriented to and provided with copies of relevant vocal health guidelines (specific to each workplace), handouts, and brochures.

It is recommended that all group seminar and workshop sessions, if possible, should be conducted within fitness facilities within spaces dedicated to group fitness. Using these venues for education and training help highlight to industry leaders, workplace management, and GFIs the environmental challenges associated with voice use while exercising. Room size will vary depending on the facility.

Group seminar and workshop sessions are great times to engage industry leaders and workplace management. Some management will have first-hand experience instructing group fitness classes, whereas others will come from alternative fitness professional or business backgrounds and may not necessarily understand the nature and demands of a GFI. By involving these individuals in seminars and workshops, they gain a greater understanding of the demands of the GFI role and how they can provide appropriate supports for their GFIs so that they may continue to deliver world-class fitness experiences to the public.

During group seminars and workshops, GFIs who identify and/or report voice concerns should be encouraged to pursue formal assessment and seek further tailored voice education and training through small group practical sessions and/or individualized sessions with a SLP.

Small Group Practical Sessions

Small group practical sessions are designed to be delivered to GFIs who have similar vocal and physical demands when instructing exercise classes (i.e., teach the same program of exercise; e.g., all GFIs enrolled in the sessions will be conducting programs that require weight lifting). Typically, GFIs attend two to four sessions over a few weeks or months. These sessions can be repeated annually to reinforce and reinvigorate the GFIs' commitment to vocal health. Practical sessions designed around task-specific vocal performance (e.g., providing verbal instruction while weight lifting) can be conducted within a clinical or gym setting depending on space requirements and equipment availability. Sessions include a vocoergonomic assessment and voice evaluation, general voice education, and task-specific education and training. This service delivery model affords greater one-on-one education and training, especially for those who may have voice concerns (pre-emptive or existing). However, education and training provided in this format are not sufficient for treatment of occupational voice disorders.

Individualized Education and Training

This type of education and training is tailored to an individual GFI's vocal function at the time and the vocal demands of the exercise type being taught. Although this model of education and training is often reserved for GFIs presenting with a diagnosed voice problem, this program may also be suitable for GFIs seeking more personalized preventative voice education and training. Subscription to this course is voluntary, does not take place in occupational working hours, and is typically conducted by a SLP working in private practice. Course/therapy fees are paid by the individual GFI. Sessions typically run for 30 to 60 minutes, with one session per week for approximately 6 weeks. The frequency and duration of therapy are often adjusted depending on the GFI's vocal presentation. For this education and training program to be successful, significant GFI motivation, compliance, and insight are required. Furthermore, successful outcomes depend on accurate and comprehensive information regarding laryngeal structure and function, the SLP's diagnostic skill, the selection of appropriate treatment techniques, and the way in which the program is executed. Education and training should encompass all determinants of vocal health status, not simply focus on the reduction of occupational vocal load.

Vocal Health Program

All of the proposed service delivery models contain overlapping elements. Specific information regarding the components and content applicable to each model of education and training is provided below.

Vocoergonomic Assessment and Voice Evaluation

Service delivery models: Small group practical sessions, individualized education and training

As group seminars and workshop sessions do not afford much one-on-one interaction, vocoergonomic assessment is limited to observation of the environment, and no voice evaluations are conducted as part of this service delivery model. However, prior to the commencement of small group practical sessions or individualized education and training, a thorough battery of assessments should be carried out, the results of which will inform the direction and content of education and training/therapy sessions. The SLP leads an assessment of work design (types of classes taught, number of classes/day or week, etc.), workplace design, and GFI behavior (e.g., health condition, life habits, vocal skill and experience, psychosocial and personality factors). Components include the following:

1. Observation of the environment (i.e., workplace design) when being used and not being used for the purposes of exercise instruction (essential). Specifically, the SLP evaluates environmental noise and sound competition, air quality and temperature/climate control, room acoustics, and other ergonomics (e.g., use, quality and condition of sound systems, microphones, exercise equipment). In preparation, the SLP reviews any internal documentation regarding policy and procedures (e.g., GFI manual), interviews appropriate members of management, and surveys the GFIs in relation to their general occupational dynamics (e.g., work design and GFI behavior). The aim of this observational analysis is to identify potential occupational risk factors for voice problems so that these can be improved upon or compensated for before and/or during education and training.
2. Case history and self-reported voice evaluation (essential)—a general voice case history should be completed. Use of a biographical and vocal health questionnaire (Appendix 4–1), administered in print or electronically, can help map the vocal demands and vocal concerns of the group of GFIs. A Voice Handicap Index (Jacobson et al., 1997) can also be completed prior to attending the initial assessment session. Completion of the Reflux Severity Index (Belafsky, Postma, & Koufman, 2002) is also recommended.

Box 4–1

Case 1

During an assessment of work and workplace design in preparation for small group practical training, there was concern among the eight GFI participants that they often found themselves shouting when they were teaching. They felt that this was due to two reasons: (1) the microphone often was not working (~60% of the time), and (2) when the microphone was working, they couldn't hear themselves clearly over the music and other environmental noise (100% of the time).

Looking at the workplace design, there was only one microphone available, settings on the sound system were suboptimal (with the GFIs admitting that they often changed the settings in an attempt to improve the mix of microphone and music levels), and all speakers were facing toward the exercise participants. There was no formal music or microphone policy in place at the facility.

At this point, the manager of the facility and the group fitness manager were invited to participate in an open discussion with the GFIs regarding the development of a music and microphone policy. The SLP acted as an interface between management and the GFI team to ensure that everyone had their opinions and ideas heard and that the recommendations decided upon were aligned with vocoergonomic factors that promoted maintenance of vocal health.

Agreed upon actions included the following:

- Development and implementation of a music and microphone policy that outlined the responsibilities of GFIs and management.
    - ☐ The GFIs wanted consistent access to working microphones. Management agreed to purchase an additional microphone and all GFIs and management staff underwent practical hands-on training on how to troubleshoot common microphone issues and how to responsibly handle the equipment. All stakeholders agreed that in the event that a working microphone was not available, GFIs could choose whether they wanted to teach their scheduled classes (and forfeit income if they decided to not teach while the microphone was not operational) or alter the exercise format (e.g., use more visual cues than usual, shorten the duration of classes) so that vocal load was reduced. Management also agreed that any microphone faults would be dealt with expeditiously, with audio-engineers assessing and repairing any faults within 24 to 48 hours.
    - ☐ A sound engineer was called in to conduct testing of the sound system to ensure its optimal functioning (i.e., appropriate sound levels [treble and bass + microphone versus music]). Instructors agreed that in the event of sound system malfunction they would alert the management team, and would refrain from changing the system's settings.

- Management agreed to purchase and install a foldback speaker (i.e., a speaker that is aimed at the GFI rather that at the exercise participants) so that GFIs were able to hear what the participants were hearing and thus monitor their own vocal volume.

Outcomes: Within 1 month, all actions were finalized. All GFIs reported increased job satisfaction having worked with management to problem solve and implement workplace design solutions. GFIs also reported increased confidence that working equipment would be available to them and any breakdown would be rectified as soon as possible. Three months post-implementation, and at completion of the small group practical sessions, all GFIs reported having access to a working microphone on all teaching occasions, with the only issue encountered being that body-pack transmitter batteries were not always charged. GFIs also reported that they were better able to monitor their vocal loudness during exercise instruction which had further helped them incorporate other elements of vocal education and training into their teaching practices.

3. A baseline audio-perceptual and visuo-perceptual assessment conducted under normal conditions (i.e., in nonexercise conditions) (essential)—a standardized perceptual evaluation tool (e.g., GRBAS [grade, roughness, breathiness, asthenia, strain], CAPE-V [Consensus Auditory-Perceptual Evaluation of Voice]) can be utilized. All GFIs should undergo an individual 5-minute voice assessment conducted by the SLP. In order to obtain data regarding maximum phonation time, respiratory behavior, pitch and loudness, resonance, resistance, flexibility, vocal quality, phonatory effort (muscle tension and anchoring), articulation, fluency, and speech rate, the following vocal tasks should be used:
   - sustained phonation using modal pitch and loudness on /a/ (three trials);
   - counting one to five (minimum loudness without whispering up to maximum loudness without shouting);
   - pitch glides or steps up and down a scale (three trials);
   - a 1-min monologue; and
   - passage reading (e.g., Rainbow Passage; Fairbanks, 1960).

4. Audio-perceptual and visuo-perceptual assessment of a simulated or live performance in the group fitness environment (essential). In small group practical training, each GFI completes a simulated performance that includes a class introduction and 3 to 5 minutes of exercise instruction within the group fitness environment, with the SLP performing auditory and visuo-perceptual assessment. When preparing for individualized education and training, simulated performance can be used for assessment; however, live performance is preferable. During each performance the SLP evaluates the following:
   - voice quality (a standardized perceptual evaluation tool [e.g., GRBAS, CAPE-V] can be utilized);

- general body position, identifying the presence of extraneous tension that may influence vocal performance;
- frequency and duration of voice use in relation to exercise being performed and proportion and types of nonverbal cues used; and
- music and background noise level.

Each performance is audio- and video-recorded.

The GFIs are also required to perform a self-assessment of their vocal performance. The SLP works with GFIs to develop auditory awareness so that they are able to identify features of voice quality that are undesirable. This can be completed by repeated analysis of high-quality audio and video recordings captured before and during exercise performance. This process aims to improve self-monitoring and increase proprioceptive awareness.

5. Ambulatory phonation monitoring during live performance in the group fitness environment (desired). As well as participant noise, the instructor's voice must compete with loud background music, often in large rooms with poor acoustics (Rumbach, 2013a). Research has shown that high-intensity music increases a consumer's enjoyment and motivation during fitness classes (Wilson & Herbstein, 2003), and so it is not surprising that it is strongly entrenched in the culture of the industry. To compete with environmental noise, a speaker's voice will increase in amplitude, frequency, and overall phonation time (Sodersten, Ternstrom, & Bohman, 2005). Accordingly, the majority of GFIs report their voice during instruction to be louder (65%) or much louder (18%) than their normal speaking voice, despite using amplification (Rumbach, 2013a). GFIs who report voice problems use a louder voice and phonate for a higher percentage of time in comparison to instructors without voice problems (Wolfe, Long, Youngblood, Williford, & Olson, 2002) and acoustic examination of vocal function in GFIs has shown statistically significant increases in fundamental frequency and intensity using pre-post instruction measures (Dallaston & Rumbach, 2016). This excessive vocalization is known as vocal loading and can lead to adverse change in vocal fold (VF) condition, including VF edge irregularity, VF edema, and VF erythema (Mann et al., 1999). Prolonged vocal loading may lead to the development of chronic voice disorders (Vilkman, 2004).

The Ambulatory Phonation Monitor (APM) is a portable, unobtrusive device that consists of a small accelerometer (throat sensor), connected via cable to a microprocessor (hardware module) that can provide long-term, continuous tracking of vocal parameters such as phonation duration, fundamental frequency, and intensity. The APM pre-processes and stores data that can then be downloaded and analyzed "off-line" using companion PC software (see Figure 4–2 for example of APM data display). Furthermore, some APM equipment has biofeedback capability, providing instantaneous feedback via vibration when "safe" limits are exceeded and/or target phonatory behaviors are not maintained. The feedback feature, if available, is expected to improve compliance with vocal rehabilitation programs, facilitating the carryover and/or generalization of behaviors established in individualized education and training sessions to the teaching environment.

It is important to note that although the APM is designed to be used during everyday activity, the exercise undertaken

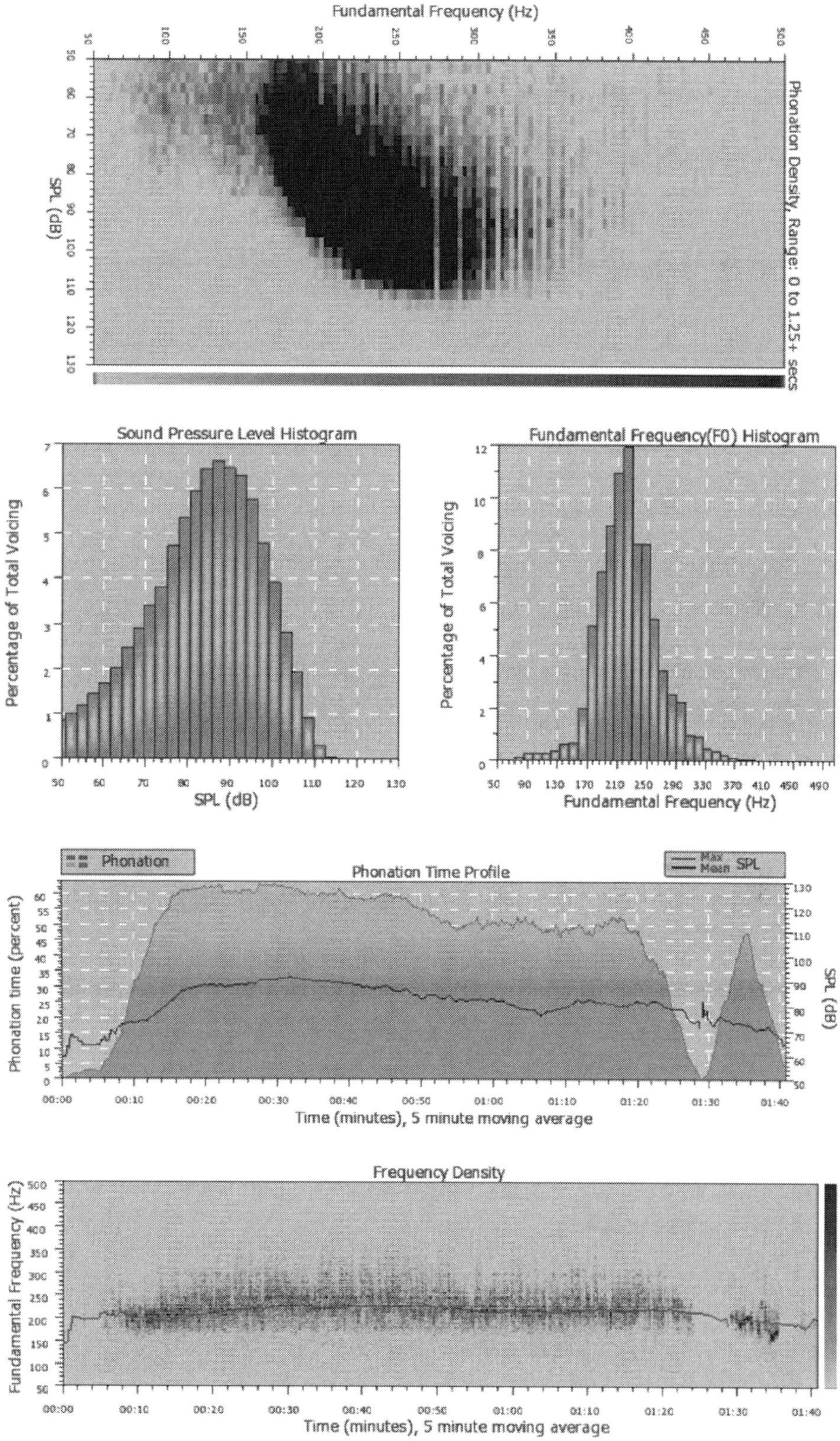

Figure 4–2. *Example of the APM data display from the Ambulatory Phonation Monitor Model 3200 (KayPENTAX) which was collected during one period of exercise instruction for a GFI.*

as part of the GFI role exceeds the degree of activity considered "normal." Therefore, there are a number of considerations to make when using APM with this population. The microprocessor can be belt-worn, with the throat sensor (accelerometer) glued to the GFI's neck in the area above the sternal notch and below the larynx. To ensure that the throat sensor remains attached during exercise and data collection, sweat-resistant tape should be used as an additional security measure. Furthermore, to avoid straining the cable connection to the sensor, the cable should be securely taped to the GFI's neck. The sensor cable should be further secured with tape under the GFIs' garments, exiting at waist level, to avoid the throat sensor being pulled off and/or extraneous tension being placed on the cable. Typically, the sensor cable should be draped around the users' neck and taped below the base of the neck. As GFIs may be required to lie down on their back to perform exercise (e.g., abdominal crunches), the cable may be taped to the front of the body in some circumstances. SLPs may choose to evaluate vocal load as it relates to a period of exercise instruction only, commencing data collection 1 hour prior to exercise instruction and completing data collection 1 hour post-exercise instruction, instead of data collection occurring across an entire day.

6. Referral to an otorhinolaryngologist (ENT) for laryngoscopy ± stroboscopy (essential for GFIs with pre-existing vocal complaints or those who present with any level of dysphonia). Some GFIs may have already undergone laryngoscopy prior to commencing SLP-delivered education and training/therapy sessions. In cases where ENT evaluation has not been sought, SLPs should play an active role in educating GFIs regarding what they can expect during ENT assessment, what potential results may be, and how the information captured will contribute to their ongoing care. It is likely that GFIs may show some apprehension toward undergoing a "medical procedure"; therefore, it is important to make sure that fear and anxiety are kept at bay. It is well known that patient anxiety attributable to medical procedures can be significantly reduced by providing improved education prior to the procedure (e.g., Luck, Pearson, Maddem, & Hewett, 1999; Marteau, Kidd, & Cuddeford, 1996).

   In Australia, ENT examinations can be conducted in both the private and public health care sectors. Although GFIs are able to access laryngoscopic voice assessments free of charge through the public health system, waiting lists can be very long. Therefore, GFIs are encouraged to see an ENT privately if it is not cost prohibitive. The cost of the procedure typically ranges between \$140 and \$205, of which Medicare (the federal health insurance program) will cover between 75% and 95%, with the "out-of-pocket" cost being approximately \$90 or less for the endoscopy component of the consultation.

For GFIs participating in individualized education and training, all baseline assessment measures are repeated at the completion of the program, with further follow-up occurring at 6 months' post-completion. GFIs are able to access further intervention, at their own expense, if required.

Education and Explanation of Vocal Anatomy and Physiology

Service delivery models: Group seminar and workshop sessions, small group practical sessions, individualized education and training

As the fitness industry is concerned with whole-body wellness, it is likely that voice training will be more successful if it aims to increase stakeholders' awareness of how caring for the vocal mechanism will contribute to their overall health. Understanding normal anatomy and phonatory behavior and the nature of occupational voice difficulties is paramount. Discussion includes but is not limited to an explanation of vocal anatomy and physiology using a simple theoretical model (e.g., Power-source-filter; see Appendix 4–2), anatomical diagrams and models, videostroboscopic images of normal vocal fold anatomy and function, and self-palpation of gross laryngeal structures (i.e., locating the thyroid cartilage to provide approximate location of vocal folds). Videostroboscopic images of screaming, whispering, coughing, and throat clearing are used to illustrate how these types of vocal behaviors deviate from normal and thus may contribute to the formation of habitual voicing patterns and development of chronic voice difficulties. For GFIs undergoing individualized education and training, an understanding of normal phonatory behavior and how their own voice production differs from this may provide context for the chosen treatment approaches prescribed and increase motivation and compliance.

General Vocal Health and Hygiene

Service delivery models: Group seminar and workshop sessions, small group practical sessions, individualized education and training

Verbal and written information regarding basic vocal hygiene is provided. An example of written material provided can be found in Appendix 4–2. Discussion includes, but is not limited to,

- awareness and avoidance of vocally abusive behaviors;
- the importance and effects of hydration;
- awareness of lifestyle factors (e.g., sleep, smoking, consumption of caffeinated and alcoholic beverages) that may contribute to voice difficulties;
- the importance of voice rest;
- information regarding the importance of postural alignment; and
- vocal first aid for use during periods of illness or acute voice change.

Conducting a question-and-answer session is encouraged. During discussions of vocal health it is important to make sure all GFIs are aware that any degree of perceptual or sensory voice change places limitations on an individual's vocal clarity and intensity. This may restrict an instructor's ability to cue participants to perform the physical exercises being prescribed in a safe manner, potentially placing exercise participants at greater risk for injury. A decreased ability to use the voice effectively to motivate and engage participants may also lead to decreased participant enjoyment/satisfaction.

Microphone Training and Troubleshooting

Service delivery models: Group seminar and workshop sessions, small group practical sessions, individualized education and training

The majority of group fitness facilities have microphone and amplification systems in place, yet research has elucidated that despite having access to microphone systems, GFIs appear to be continuing to increase their vocal volume above normal speaking level while amplified and that GFIs are often required to teach with an unamplified voice due to sound system and microphone breakdown (Rumbach, 2013a, 2013b; Rumbach et al., 2015). It appears that GFIs not only need formalized training on proper techniques for microphone use but also need consistent access to good-quality sound systems and microphones that are in working order.

During this part of education and training, instructors are given the opportunity to familiarize themselves with the equipment available; receive instruction and feedback on optimal microphone positioning, microphone care, and troubleshooting; and learn/practice how to evaluate intensity of their amplified voice and music. Please note that details of microphone care and troubleshooting will vary depending on the equipment being used; however, some general points for discussion are provided below. Workplace management should also learn about the importance of having a good sound system, a working microphone with a headset and receiver, and high-quality speakers.

Discussion includes, but is not limited to the following:

- Microphone system requirements
    - ☐ Sweat-resistant headset cardioid condenser microphone and receiver attached to a good sound system with high-quality surround-sound speakers.
- Optimal microphone positioning
    - ☐ When worn, optimal microphone placement is 1 to 2 inches from the corner of the mouth. Positioning the microphone directly in front of the mouth is not advisable as it will likely result in plosive distortion, amplification of breath sounds, or spitting into the microphone capsule while teaching.
- Microphone care
    - ☐ Do not blow into the microphone to test it. If the microphone being used has a foam windscreen, ensure that it is secured to the microphone capsule.
    - ☐ Do not bend the microphone boom arm as you risk damaging internal connections—mold the head frame gently to your head by using constant, even pressure.
    - ☐ Do not use medicated or alcohol wipes to clean the microphone as these may disintegrate the microphone capsule. Clean the headset with a dry towel, wiping away from the microphone capsule.
- Microphone troubleshooting
    - ☐ Feedback (i.e., a squealing, screeching, or howling sound) occurs when the microphone volume level is too high, the music is too loud for the microphone, or when you are standing too close to the speakers. Feedback can often be eliminated by turning the microphone volume down or moving away from the speakers. Turn all music off and adjust the microphone level to the point where the voice sounds dry and natural, with no "ringing" sounds. Once the microphone volume is set, the music volume can be increased until the correct balance of voice over music is achieved. Higher-quality speakers may also reduce the likelihood of feedback. Treble and bass controls should be equal, as an exaggerated treble setting on the sound mixer or amplifier can also cause feedback.
- The adoption of music and microphone policies
    - ☐ The microphone volume should be 10 dB louder than the music volume so that the voice is able to be heard; music intensity

should measure no more than 90 dB (IDEA Health and Fitness Association, 2003). As volume controls on the music and microphone amplifiers are not accurate means for measuring sound intensity, fitness facilities are urged to use a Class 1 or 2 sound-level meter near the center of the front of the room in order to measure music and voice sound levels during fitness classes.

- ☐ Instructors should have consistent access to working microphone and amplification systems. In the case of system malfunction, instructors should not be expected to teach with their voice unamplified. Changes to class structure and format should be made to accommodate safer voice use while the system is undergoing repair. Systems should be repaired within a reasonable time frame (<5 working days, preferably within 24 to 48 hours).

Vocal Warm-Ups

Service delivery models: Small group practical sessions, individualized education and training

A series of warm-up exercises are introduced using modeling and feedback. These include but are not limited to stretches for the head and neck alongside semi-occluded vocal tract exercises (e.g., straw phonation, lip and tongue trills).

Practical Vocoergonomic Training

Service delivery models: Small group practical sessions, individualized education and training

Practical training incorporates a series of occupational-based actions that are supported with didactic interactions and written materials. Discussion and demonstration includes but is not limited to the following:

- *Teacher-centered versus student-centered instruction*—Exercise participants value both teacher-centered and student-centered learning experiences and GFIs should adopt both teaching styles. The GFIs' role during teacher-centered instruction is to provide information to the exercise participant, with the emphasis being placed on correct execution of movement and movement patterns/combinations. The GFI typically teaches from a stage and does not leave the front of the room. In contrast, during student-centered instruction, the GFIs' role is to coach and facilitate the experience, with the emphasis being placed on moving and learning together from experience. The GFI can move around the room and make contact with all participants during the class. Although some branded or "off-the-shelf" fitness products may favor one type of instruction over the other, GFIs are encouraged to consider both teaching approaches and how they can be incorporated into their day-to-day teaching of group exercise programs.
- *The importance of scripting and execution of verbal cues at points in the exercise task that minimize strain on the vocal system.* Simultaneous exercise represents an additional stressor on the vocal mechanism in GFIs. Voice production is most efficient when all components of the vocal mechanism (the breath, vibration, and resonance) work in

coordination to achieve phonation at minimal musculatory effort (Colton, Casper, & Leonard, 2011). However, simultaneous exercise causes a shift in both respiratory behavior and laryngeal function that results in an increase in the effort (both perceived and physiological) necessary for phonation (Sandage, Connor, & Pascoe, 2013).

Many exercise routines feature choreographed movements that alter the position of the head, neck, or torso. Extended, flexed, or twisted head positions are not optimal for voice production, as the muscles and structures of the larynx and pharynx become constricted or compressed by extrinsic laryngeal muscles and curvature of the cervical vertebrae (Rubin, Mathieson, & Blake, 2004; Shewell, 2009). The voice during suboptimal head positions may be perceived as strained or narrow (Shewell, 2009). Movements that curl the spine and roll the shoulders (e.g., abdominal crunches) compress the lungs, limiting capacity to supply adequate breath support for speech (Shewell, 2009). Inadequate breath support for speech may result in difficulty projecting the voice and vocal fatigue. Furthermore, during the initiation of strenuous movement, such as lifting weights, the muscles of the larynx engage to close or "bear down," trapping the air within the thoracic cavity, stabilizing the ribs, and enhancing the efficiency of the upper limbs (Naito & Niimi, 2000). Initiation of voice during this adducted state of the vocal folds, which may be accompanied by considerable muscle tension, may result in an abrupt, explosive onset of phonation, which is associated with vocal abuse (Colton et al., 2011).

The need for increased ventilation during exercise is responsible for additional changes to the physiological parameters of voice production in GFIs. Breathing patterns necessary to meet metabolic needs during exercise interfere with respiratory control necessary for controlled phonation (Baker, Hipp, & Alessio, 2008; Doust & Patrick, 1981). This is evident by the observation that speech during exercise is louder and more tremulous, with increased pitch and breathiness (Doust & Patrick, 1981). A decrease in upper airway temperature secondary to increased ventilation rate has also been observed (Sandage et al., 2013). The effect of temperature change on the vibration of the vocal folds and function of the laryngeal musculature is not clear, though it is hypothesized that a reduction in temperature may impair contractile function (Sandage et al., 2013). Additional physiological changes to the larynx during exercise include dilation of the glottis, anterior laryngeal rotation, and flattening of the epiglottis against the base of the tongue (Beaty, Wilson, & Smith, 1999). These changes are thought to increase airflow and minimize turbulence and airway resistance (Beaty et al., 1999). However, the specific effect on the efficiency of phonation is yet to be explored.

Awareness should be drawn to the following:

- ☐ *Importance of postural alignment and how misalignment may contribute to voice difficulties.* GFIs are taught how exercise may alter voice production and how the effects of these postural changes can be minimized, compensated for, or avoided. Examples of practical teaching tips are outlined in Case 2 (Box 4–2) and Case 3 (Box 4–3).
- ☐ *How to let the music speak and maximize power of physical instruction instead of having complete reliance on verbal cueing.* Music is often a vital component of a group fitness environment. Music can provide participants with positive physiological and motivational constructs for exercise (Harmon & Kravitz, 2007). Music accompaniment can reduce participant-reported fatigue, increase levels of psychological arousal, improve motor coordination, and promote relaxation (Karageorghis & Terry, 1997; Szabo, Small, & Leigh, 1999; Szmedra & Bacharach, 1998). Therefore, GFIs need to understand how to work with the music being used in their classes. Cues need to be delivered with appropriate timing to ensure participant success. Furthermore, GFIs' cueing methods should accommodate

Box 4–2

Case 2

I regularly work with GFIs who teach weight-based resistance training at a moderate to high intensity. As they are holding weights to exercise, they have limited capacity to use their hands to safely deliver nonverbal, visual cues and thus rely on their voices to ensure that participants know what they are doing and when to do it. However, GFIs can be provided with guidance on how to maximize their vocal safety when delivering verbal cues. Typically we instruct GFIs to avoid giving verbal cues at the height of physical exertion, when the Valsalva maneuver (i.e., forced exhalation against a closed glottis used to increase intra-abdominal pressure, creating more support for the lower spine) is being performed. For example, when performing any variant of a squat, verbal cues should be delivered as the GFI descends into the movement, not as they ascend with exertion.

The SLP observes a live class to determine what exercises are typically performed and the GFIs' teaching behaviors. Education and specific training are then provided, with GFIs being asked to start applying this when teaching their classes. The following sessions, each administered a month apart, focus largely on developing body awareness (focusing on the larynx) during simulated teaching. Negative practice is used to reinforce the desired behavior. GFIs are videoed during live performance with feedback being provided by the SLP, as well as peers with industry experience, to ensure the integrity of the exercise and the quality of the experience for exercise participants is maintained.

Box 4–3

Case 3

I was asked to provide some practical teaching tips to a group of six yoga instructors who reported that their voices were generally tired at the end of classes. Prior to enrollment in the training, each GFI submitted a videoed performance of a live class. The main objective for the practical training sessions was to draw awareness to the larynx and educate how head and neck position, when it moves away from anatomical position, can contribute to negative effects on the voice. The sessions focused on allowing the GFIs to find the balance between teaching well and vocalizing well. In addition to introducing a range of basic vocal exercises (straw phonation, high-pitched blowing, resonant hum) and recommending they utilize a microphone when instructing, I encouraged the GFIs to adopt a blended teaching approach, with GFIs moving among the participants to provide one-on-one coaching and education as well as teaching from a stage, demonstrating execution of poses to the larger group, using large nonverbal visual cues to improve participant alignment. GFIs were also taught to move out of poses (returning to head, neck, and torso alignment consistent with anatomical position) to provide more detailed instruction so that there is minimal compression and constriction of the larynx and pharynx. For example, when coaching abdominal exercises, the GFI demonstrates the exercise, and once the participants have begun the desired task, sits up and provides expert coaching to correct postural alignment and exercise execution. GFIs were asked to incorporate these strategies into their teaching, and after 1 month, video-record one complete class in preparation for the next practical training session. Feedback was provided by the SLP in conjunction with other group members at the next practical training session. Simulated performance was utilized to reinforce feedback. This procedure was repeated for a further two sessions, each scheduled 1 month apart.

After three feedback and monitoring sessions, evaluations showed significant improvements across all of the aspects emphasized in five of the six GFIs. Specifically, use of follow-up nonverbal/visual cues increased by 67% and GFIs had moved away from a teacher-centered model to a hybrid approach, using four times more one-on-one interaction than observed in the pre-training videoed classes by the final feedback session. One GFI reported ongoing vocal fatigue. The evaluations conducted revealed that this GFI had not incorporated all recommendations into their teaching style over the duration of the vocal health program (i.e., increase in follow-up nonverbal/visual cues was 18% and three times more one-on-one interaction, microphone frequently not used when teaching), highlighting that commitment and motivation of the GFI to change is paramount to the program's success.

the varied learning styles of exercise participants (visual, auditory, and kinesthetic). Therefore, GFIs are taught about different types of cues and their purpose (Table 4–2), with a large emphasis being

Table 4–2. Types of Cues and Cueing Methods

	Purpose	Example	Example of Visual Cue That Can Be Used in Conjunction With or in Place of a Verbal Cue
Anticipatory	Tells the exercise participant when to do the next movement and what it will be	"We're going to march down in 4, 3, 2, march"	Hand signals for counting
Movement	Provides verbal reinforcement of a movement to enhance exercise participant confidence and success	"Turn step—up, up, down, down."	Hand signals for showing direction, turning, holding a move, indication of the leading leg
Motivational	Aims to increase participants' self-confidence, enjoyment, and enthusiasm	"30 seconds to go!" "Fight for your fitness" "Let's get it done" "That's how it's done team!" Vocal noises such as whoops, trills, yahoos, etc., may also be used.	Body positioning and effort can be used to encourage greater levels of work (e.g., demonstrating a deeper squat with a hand signal to signify "get lower"; increasing range of movement to encourage participants to work harder)
Educational	Delivers relevant information regarding the exercise and/or health and fitness topics. Educational cues can also provide information about how the body should feel during the exercise.	"Bend your knees, feel how your glutes engage further."	Educational cues are best delivered verbally. GFIs can encourage exercise participants to monitor body position and muscle activation by coupling verbal cues with hand and body signals as follow-up to the initial verbal cue.
Alignment and safety	Delivers important information on alignment and appropriate use of equipment to ensure safe execution of exercises	Lunge—"Knees bend to 90 degrees and track out over second and third toes." Extended side angle pose (Utthita Parsavakonasana): "Gently lower your hips to create a straight line from fingertip to toe."	Pointing to various parts of your own body and/or showing large changes in body position (undesirable toward desirable) to indicate proper body alignment.

continues

Table 4–2. *continued*

Further notes regarding verbal and visual cueing:
• Always use clear and concise verbal cues. Sometimes less is more—there is no need for a GFI to talk throughout the entire workout. Allow the participants to concentrate on what they are doing and give them the opportunity to enjoy the flow of the workout and the music. • Make eye contact with participants. • The most powerful visual cues are communicated through facial expression and body position and movement. Movements should be precise and controlled. Use exaggerated motion and distinctive postures to convey proper exercise technique and direction changes. Seeing the contrast between correct and incorrect position and movement, participants will hopefully be more attuned to self-correction. • Combine verbal and visual cues to create stronger learning opportunities for participants so that connections are made between the spoken words and the visual example. Also, be consistent in the visual cues that are used to develop a shared understanding with the participants. This will allow the GFI to utilize visual cues in place of repetitive verbal cues throughout the workout.

placed on highlighting the value of using nonverbal, visual cues and how these can be executed during exercise performance (i.e., using hand signals for counting and showing direction etc.), demonstrating physical alignment, physical energy, and action for participant motivation. Examples of practical teaching tips are outlined in Case 2 (see Box 4–2) and Case 3 (see Box 4–3).

Direct Voice Training and/or Treatment

Service delivery models: Individualized education and training

In individualized education and training, the program is customized by the SLP to efficiently and efficaciously address the GFI's vocal rehabilitation needs and expectations. Recommendations and selection of treatment approaches are made based on the information gathered during the assessment process and are thus tailored to the individual GFI. Management approaches for voice disorders typically overlap and involve patient education (see above) as well as behavioral modifications according to the individuals' reported and presenting symptoms. Direct voice intervention using traditional voice therapy techniques is provided in conjunction with practical vocoergonomic training (see above). The therapy prescribed is based on the GFI's presenting vocal behaviors/diagnosis—there is no "one-size-fits-all" approach. Irrespective of the GFI's presentation and the voice therapy techniques trialed, principles of motor learning should be incorporated into therapy delivery. Training techniques include, but are not limited to, optimization of postural alignment, optimization of efficient respiratory behavior (abdominal-diaphragmatic breathing), relaxed voicing with elimination of hard glottal attack (e.g., chewing, yawn-sigh, chant talk), oral-nasal resonance, and voice projection. Case 4 (Box 4–4) and Case 5 (Box 4–5) present examples of individualized education and training programs.

Box 4–4

Case 4

Georgia, a 23-year-old female, presented for a voice evaluation. She had been working as a GFI for 18 months, teaching five step-based cardio classes (moderate to high intensity, 55 min per session) per week. Georgia described the onset of her voice problem as gradual. Her main complaint was that her voice no longer sounded normal to her and that she now had difficulty singing.

Georgia had a nonremarkable medical history. She was a nonsmoker and casual drinker (one to two glasses of wine per week). Daily fluid intake was limited (<1 L of water) and she reported large caffeine consumption (5× coffee/day + energy drinks).

Voice evaluation: On our first meeting, Georgia's voice was perceptually normal. After a period of exercise instruction, perceptual evaluation revealed a slight hoarse quality (breathy, strained, and rough). Maximum phonation time (MPT) on /a/ was 14 s. Pitch and intensity profile was within normal limits, but she reported that her pitch range had become narrower in recent months.

VHI: The VHI is a 30-item questionnaire that asks an individual to describe his or her voice and the effects of the voice on his or her life using a 0 to 4 severity scale (0 = never, 4 = always). Georgia's total VHI score was 44/120 (self-perceived voice severity = moderate).

Vocoergonomic assessment: The fitness facility had a good-quality sound system with foldback. Georgia had consistent access to a working microphone. The teaching space was large, comfortably accommodating up to 50 exercise participants. Fans and air-conditioning were utilized, and environmental noise from the gym floor was largely blocked out if the fitness studio doors were closed.

Vocal Health Program:

Georgia participated in a multidimensional vocal health program implemented over 5 weeks that included

- education and explanation of vocal anatomy and physiology;
- general vocal health and hygiene education (with a large focus on increasing water intake);
- practical vocoergonomic training, focusing on scripting, increasing nonverbal visual cues, and proper use of the microphone and sound system; and
- voice therapy—four sessions (one session per week for 4 weeks)—that included
  - ☐ generalized head and neck stretches (recommended to perform minimum 2× daily, or more frequently if required);
  - ☐ vocal function exercises (2× daily practice);
  - ☐ forward resonance (hum, single words, and phrases; 2× daily practice); and
  - ☐ twang (introduced in Week 3—facilitator + short phrases; 2× daily practice).

Outcomes: Georgia's voice was perceptually normal. She reported greater vocal capability post-therapy, and that she was "her old self." She no longer presented with a slightly hoarse vocal quality following periods of exercise instruction. MPT on /a/ was 22 s, an increase of 8 s from her initial evaluation. Her VHI score decreased to 4.

Box 4–5

Case 5

Susan, a 37-year-old female, presented for a voice evaluation. She had been working as a GFI for 12 years, teaching a range of moderate- to high-intensity aerobics and weight-resistance training classes, averaging 16, 55-min classes per week. She taught classes 6 days a week (finishing at 8:30 p.m. on Monday, Tuesday, and Thursday), teaching between two and four classes per day.

Susan first experienced hoarseness and voice loss approximately 6 months before her voice evaluation. She described the onset of the problem as sudden and coincided with an upper respiratory tract infection. She continued to teach her scheduled classes while sick as she did not want to "let her participants down." Since that time, her voice had gradually improved but had not returned to "normal." She stated that her voice fatigues over the course of the day and she has difficulty projecting her voice. She reported that her voice problem negatively impacted her professional and personal life. Susan had to ask other GFIs to cover some of her evening classes so that she could rest her voice, and she found herself speaking less to her husband and two sons at home in order to preserve her voice for work.

Susan was a nonsmoker and nondrinker. Daily fluid intake was excellent (>2 L of water) and she reported minimal caffeine intake (2× coffee). She reported no current musculoskeletal issues. She reported nil significant medical history.

Laryngeal Examination: ENT examination revealed edema and erythema of the arytenoid cartilages. Stroboscopy revealed medial compression of the true and false vocal folds with a large posterior glottal chink. Mucosal wave was reduced, with thick mucus stranding across the vocal folds evident.

Voice evaluation: Voice quality was characterized by moderate strain, moderate to severe breathiness, mild to moderate roughness, and slight glottal fry. Phonation breaks and hard glottal attack were heard. Maximum phonation time (MPT) on /a/ was 8 s, which is not within normal limits for her age and gender. Modal pitch was low for age and gender. Pitch variability was within normal limits for everyday speech; however, pitch range was reduced. Modal intensity and variability were appropriate for everyday conversational speech, and range was narrow. Susan was noted to cough and throat clear throughout the evaluation.

VHI: The VHI is a 30-item questionnaire that asks an individual to describe his or her voice and the effects of the voice on his or her life using a 0 to 4 severity scale (0 = never, 4 = always).

Susan's total VHI score was 63/120 (self-perceived voice severity = severe).

RSI: Susan rated her reflux symptoms over the past month using the RSI. Her score was 29 out of 45 possible points (with a score of 13 and above indicating significant reflux disease). She indicated hoarseness, presence of an annoying cough, and throat clearing as severe problems (ratings of 5). The ENT prescribed anti-reflux medication 2 weeks prior to her first SLP evaluation; she reported her symptoms had improved since starting the medication and instituting earlier evening mealtimes and diet changes.

Vocoergonomic assessment: The fitness facility had a good-quality sound system. No foldback was available. Susan had consistent access to a working microphone. The teaching space was moderately sized, comfortably accommodating up to 30 exercise participants. Fans and air-conditioning were utilized, and there was a moderate amount of environmental noise from the gym floor.

Vocal Health Program:

A multidimensional vocal health program was implemented over 3 months, which included

- education and explanation of vocal anatomy and physiology;
- general vocal health and hygiene education focusing on cough reduction strategies throughout the day (tallying success during three 10-min periods per day); daily steam inhalations; increasing water intake before, during, and after exercise instruction; reflux management strategies and anti-reflux medication as per ENT; increasing daily periods of vocal rest);
- practical vocoergonomic training, focusing on scripting, timing, and frequency of verbal cues, increasing nonverbal visual cues, and properly using the microphone and sound system.
- voice therapy—eight sessions over 12 weeks—that included
  - ☐ generalized head and neck stretches (recommended to perform minimum 2× daily practice, or more frequently if required);
  - ☐ release of constriction (i.e., silent giggle and yawn-sigh; 2× daily practice and during periods of increased vocal strain);
  - ☐ forward resonance (hum, single words, and phrases; 2× daily practice);
  - ☐ vocal function exercises (2× daily practice); and
  - ☐ twang (introduced in Week 8—facilitator + short phrases; 2× daily practice).

Outcomes: Susan was compliant with all recommendations and voice therapy exercises. After the completion of eight sessions, Susan's MPT on /a/ was 17 s, an increase of 9 s from her initial evaluation. Modal pitch was perceptually normal for her age and gender, with expansion in pitch range also evident. Intensity range was improved, but Susan continued to have difficulty producing a clear, quiet voice. Frequency of coughing and throat clearing reduced by 75%. Her VHI score decreased to 19. Susan's RSI score reduced to 8. Perceptually, her overall quality improved, but her voice remained mildly hoarse. Susan returned to her normal teaching schedule.

"When and How Do I Get Help?"

Service delivery models: Group seminar and workshop sessions, small group practical sessions, individualized education and training

With occupational dysphonia being commonly accepted in the culture of the fitness industry, we need to raise awareness of the importance of vocal health in the fitness industry. It is likely that many instructors are unaware what constitutes a voice problem. All stakeholders should be provided with information regarding reactive and proactive indicators of voice problems. If GFIs and their employers are trained to recognize and report warning signs of voice problems, all stakeholders will be afforded the best opportunity to modify contributing factors and prevent further progression of symptoms. Warning signs of voice problems that are discussed include

- hoarseness or other changes in the way the voice sounds that last more than 2 weeks or regularly come and go;
- pain or discomfort associated with speaking;
- vocal fatigue;
- frequent need to cough or clear the throat or a feeling of a persistent tickle; and
- sudden change or loss of voice, especially if it happens during or after a class.

SLPs need to encourage GFIs to seek medical help early, and to avoid the temptation to self-diagnose using information found on the Internet, irrespective of the education and training model being utilized. Furthermore, workplace management should encourage and support instructors to seek help in a timely fashion. Although some GFIs may have already successfully navigated the health care system, the pathways for assessment and treatment for voice problems that are applicable to the health system in which you are operating should be clearly disclosed. For example, in Australia, GFIs are encouraged to visit their general practitioner for a referral to an ENT for a laryngeal examination with or without videostroboscopy. On diagnosis, the ENT may then refer the GFI to a SLP for voice therapy. Debunking the diagnostic and therapeutic process, especially for GFIs undertaking group seminar and workshop sessions, may aid in reducing anxiety for those anxious about their voice and may be what is required for GFIs to seek and accept assistance.

Conclusion

Voice education and training in the fitness industry is in its infancy. Formal voice education packages that are tailored to the needs of instructors and the industry need to be further developed, trialed, and evaluated to determine whether they may act as a successful preventtive measure and lead to changes in industry opinion regarding voice care. Early identification and treatment of voice difficulties in this population may serve to reduce the activity limitations and participation restrictions known to result from voice problems in the fitness industry. However, implementation of longitudinal vocal health programs is needed. This will only be successful if there is buy-in from all stakeholders.

When successfully executed by SLPs cognizant of the fitness industry and its demands, the service delivery models outlined within this chapter have advantages for the following:

- The GFI has his or her vocal health preserved so that he or she is able to communicate competently and clearly in classes, facilitating participant engagement, enjoyment, and safety, with overall well-being and professional performance being maintained or improved.

- The employer and fitness industry at large actively promote and support GFI well-being, contributing to increased job satisfaction, stability within the team, and longevity within the industry, which consequently improves the company and industry image in the eyes of the GFI and the everyday consumer.
- The exercise participant will be taught by GFIs who are healthy and able to competently communicate, motivate, engage, educate, and provide safe exercise instruction to them in all exercise environments.

References

Australian Bureau of Statistics. (2006). *Employment in sport and recreation, Australia.* Retrieved from http://www.abs.gov.au/ausstats/abs@.nsf/mf/4148.0

Baker, S. E., Hipp, J., & Alessio, H. (2008). Ventilation and speech characteristics during submaximal aerobic exercise. *Journal of Speech, Language, and Hearing Research, 51*(5), 1203–1214. doi:10.1044/1092-4388(2008/06-0223)

Beaty, M. M., Wilson, J. S., & Smith, R. J. (1999). Laryngeal motion during exercise. *Laryngoscope, 109*(1), 136–139. doi:10.1097/00005537-1999 01000-00026

Belafsky, P. C., Postma, G. N., & Koufman, J. A. (2002). Validity and Reliability of the Reflux Symptom Index (RSI). *Journal of Voice, 16*(2), 274–277.

Colton, R. H., Casper, J. K., & Leonard, R. (2011). *Understanding voice problems: A physiological perspective for diagnosis and treatment.* Philadelphia, PA: Wolters Kluwer Health/Lippincott Williams & Wilkins.

Dallaston, K., & Rumbach, A. F. (2016). Vocal performance of group fitness instructors before and after instruction: Changes in acoustic measures and self-ratings. *Journal of Voice, 30*(1), 127.e1–127.e8. doi:10.1016/j.jvoice.2015.02.007

Doust, J. H., & Patrick, J. M. (1981). The limitation of exercise ventilation during speech. *Respiration Physiology, 46,* 137–147.

Fairbanks, G. (1960). *Voice and articulation drillbook* (2nd ed.). New York, NY: Harper and Bros.

Fitness Australia. (2012). *Fitness Industry Workforce Report 2010–2020.* Retrieved from http://www.fitness.org.au/articles/fitness-industry-workforce-report-2010-2020/14

Fitness Australia. (2014). *Position statement: Scope of practice for registered exercise professionals.* Retrieved from http://fitness.org.au/articles/policies-guidelines/scope-of-practice-for-registered-exercise-professionals/26/38/20

Fontan, L., Fraval, M., Michon, A., Dejean, S., & Welby-Gieusse, M. (2017). Vocal problems in sports and fitness instructors: A study of prevalence, risk factors, and need for prevention in France. *Journal of Voice, 31*(2), 261.e33–261.e38. doi:10.1016/j.jvoice.2016.04.014

Harmon, N. M., & Kravitz, L. (2007). The effects of music on exercise. *IDEA Fitness Journal, 4*(8), 72–77.

Heidel, S. E., & Torgerson, J. K. (1993). Vocal problems among aerobic instructors and aerobic participants. *Journal of Communication Disorders, 26*(3), 179–191. doi:10.1016/0021-9924(93)90007-W

IDEA Health and Fitness Association. (2003). IDEA Code of Ethics: Group fitness instructors. *IDEA Fitness Edge, 2004*(5). Retrieved from http://www.ideafit.com/fitness-library/group-fitness-instructors

Jacobson, B. H., Johnson, A., Grywalski, C., Silbergleit, A., Jacobson, G., Benninger, M. S., & Newman, C. W. (1997). The Voice Handicap Index (VHI): Development and validation. *American Journal of Speech-Language Pathology, 6*(3), 66–70. doi:10.1044/1058-0360.0603.66

Karageorghis, C. I., & Terry, P. C. (1997). The psychophysical effects of music in sport and exercise: A review. *Journal of Sport Behavior, 20*(1), 54–68.

Long, J., Williford, H. N., Olson, M. S., & Wolfe, V. (1998). Voice problems and risk factors among aerobics instructors. *Journal of Voice, 12*(2), 197–207.

Luck, A., Pearson, S., Maddem, G., & Hewett, P. (1999). Effects of video information on pre-colonoscopy anxiety and knowledge: A randomised trial. *Lancet*, *354*, 2032–2035.

Mann, E. A., McClean, M. D., Gurevich-Uvena, J., Barkmeier, J., McKenzie-Garner, P., Paffrath, J., & Patow, C. (1999). The effects of excessive vocalization on acoustic and videostroboscopic measures of vocal fold condition. *Journal of Voice*, *13*(2), 294–302.

Marteau, T. M., Kidd, J., & Cuddeford, L. (1996). Reducing anxiety in women referred for colonoscopy using an information booklet. *British Journal of Health Psychology*, *1*, 181–189.

Mathieson, L. (2001). *Greene and Mathieson's the voice and its disorders*. London, UK: Whurr.

Naito, A., & Niimi, S. (2000). The larynx during exercise. *Laryngoscope*, *110*(7), 1147–1150. doi:10.1097/00005537-200007000-00015

Newman, C., & Kersner, M. (1998). Voice problems of aerobics instructors: Implications for preventative training. *Logopedics Phoniatrics Vocology*, *23*(4), 177–180. doi:10.1080/14015 4398434086

Rubin, J. S., Mathieson, L., & Blake, E. (2004). Posture and voice. *Journal of Singing*, *60*(3), 271–275.

Rumbach, A. F. (2013a). Vocal problems of group fitness instructors: Prevalence of self-reported sensory and auditory-perceptual voice symptoms and the need for preventative education and training. *Journal of Voice*, *27*(4), 524.e11–524.e21. doi:10.1016/j.jvoice.2013.01.016

Rumbach, A. F. (2013b). Voice problems of group fitness instructors: Diagnosis, treatment, perceived and experienced attitudes and expectations of the industry. *Journal of Voice*, *27*(6), 786.e1–786.e9. doi:10.1016/j.jvoice.2013.03.012

Rumbach, A., Khan, A., Brown, M., Eloff, K., & Poetschke, A. (2015). Voice problems in the fitness industry: Factors associated with chronic hoarseness. *International Journal of Speech-Language Pathology*, *17*(5), 441–450. doi:10.10 16/j.jvoice.2013.03.012

Sandage, M. J., Connor, N. P., & Pascoe, D. D. (2013). Voice function differences following resting breathing versus submaximal exercise. *Journal of Voice*, *27*(5), 572–578. doi:10.1016/j .jvoice.2013.04.001

Sapir, S., Atias, J., & Shahar, A. (1990). Symptoms of vocal attrition in women army instructors and new recruits: Results from a survey. *Laryngoscope*, *100*, 991–999.

Sapir, S., Keider, A., & Mathers-Schmidt, B. (1993). Vocal attrition in teachers: Survey findings. *European Journal of Communication Disorders*, *28*, 177–185. doi:10.3109/13682829309041465

Shewell, C. (2009). *Voice work: Art and science in changing voices*. Chichester, UK: Wiley-Blackwell.

Smith, E., Taylor, M., Mendoza, M., Lemke, J., & Hoffman, H. (1998). Functional impact of nodules: A case comparison study. *Journal of Voice*, *12*, 551–558.

Sodersten, M., Ternstrom, S., & Bohman, M. (2005). Loud speech in realistic environmental noise: Phonetogram data, perceptual voice quality, subjective ratings, and gender differences in healthy speakers. *Journal of Voice*, *19*(1), 29–46. doi:10.1016/j.jvoice.2004.05.002

Szabo, A., Small, A., & Leigh, M. (1999). The effects of slow- and fast-rhythm classical music on progressive cycling to voluntary physical exhaustion. *Journal of Sports Medicine and Physical Fitness*, *39*(3), 220–225.

Szmedra, L., & Bacharach, D. W. (1998). Effect of music on perceived exertion, plasma lactate, norepinephrine and cardiovascular hemodynamics during treadmill running. *International Journal of Sports Medicine*, *19*(1), 32–37.

Vilkman, E. (2004). Occupational safety and health aspects of voice and speech professions. *Folia Phoniatrica et Logopaedica*, *56*(4), 220–253. doi:10.1159/000078344

Wilson, W. J., & Herbstein, N. (2003). The role of music intensity in aerobics: Implications for hearing conservation. *Journal of the American Academy of Audiology*, *14*(1), 29–38. doi:10.37 66/jaaa.14.1.5

Wolfe, V., Long, J., Youngblood, H. C., Williford, H., & Olson, M. S. (2002). Vocal parameters of aerobic instructors with and without voice problems. *Journal of Voice*, *16*(1), 52–60. doi:10 .1016/s0892-1997(02)00072-3

World Health Organization. (2001). *International classification of functioning, disability and health: ICF*. Geneva, Switzerland: Author.

APPENDIX 4–1

Voice Screening Questionnaire

Name: ______________________________ Date of Birth: ____/____/________

Length of time working as a group fitness instructor: ________ years ________ months

Is group fitness instructing your primary occupation? ☐ Yes ☐ No

If no, please specify main form of paid employment: ______________________

Group fitness schedule:
Please list all of your permanent/regular classes. Provide start times and type of exercise program (e.g., 6 a.m. Yoga).

Monday	Tuesday	Wednesday	Thursday	Friday	Saturday	Sunday

What is the average duration of each class?

☐ 30 minutes ☐ 45 minutes ☐ 1 hour ☐ Other: ___________

Have you received any formal voice education and training? ☐ Yes ☐ No

If yes, please detail what education you have received regarding voice care:

____

____

____

Do you use a microphone while instructing? ☐ Yes ☐ No

Do you drink water while instructing? ☐ Yes ☐ No

Do you drink other fluids while instructing? ☐ Yes ☐ No

If yes, please specify: ______________________________

Indicate the extent to which the following statements apply to you:

	Never	Sometimes	Always
My voice sounds hoarse/croaky, husky, etc.			
My voice sounds breathy.			
I feel that using my voice takes effort.			
My voice sounds lower than normal.			
My voice sounds higher than normal.			
My voice breaks or cracks.			
I have difficulty producing a soft voice.			
I have difficulty producing a loud voice.			
My voice tires/fatigues.			
I lose my voice.			
My throat feels dry.			
My throat feels sore or aches.			
I have a tickle in my throat.			
I feel as if I have a lump in my throat.			
I frequently need to cough and/or clear my throat.			

Have you noticed any changes in your voice and the way it sounds since you began working as a group fitness instructor? ☐ Yes ☐ No

If yes, please describe the way your voice has changed:

____

____

____

Do you believe that you have a voice problem? ☐ Yes ☐ No

If yes, how severe is the problem? 1 *Slight* 2 3 4 5 *Severe*

Are you currently worried about your voice? ☐ Yes ☐ No

Have you ever been officially diagnosed as having a voice problem? ☐ Yes ☐ No

If yes, what was the diagnosis? ____________________________

Provide information regarding any treatment you may have received:

____

____

____

Do you routinely use any strategies or exercises to care for your voice? ☐ Yes ☐ No

If yes, please detail:

____

____

____

HEALTH AND LIFESTYLE

Do you currently smoke? ☐ Yes ☐ No

If yes: On average, how many cigarettes do you smoke each day? ______________

How long have you smoked? ________ years ________ months

On average, how many glasses/cups of each of the following nonalcoholic drinks do you consume in one (1) day? For any drinks that you do not consume, please respond with a "0."

Coffee (including coffee-flavored milk) ________

Tea (with caffeine) ________

Cola soft drinks ________

Energy drinks ________

Herbal tea, juice, cordial, non-cola soft drinks ________

Water (including plain mineral water and soda water) ________

On average, how many standard alcoholic drinks do you consume per week? For any drinks that you do not consume, please respond with a "0."

Note: One standard drink = 100 mL wine, 285 mL beer, 30 mL spirits, 60 mL sherry.

Wine ________

Beer ________

Spirits ________

Sherry ________

On average, how many hours of sleep do you get each evening? _______ hours

Is your weight stable? ☐ Yes ☐ No

If no: Are you purposely trying to lose or gain weight? ☐ Yes ☐ No

How much have you lost/gained? _________ kgs

Over what time? ________ years ________ months

Do you currently suffer from any of the following?

☐ Asthma

☐ Allergies: ____________________

☐ Reflux (indigestion, acid regurgitation, acidic/metallic taste in the mouth)

☐ Musculoskeletal problems: ____________________

☐ Thyroid issues

☐ Hormone issues (e.g., irregular menstruation, menopausal)

☐ Anxiety/panic attacks

☐ Depression

☐ Other chronic medical condition/s: ____________________

Are you taking any medications (over the counter or prescription) regularly?

☐ Yes ☐ No

Name of medication	How often?	Length of time you have taken the medication (in months)	Reason for taking medication

Is there anything else you think we should know or would like to discuss?

____

____

____

____

APPENDIX 4–2

Keeping the Voice Fit: A Vocal Health Guide for the Group Fitness Professional

Every person's voice is unique. It is an essential tool of the trade and allows us to guide our group fitness participants to do the right thing at the right time and to educate and motivate them toward accomplishing their goals. A number of reports (Heidel & Torgerson, 1993; Long, Williford, Scharff Olson, & Wolfe, 1998; Newman & Kersner, 1998; Wolfe, Long, Conner Youngblood, Williford, & Scharff, 2002) place group fitness instructors at risk of developing voice problems as a result of the heavy vocal loading associated with the profession. It is our job to make sure we keep our vocal cords healthy and fighting fit! This article aims to (a) describe the components of the voice system; (b) provide you with some tips on how you can keep your voice healthy; (c) make you aware of potential signs and symptoms of voice problems, and (d) explain where you can go to get help for any voice concerns.

How Does the Voice Work?

There are three main components of the voice system (the resonators, the larynx, and the lungs) that must work together to produce voice (Figure 4–3).

The Resonators (Nose, Throat, Mouth, Lips, and Sinuses) = The Amplifiers

- They amplify and project the voice.
- They shape sound into speech.

The Larynx (Voice Box) = The Source

- The vocal cords are small, mobile, and muscular and lie within the larynx.
- Sound is generated when a constant, smooth stream of air passes up through the cords during exhalation and the cords come together and vibrate (Figures 4–4 and 4–5).

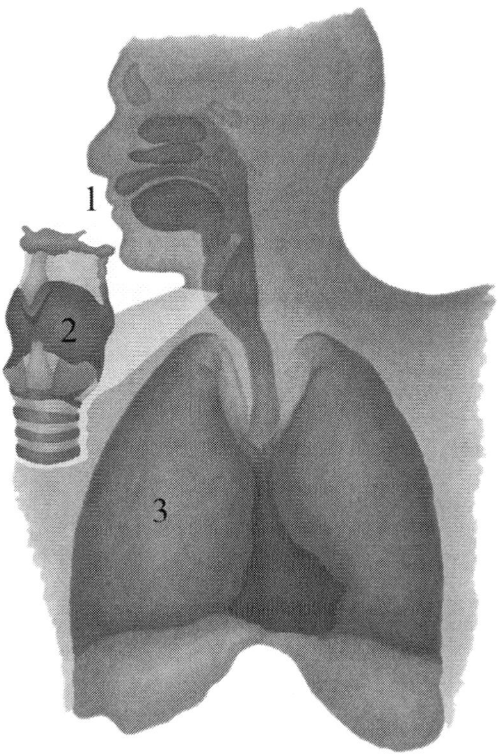

Figure 4–3. *(1) The resonators; (2) the larynx; (3) the lungs. (Illustration by Shannon Chapman [BSpPath].)*

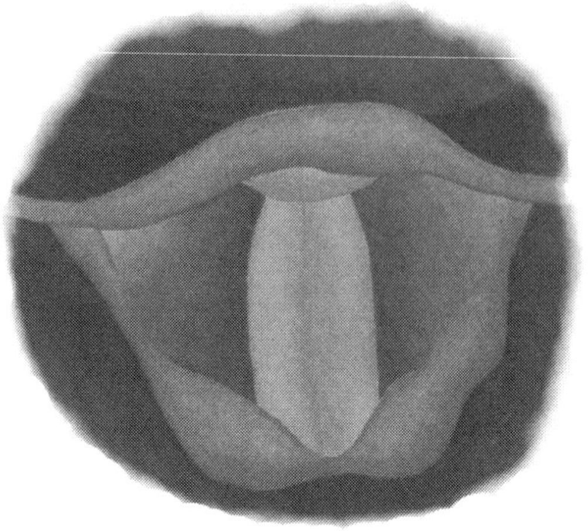

Figure 4–4. *As you exhale, the vocal cords come together and vibrate to produce sound. (Illustration by Shannon Chapman [BSpPath].)*

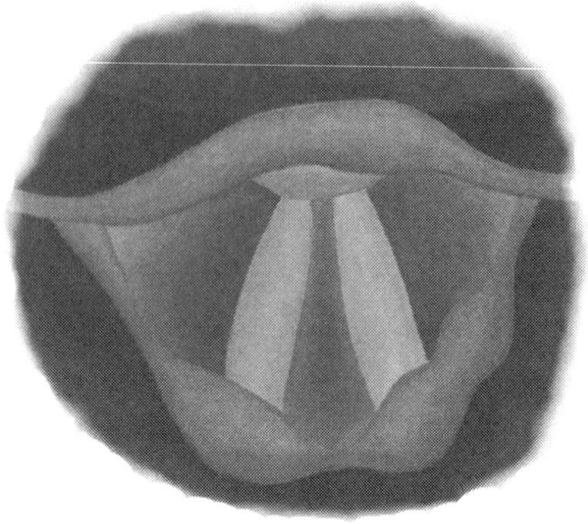

Figure 4–5. *The vocal cords are open on inhalation. (Illustration by Shannon Chapman [BSpPath].)*

- Adjustments in the position and length of the vocal cords (they are stretchy like rubber bands) create changes in vocal loudness, pitch, and inflection.

The Lungs = The Power

- Breathing is the foundation of the voice system.

What Can I Do to Help Keep My Voice Healthy?

Appropriate levels of vocal care and attention to vocal hygiene are a vital step in preventing voice problems. Paying attention to vocal hygiene is also an essential part of vocal rehabilitation. Remember, your voice is a reflection of your overall health. The following recommendations can be incorporated into your lifestyle to help keep your voice in good shape. However, these tips are by no means an exhaustive list and do not guarantee vocal safety.

Avoid Common Vocally Abusive Voicing Patterns

- Speaking/singing with excessive loudness
- Speaking/singing with excessive high or low pitch
- Speaking/singing with excessive laryngeal and neck muscle tension
- Yelling or screaming
- Forced, strained, or effortful speech/singing
- Vocalization during effortful closure of the larynx (e.g., grunting, coughing, throat clearing)

Stay Hydrated

Vocal cords that are well hydrated are less likely to produce a lot of friction when vibrating to produce sound. To keep the vocal cords hydrated there are three approaches to consider:

- *Drink water.* When we drink fluids it helps to hydrate the entire body, but it can take as long as 24 hours for the fluids to circulate and hydrate the body's tissues. Therefore, it is important to have at least eight glasses of water per day to keep the body's cells well nourished. However, drinking to "wet the cords" or lubricate them directly is not possible. Before the fluid reaches the vocal cords it actually gets swallowed and sent down into the esophagus. The closest fluid gets to the vocal cords in a normal person is about 1 inch above the vocal cords. When water does hit the vocal cords a cough reflex is triggered to expel any material that may have entered or is about to enter our airway—it is the response that we associate with something "going down the wrong way." If the body as a whole is dehydrated, then the vocal cords fatigue faster, get damaged more easily, and take longer to recover.
- *Inhale steam.* The only way we can get moisture to the vocal cords directly is through breathing it in. Everything that you breathe in touches the vocal cords on the way into your lungs, so breathing in steam essentially bathes the vocal cords in moisture. Use a portable inhaler from the pharmacy, take a hot shower and inhale the steam, visit the gym steam room, or use a vaporizer/humidifier in your bedroom at night.
- *Avoid drying agents* such as alcohol, caffeine, and some medications.

Know Your Enemies

Smoking, alcohol, caffeinated beverages, and reflux.

- When you inhale smoke your vocal cords become inflamed and swollen with extra fluid as the body tries to protect itself from the heat and chemicals in the smoke. Even if you do not smoke, stay away from others that are blowing it in your direction.
- Drinks that have a diuretic effect (i.e., encourage your body to pass out water) may dry out your vocal cords. The most common diuretics are alcohol and caffeinated beverages (e.g., coffee, energy drinks). You may not want to eliminate these from your lifestyle and you do not have to. Minimize, or at least compensate for the alcohol and caffeine consumption with extra water so that you maintain systemic (and therefore vocal cord) hydration. One cup of coffee = one extra glass of water.
- Gastroesophageal reflux, or acid coming up from the stomach and into the throat, is a common irritant for the vocal cords. Some people may experience reflux as heartburn or indigestion; others may not experience any obvious symptoms. The larynx, unlike the stomach, is not lined with specialized cells that stop the acid from burning. Reflux that occurs at the level of the larynx (laryngopharyngeal reflux) can cause hoarseness and excess phlegm, which is a result of the vocal cords being swollen. You can minimize the possibility of having laryngopharyngeal reflux by not exercising or going to bed right after eating. Eat after your classes if possible, and if

you teach late at night, try having a smaller meal for dinner and stay up for few hours after eating before heading to bed.

Enjoy Voice Rest

We live in a society where we can talk to anyone, anywhere, at any time. No longer do we have periods of quiet time built into our daily schedules. All professional athletes have rest days built into their training. The same principle should apply to voice care as you are a vocal athlete. Take multiple short breaks (10–15 minutes) throughout your day to enjoy silence. Your voice will stay healthier when allowed frequent opportunities to rest, recover, rehydrate, and relax.

If You're Sneezy, Take It Easy!

When you get sick, the bad guys (e.g., viruses, bacteria) invade the cells that line the nose, mouth, and throat. Your body sends extra fluid, blood, and immune cells to the area to fight off infection, which is why these areas get swollen. When the vocal cords get swollen, they vibrate more slowly, and sometimes unevenly. This is what gives you the lower, raspier sounding voice you have when you have a cold. Repeated coughing can also irritate your vocal cords and make them more swollen. A blocked nose will change your resonance so your voice may sound dull. Trying to sound normal and pushing to get a good voice under these conditions will give you more trouble in the long run. When you are sick, avoid voice use during strenuous physical exercise. It may be necessary to have a few days of voice rest, lots of sleep, fluids, and steam so that your body and voice can recover. Also, be mindful of the medications you are taking and what the possible side effects on the voice might be. Some throat lozenges contain ingredients designed to temporarily numb the throat. These chemicals may actually irritate the vocal cords, and you are also more likely to overuse your voice if the "stop" signal, in the form of a sore throat, is gone. If you have an acute sore throat related to a cold use these types of lozenges if necessary, but make sure you avoid prolonged talking during that time. If the problem is the sound of your voice, using lozenges and sprays will not help.

Warm Up the Voice

Just as you would not run a race without warming up your muscles first or start a class with a peak track, it is important to warm up the voice before a vocal workout. Generally for optimal effect, a vocal warm-up should be done no more than an hour before the vocally demanding event. Some people might ask why they need to warm up their voice when their voice seems to be going okay without the need for a specific vocal warm-up. The answer lies in what your vocal needs and habits are. A warm-up is just part of the process in optimizing vocal efficiency and is recommended for everyone. Even a quick warm-up immediately before speaking is better than nothing. Daily diligence may be your best line of defense against injury.

Sleep Is Your Best Friend!

Simple fatigue can lead to vocal strain. Adequate sleep (7–8 hours per night) may be an important part of your voice care plan. Sleep is the body's chance to revitalize by building new cells to replace worn-out tissues and restore both equilibrium in metabolic and mental states. Your voice benefits from all of this.

Specific Voice Tips to Use When Teaching

Make the Most of Your Microphone!

Remember to let the microphone do its job—it is there to make you louder, not clearer. The amplification of sound actually causes a small reduction in speech clarity so make sure you continue to speak with clear diction. When using a microphone you do not really need to "project" or yell; you can speak at a comfortable level. This does not mean that your voice is going to sound boring; use intonation and inflection and good resonance as well as facial expression to make your voice sound full, rich, and interesting. Another thing to remember is that your microphone should be 10 dB louder than your music volume so that you are heard (IDEA Health and Fitness Association, 2003).

Reduce the Competing Background Noise When Possible

It may be too hot to turn the fans or air conditioning off or down. The participants in the back row may always chat for the entire duration of your class. Your music may be booming from the speakers overhead. Be creative in your problem solving. Turn the fans on after the first three tracks and turn them off during the abs and cool down, politely ask people to be quiet, and turn the music down just a notch. If you find yourself raising your voice to an uncomfortable level, do something about it!

Keep Your Cues Simple and Increase Your Use of Nonverbals When You Can

Also, use short periods of silence to rest your vocal cords. We often panic that if we are not talking all the time, it means we are not talking enough. Once you have set your participants up and they are doing well, forget about searching for something to say and let the music have a chance to speak—remember the music plays an important part in creating fitness magic, too!

Avoid Using Unconventional Vocal Noises

Grunts, woohoos, squeals—or audible expulsions of breath. These actions can cause vocal cord trauma. When exercising, breathe as silently as possible—the sound of turbulence in your throat means that your airway is not completely open and your vocal cords may be getting roughed up or unnecessarily dry from the air passing up through the vocal cords. Deliberately constricted, audible "ujaya" breathing can be stressful to the voice if done incorrectly, with the constriction being placed low in the throat. If you practice ujaya breathing, protect your voice by focusing the turbulence and heat of ujaya closer to the soft palate. When in doubt, keep your breathing silent to protect the vocal cords from air turbulence, dryness, and fatigue.

Do Not Hold Your Breath While Doing Any Type of Exercise

Breath holding forcibly closes the vocal cords. The sheer force of this sudden and violent adduction of the cords can contribute to vocal cord tissue change and maladaptive patterns of behavior for the laryngeal musculature. When lifting weights, do not hold your breath, even if it means lifting less weight. Do not exhale on exertion; start exhaling before the push.

Role Model Great Posture and Stay in Your Set Position!

Postural misalignment is a common cause of muscle tension in the larynx (Schneider, Dennehy, & Saxon, 1997). Postural misalignments that may result in voice problems include hyperextension/hyperflexion of the neck and jaw, "slouching" of the spine, raising the shoulders, and an exaggerated position of the pelvis.

Avoid Exercising When Injured—This Includes Vocal Injury!

Just like you would not do propulsive lunges with a broken ankle or a clean-and-press with a dislocated shoulder, if the voice is injured you need to let it rest and heal before sending it back to work. We often push ourselves to continue exercising when injured, but this mentality is not conducive to a speedy recovery and can lead to chronic injury. This applies to injured vocal cords as well. Without taking time out from heavy voice use (i.e., teaching) you may be setting yourself up for a long-term voice difficulty. Another thing to keep in mind is that the vocal cords themselves do not contain any nerve endings, so by the time you feel discomfort in your throat or hear a difference in your voice the damage has already been done. If the show must go on, take all precautions necessary to protect your voice during this time—use all of the tips provided. Remember, pushing yourself to sound normal before you have recovered completely increases your risk of vocal damage and forming bad vocal habits.

Is There a Problem With My Voice?

Most voice problems are caused simply by how and how much the voice is being used. Listen and feel what your voice is telling you. The vibrating edges of the vocal cords that come together to generate sound can become bruised, swollen, or scarred, which will change how your voice sounds or feels. Changes in the sound and comfort of your voice that do not go away or frequently reoccur are important to notice as these may be indicators that something might be wrong. Some warning signs of a voice problem include

- hoarseness or other changes in the way your voice sounds (e.g., lower pitch) that lasts more than 2 weeks or regularly comes and goes (e.g., during or after teaching a class);
- pain or discomfort associated with talking;
- vocal fatigue (i.e., tiredness in the throat);
- frequent need to cough or clear the throat or a feeling of a persistent tickle; and
- sudden change or loss of your voice, especially if it happens during or after a class.

Are you changing the way you use your voice to accommodate for a problem?

Where Do I Go to Get Help?

There is a lot of information on the Internet about the voice and potential problems and pathologies. Avoid the temptation to try to self-diagnose. If you are concerned about your voice and how it sounds and feels, do not panic. Anxiety can make a voice problem worse. You need to remember that voice problems cannot be diagnosed or judged accurately by the way your voice sounds or feels to you. The only way to make a true diagnosis is by visiting an ear, nose, and throat specialist (ENT) for an instrumental examination of the vocal cords. Visit your general practitioner and request a referral to see an ENT for a thorough examination of your vocal health.

References

Heidel, S. E., & Torgerson, J. K. (1993). Vocal problems among aerobic instructors and aerobic participants. *Journal of Communication Disorders, 26*, 179–191.

IDEA Health and Fitness Association. (2003). IDEA Code of Ethics: Group fitness instructors. *IDEA Fitness Edge, 2004*(5). Retrieved from http://www.ideafit.com/fitness-library/group-fitness-instructors

Long, J., Williford, H. N., Scharff Olson, M., & Wolfe, V. (1998). Voice problems and risk factors among aerobics instructors. *Journal of Voice, 12*(2), 197–207.

Newman, C., & Kersner, M. (1998). Voice problems of aerobics instructors: Implications for preventative training. *Logopedics, Phoniatrics, Vocology, 23*, 177–180.

Schneider, C. M., Dennehy, C. A., & Saxon, K. G. (1997). Exercise physiology principles applied to vocal performance: The improvement of postural alignment. *Journal of Voice, 11*(3), 332–337.

Wolfe, V., Long, J., Conner Youngblood, H., Williford, H., & Scharff Olson, M. (2002). Vocal parameters of aerobic instructors with and without voice problems. *Journal of Voice, 16*(1), 52–60.

SECTION IV

Practices and Outcomes of Experts From South America

CHAPTER 5

Speech-Language Pathology Services for Professional Television Broadcasters

Vanessa Pedrosa

Summary

Broadcasters need to communicate with clarity and credibility. These traits are often not natural for the communicator. Speech therapy is responsible for assisting professionals to develop this potential, while adding quality, audience, and value to their shows, newscasts, and the network. When the network invests in the communication quality of its professionals and tailors this communication to its target audience by means of research and speech therapy, the financial and audience return is measurable.

Clarity means intelligible communication, with an easily and clearly delivered voice. Credibility means offering reliability to the viewer—that is, earning trust by what is said and how it is said.

A good media professional must know how to use the language, ideas, and sentence organization precisely and how to synthesize and use the aspects of expressiveness of communication such as voice, articulation of speech sounds, speech rate, modulation of speech, breathing, body (gestures, posture, and facial expressions), language, and vocabulary. All of these aspects need to deliver spontaneity and naturalness on the video and are carefully developed in conjunction with the speech therapist.

The objective of this chapter is to describe speech therapy and training for television and Internet journalists, television host, and sports journalists.

The focus of the work is to develop professional communication with clarity and credibility, enhancing communication style more naturally. The author conducted this work for Brazilian television networks in São Paulo, Rio de Janeiro, and other Brazilian cities.

Progression of Communication Styles in Television and Journalism in Brazil

Television has developed the ability to integrate and to articulate various communication styles in its programming. This potential has made television the main outlet for mass communication. The purpose of journalism is to inform and to win larger audiences and, therefore, substantial revenues (Temer, 2009).

Television in Brazil began in 1950. The first daily news program aired 2 days after broadcasting began, and so did the main Brazilian television news program of the 1950s, "The Esso Reporter" show (Maia, 2011). The news was very simple and was influenced by radio style—rapid, nasal, and resonant speech. The voice of the presenter was tense, serious, and high pitched with very marked emphasis.

In the following decades, television took on its commercial character and the search for ratings. Video recorded outside of the studio made it technically possible to record a standup for the news. The education and experience of television professionals shifted to those of print journalism from those of radio as had been the initial trend. Newscasters had degrees in printed journalism and were no longer from radio (Maia, 2011).

In 1964, Brazil suffered political turmoil with a military coup. This event established censorship in journalism and prohibition of activities or demonstrations on topics of a political nature. As a consequence, news programs went back to being presented by announcers rather than journalists in order to avoid any opinion or interpretation of the news. This imposition lasted until 1978 (Secchin, 2007).

However, there were advances in aesthetics and camera technology, studios, and broadcasting of stand-up via satellite (also called *link*). The role of the reporter grew, so television news was able to participate directly in covering the facts.

Television news programs were mostly presented in anchor-desk format, with a strict script and story formulation and no improvisations. In this style of television news, it was very important for the professionals to have a good appearance and a beautiful voice, without emotional involvement or opinion about what was being reported. The news was read without tonal variation, maintaining a monotonic and even tone (Rezende, 2000).

Newscasters had an inexpressive way of communicating, a resonant voice, and a certain distancing from the viewer, with a strong influence from radio communication again. Most television newscasters had to have a strong, deep voice with nasal resonance. Diction was very pronounced, and there was little concern with the body. Hand gestures and facial expressions were not a point of concern for television newscasters. The drafting of the script that was read on the news and in television presentations has been progressively simplified and has become closer to spoken communication throughout the years (Kyrillos & Cotes, 2008).

In 1974, the first Brazilian speech therapist was hired by a network to provide vocal training to its professionals. Glorinha Beuttenmüller was hired for her experience with speech therapy for the blind. She proposed that speech should not be delivered only with the voice but also with the entire body. This work spread throughout the journalism offices of all Brazilian states with the goal of minimizing speech distortions and accents across the different regions of Brazil (Memória Globo, 2009)

At the end of the 1970s, journalists started to become important again in television news, with the political changes and the need to focus more on content. Government censorship softened, and television news programs needed to provide information more freely (Castilho, 2015). In 1980, the first television news program that prioritized expert journalists' commentary and analysis of the facts appeared.

In 1988, a new type of newscaster appeared. A journalist was responsible for guiding, presenting, and commenting on the news (Porto, 2009). The anchor's communication style was based on commentary previously prepared and read or improvised. Anchors developed catchphrases to indicate their opinions on a fact or a story. Speech was highly modulated and emphatic.

In the beginning of the 1990s, there was an important shift in television communication. The images became more precise, which in turn created a greater concern with the presenter's physical appearance. Another change was a softening of the stereotypical standard. The voice did not have to be so resonant anymore, and diction became more natural (Kyrillos & Cotes, 2008). The huge technological advances in the 1990s allowed newscasters to report live, with footage and news from several countries. Information started to be delivered more dynamically to the viewer. It was possible to transmit air raids live. Good examples of this are all sports events and any important event that is transmitted live all over the world such as the terrorists' attack on September 11, 2001. Speech therapy worked in tandem with these changes to assist communicators in better exploring the voice, speech, and expressiveness in each communication concept, as well as working with vocal health (Kyrillos & Cotes, 2008).

The Internet and its huge expansion in the 2000s altered the standards of communication in television—not just in Brazil but throughout the world. A news story on television is no longer news when it goes on the air. News spreads across the world through the Internet all day long, and most of the population already has access to this news in real time. This change in perspective, whether the news is new or not, changed the language on television (Krotoski, 2011). Telling the facts of a story, adding value and commentary to the news, was one of the alternatives journalism found to make a story interesting even if it was not new.

During current newscasts, the studio environment and newsroom have real and virtual sets; studios are integrated with newsrooms, resources, screens, interactive screens, laptops, tablets, and teleprompter controls, among other tools, at the presenter's discretion. These affect the newscasters' dynamics, making their language, communication, and interaction processes more direct, spontaneous, and natural. These changes directly affect expressiveness because of the level of movement of the newscaster and of the reporters in the field, as well as their posture, and the different demands of each person and piece of equipment. In regard to expressiveness, the newscaster has started performing other interactions. It is natural that the voice, speech, language, and posture take on new formats that are more natural, dynamic, and conversation-like (Silva & Penteado, 2012).

New technology allows for the generation and multiplication of simultaneous informative lines of content, and television professionals must be prepared to produce distinct content and deal with the new technology—that is, they must rethink their way of working television news (Becker & Teixeira, 2009). Therefore, there were drastic changes in speech therapy approaches and work philosophy when dealing with television journalism.

The preferred vocal traits (Behlau et al., 2005) for television journalism underwent a period of profound transformation. This transformation stems from the need to connect, to grab the attention of an audience that has an interactive, dynamic, and ever-changing world at its disposal. The spread of digital technologies and the resulting convergence in the fields of communication, computers, and telecommunications are changing the journalism profession.

With the advent of major Internet video networks, anyone can make his or her own news story and post it online. Communication is becoming less formal and more geared toward telling stories creatively, directly, and interactively.

After more than 50 years of major accomplishments, the old method of television production is showing obvious signs of change. Television news narration has evolved from the concern with intelligibility produced by hyperarticulation while reading the news to the concern with interaction with and engagement in the authorship of the news. Speech therapy evolved as a science and professional field dealing with not only the attributes of vocal quality but also many other communication characteristics. Journalism evolved as a work philosophy as well as in relation to technical innovations that influenced production routines and the journalism profession. The current technology allows for almost instantaneous content development. This forces television professionals to be ready to read the facts and tell the stories more originally and without prior script development.

Today, the goal of a more natural communication, without excess vocal resonance, forces video professionals to think differently. They need to read the news with a more natural and unaltered voice. The language chosen is less formal, and accessible to different audiences and ages.

Introduction of Speech-Language Pathologist Services to Television Networks

In 2004, a Brazilian television network started profound programming changes in order to renew its journalistic standard (the format of its news programs, the language used, and the communication of professionals), boost quality and credibility with its viewers, improve content and image, and improve the format of the news programs. Hiring a speech therapist for its main network in São Paulo was part of the changes. As the network's senior speech-language pathologist (SLP), the author was asked to create a communication identity for the news programs, plan the communication style for each news program, and develop strategies for maintaining this quality. Although the investment returns of the network's improved communication quality cannot be measured directly, it is worth mentioning that network's earnings and ratings have tripled in the last 10 years. These earnings are, no doubt, the outcome of the strategic changes made by the network in its quest for quality and credibility.

Today, almost all Brazilian networks understand that the work of the speech therapist is crucial to achieving exceptional broadcasting quality. The in-house network's SLP is responsible for observing every detail that may either add value (e.g., naturalness in communication, quality of the articulation, etc.) to or remove value (e.g., less of expressiveness or wrong expressivity) from the information provided, the shows, and the people involved. In addition, SLP services improve the quality of life of the network's professionals. The speech therapist knows the television broadcasters' voices and cares for their vocal quality as well as helping them develop their skills in line with their career paths. For example, a broadcaster who is interested in switching shows can work on developing certain communication skills such as orality, improving voice quality and fluency. The speech therapist's job includes studying the style of television communication across time and understanding the targeted purpose of the shows because each program has a specific language according to editorial profile and public (e.g., morning news programs are more talkative, and night news programs are more formal).

It is important here to define style. Style is the character that journalists apply to television news. The style of communication is a predominant form of expression at a specific moment, and this concept is also associated with tendency. In a broader way, style is the standard of language, aesthetic, and technical expression of journalism (Sterling, 2009). The SLP analyzes each television professional's individual style and communication characteristics, studying the type of audience (e.g., statistical profile of viewers, such as age, education, income, preferences, etc.) and being clear regarding management's expectations (e.g., more dynamic program, less reading from scripts, more spontaneous communication, etc.). Style is a broad description of the communication of the individual. In general, it reflects a group of language features, both verbal and nonverbal (Sterling, 2009). These features are more or less constant and enable the identification of the speaker.

The in-house network's SLP is responsible for providing detailed descriptions of the television professionals' communication profiles, as well as profiles of the network's shows. A follow-up detailed SLP service proposal for each video professional is then outlined.

These services grow with the growth of the network. In 2004, the aforementioned television network had five daily news programs (two local and three national), one weekly documentary news program, one Sunday show, and one weekly sports show. This network has expanded its journalism programming in total amount of hours and amount of shows. Each program has its own language and pace and focuses on different news stories and audiences. SLP services have to address the individual needs of each show and each professional.

Very few television broadcasters (reporters, newscasters, and host) have voice problems, so quality and vocal health are not the main work of an in-house television network SLP. A broadcaster who works on video does not necessarily need to have a clear voice. However, broadcasters must maintain the voice qualities they already possess or try to improve them.

Growth of Speech-Language Pathologist Services to Television Networks in Brazil

After 2 years of SLP services provided exclusively for the aforementioned open television (free viewing access) main network in São Paulo, it was necessary to expand the knowledge and experience gained to all of the other networks affiliated with the main network. The level of quality achieved by the main network in television news communication needed to be extended to the other affiliated networks throughout Brazil.

This expansion took 5 years of regular visits to the affiliated television news networks in Brazil, as well as offering training for the television broadcasters and providing lectures addressing the role of communication quality in television shows for newscasters and re-porters. Direct support was given biweekly in Belo Horizonte, Brasília, Rio de Janeiro, and Santos to the same kinds of professionals. The support involves speech therapy assistance to professionals with training in the communication characteristics established by the network and improvement of individual communication characteristics. Training includes different communication skills such as improvising live, ways of commenting during the newscast, how to read off teleprompters, and all aspects of communication. This effort led to the hiring of speech therapists by the affiliated network in these cities, as well as in other cities, such as Balneário Camboriú, Curitiba, Maceió, Manaus, Porto Alegre, and Salvador.

In order to coordinate the work with this team, the network and the author supervise annual meetings. Currently, SLPs working for this network conduct annual on-site meetings with the SLPs working in all the networks in different cities in Brazil, as well as holding periodic online meetings. These meetings allow for learning from each other's experiences and standardizing the services provided for all television broadcasters in the network.

Speech-Language Pathologist Service and Network Relationship (Employment Options)

Another important issue concerning speech therapy work is the form of the contract between a professional speech therapist and the network. The contract format between the speech therapist and the network will depend on the proposal offered. The contractual form may be one of the following:

- When the network officially hires and employs the SLP, an employment contract is used and must comply with the Consolidation of Labor Laws, a set of legal regulations governing workers' rights in Brazil.
- When the network hires the speech therapist as a service provider, an outsourced contract is used. In this case, the contract is renewed annually or for a longer period agreed on by both parties.

The work week is defined according to the demands of the broadcasters. Many factors are taken into account, such as the actual service time involving the speech therapist and the television broadcasters; the preparation time for such services; the time invested in monitoring the broadcasters' programs to evaluate communication performance; and time for meetings with the managers, news directors, and program directors to discuss journalism guidelines and each professional's communication performance. It is also important to factor in time for emergencies such as laryngitis, sinusitis, and flu that affect voice quality.

The determination of the work week depends on the needs of the professionals with whom the SLP will be working. It is very important to bill not only for the time spent between speech therapist and broadcaster but also for the preparation time for the sessions; the time viewing the shows; and the periodic meetings with management, journalism directors, show directors, and editors of the news programs, and so on. Group narration workshops also are conducted, as well as participation in pilots. A pilot is an audition that a candidate or a presenter does in order to present a different show. The pilot is an audition to find out whether the candidate fits into the show's format and also to test whether all the technical aspects of putting the show on the air are working properly. SLPs also may evaluate new candidates before hiring, participate in show recordings, assist with vocal warm-ups before the shows, assist with preparation for communication about merchandising, and train interns.

A speech therapist's work directly affects the quality of video communication, which requires a wide range of skills. SLPs working for television networks are expected to take courses in sports commentator training, television news presentation, narration for commercials, institutional video narration, and training for actors. These courses help them understand the special needs of television networks and the best techniques to help them work and grow.

The Role of the Speech-Language Pathologist in Networks

Speech therapy services target verbal expressiveness (improved use of language in terms of the types of words used during speech, sentence length, and improvised speech), nonverbal expressiveness (pitch, vocal loudness, modulation, pauses, speech rate, articulation of word sounds, etc.), corporal expressiveness (standing or seated body posture and body movement in front of the camera, inside or outside of the studio), and facial expressions (emotion related, topic related, and video aesthetic related).

Several elements can interfere in spoken language, and the SLP can help work on these. These elements can include regional factors such as accent and variations in language use; cultural factors such as academic and cultural training; contextual factors such as the situation, the subject, or the news program presented; and natural factors such as age and sex. It is very natural for a new journalist to have patterns of speech, articulation, and vocabulary different from those of a more experienced journalist, and SLP intervention is needed to encourage maturation.

The speech therapist is also responsible for helping the journalist improve his or her style and communication skills and fit those into the desired type of television show. The speech therapist's job is focused on developing natural communication, focused on orality in a simple and direct manner.

Different Formats and News Programs That the Author Advises

Television news programs that focuses on local or national police stories have a conversational narrative, with the broadcaster's monologue interpreting the story, as well as dramatizing and providing personal opinions on the story. Some broadcasters can choose to use a teleprompter to read but focus mainly on spontaneous narrative and their skills to communicate naturally.

Another show may be lighter, blending stories about main facts with behavior trends. It may be presented by one or more than one host, which allows for a dialogue between them. The narrative must be creative, varied, and natural. The host rarely uses a teleprompter and has a lot of room to comment and add his or her own style of natural speech.

The national news programs have anchor-desk formats with two broadcasters, but there some news programs can have one or more broadcasters reading from a teleprompter. The stories are more standardized in structure and have a short duration. It is natural that the reporters and newscasters have a more balanced tone of voice and speed. The newscasters seldom comment on the stories.

Documentaries have a presenter introducing the subject without headlining the story. A tone of suspense is very common to the narration. The teleprompter is always used. The stories are long and well produced, with intense research and investigation of the subject. Documentaries may be about any subject, from interesting stories about people and places to stories about police investigations.

Digital magazine broadcasters have the most challenging form of presentation. The script narrated by the presenter is called the *head. Heads* are very short and demand a high level of interpretation for the topic to make sense to the viewer, whereas news reports are long, and the narration is very expressive. A lot of vocal resistance is required to record the long offs. Off is the text read by the journalist and covered by images; the narrator does not appear on the video. Recording offs for stories for digital magazines and documentaries can take more than an hour.

The story must be read by the reporter in a few different ways, depending on the chosen strategy. The most common structure of the story is off-stand-up-off. Using this structure can make a story that is a few seconds long last several minutes. The off is when the reporter reads and records the previously written script, and then later the audio is synchronized with the video. The off is written, read, and recorded by the reporter inside a special booth for this type of recording or straight to camera inside the news van. Usually, a head-and-shoulders shot featuring the reporter talking into the camera at the scene of the news event is often used as a transition or at the beginning or ending (UNESCO, 2016). It is when the reporter signs the piece. Most of the time, the journalist is on the scene of the news event and takes the opportunity to show some important images. It is during the stand-up that the reporter provides the most important news of the entire piece. The reporter may use a narration style with a voice that is more naturally expressive, with a normal speech rate, or with a more exaggerated expressiveness and slower speech rate.

The link (the stand-up for the reporter goes live from any other place, city, or country) is also very common. Reporters ready to segue must have vocal control in noisy places, precise diction, and good auditory figure-ground discrimination and selective hearing (central auditory processing skills). They also must coordinate speech with information they are receiving in the insert earphone about what needs to be said and how long they have, as well as the ability to narrate a fact in a short segue time. A segue can last from a couple of seconds to several minutes, depending on the importance of the fact.

Another format is the booth. In booth broadcasting, a reporter is used as support for the presenter. The reporter is not seen but narrates the news live from inside the booth without a previously prepared script. The voice of this reporter goes over the images presented. This strategy is widely used in breaking news, when the presence of an on-site reporter may not be possible. The booth format normally is used for news on traffic, accidents, and weather conditions. In these two news, the link and the booth, show formats, an improvised narrative is very common and requires an extensive vocabulary from the presenter, as well as knowledge of the city, the main facts of the day, and ease of communication.

Targeted Population

Speech therapy services for television broadcasters in Brazil are common practice today. It is offered for many open television (free viewing access) and cable television (paid viewing access) networks, as well as Internet television, institutional television networks such as TV Câmara, TV Senado, and private companies.

The professionals targeted are television news professionals, reporters and newscasters, live shows hosts, recorded shows hosts, sportscasters, and commentators. This author is the SLP responsible for one of the largest open television networks in Brazil. The office is in the main network in Brazil, and the author coordinated the work of all of the other speech therapists in the network's affiliate networks throughout Brazil. This particular network has 50 newsrooms spread across the country. Professionals receiving speech therapy services are men and women as young as 22 and as old as 80. They all have undergraduate degrees, mostly in journalism or in radio and television. A few hosts had other jobs before becoming television presenters. Some were models, business managers, economists, and so on. These professionals cover the many television news programs, journalistic documentaries, sports, and entertainment shows.

The network has local and national news programs with different formats and goals as described before. These professionals have a workload around 8 hours per day. Many of them have other vocal activities aside from their jobs. The most common are singing, event hosting, teaching classes, and other profession-related activities at other companies.

Speech-related complaints are shortness of breath while reading, expressiveness difficulties, improvisation difficulties, and hoarseness. The usually health complaints are stress, stomach pain, insomnia, rhinitis, sinusitis, and back pain.

Vocal Demands

Newscasters do not have vocal demands as high as those of a singer or a sportscaster, in most cases, and that is why it is worth describing a newscaster's activities separately. Daily television news reporters do not have to talk excessively. The most demanding on the professional's voice is recording the off. Many professionals like using a highly resonant voice, not very natural, which demands more of the voice quality and health of the vocal folds. However, this vocal behavior is becoming less popular. Younger professionals already use a more natural narration style involving less muscle tension.

The professional is exposed to the adversities of a news story, such as visiting a high-crime area and visiting places with risk of contamination such as hospitals or potentially dangerous places such as fires, factories, rain, floods, hot sun, cold weather, and so on. The daily stress is intense for this professional who must deliver between one and three news stories a day. This stress and the exposure to the dangers of the profession make vocal problems a frequent occurrence associated with emotional or health conditions such as the flu, colds, laryngitis, pharyngitis, or sinusitis.

Special reporters, in general, produce one story during several days. They have many scheduled interviews and may travel, but they are also exposed to the same stressful factors. However, they have a longer production time for a story. Their stories are long, and off recordings can last up to 1 hour in the recording booth, which requires emotional control and intense use of the voice.

Reporters who do international coverage do daily stories and specially produced stories. Their challenges have to do with time zone differences between the country where they work and the network's headquarters. A reporter in Japan has around a 12-hour difference. International reporters must produce their stories during the normal workday and communicate with the network headquarters at night. These changes are harmful to the voice. War correspondents are subjected to adverse situations such as emotional problems, stress, exposure to airborne chemicals, precarious access to food, and other challenges. My work with foreign correspondents is done via Skype, and the session dynamic follows the same structure as that for those who are physically present (ASHA, 2012).

The reporter may also have to do live segments during the news program, as previously mentioned. In these cases, the reporter has to gather the information, organize the script or the highlights of the information, and talk live with the anchor in the studio. The reporter tells the story that was either improvised or memorized. The style the author suggests for the professionals who do links is that they never memorize the script but rather organize the subject in such a way that they can tell the story in a few words in a few seconds or up to a few minutes. The link is also a great source of stress because the reporter talks live while receiving instructions from the video director at the network. The instructions can be about the time limit they have to talk and when to wrap it up. These instructions are given via an earpiece or headphones they wear during the entire broadcast. The intensity of the reporter's speech varies depending on where the reporter is to record or do a link.

Presenters have different vocal demands. Their routing on arriving at the network is to do hair, makeup, and wardrobe for the news. They attend several meetings and set the subjects of the day, study these subjects to make comments or add information during the broadcast, and deliver the news. A news program can last anywhere from 30 minutes to several hours, as is the case with digital magazines. The stress of live new shows is very high because of the high level of attention for a long period of time. The newscaster's vocal problems are more related to prolonged vocal stress. The newscaster's speech intensity can be normal in more traditional news programs and more intense in shows with high factual content.

The sportscaster is the professional with the highest quality demand. Sportscasters talk for long periods of time, usually at a heightened intensity. Sports such as soccer demand a lot more of the sportscaster's voice. Sports such as tennis require speaking for long periods of time, but with less emotion and intensity. However, vocal quality is a higher requirement in the routines of these professionals. A sportscaster's routine starts when entering the broadcast booth, which may be at the studio or at a stadium or sports arena. The ergonomics of these places vary greatly. It can be a comfortable space, roomy and with good acoustics, or it can be the complete opposite. During major sporting events such as the Olympics, sportscasters have an intense routine, broadcasting several matches throughout the day for several days. They are true vocal athletes.

Training for Regular Sportscaster Routines

A sportscaster's daily vocal preparation addresses vocal hygiene, detection of possible harmful vocal agents, vocal correction exercises to improve resonance or vocal quality, warm-up exercises, cool-down exercises, speech performance to improve articulation of the speech sounds, proper sports vocabulary, expressiveness, speech duration and coordination of this duration with plays from a specific sport, and buzzwords. Vocabulary is an important aspect of training. Sportscasters need to develop a specific vocabulary for each sport.

It is very important for the speech therapist periodically to watch the sports broadcasts on set (while being recorded live on set) and on television. Live observation of the performance allows for the following assessments:

- Body positions that affect vocal projection and voice health such as wrong posture of the head or of the body. Cervical tension and muscle tension in the neck during a game can produce skeletal muscle tension syndrome.
- Body movements, such as leg swings and head position, that affect communication. These movements undermine a good voice and can represent anxiety.
- Ergonomically inadequate chairs, tight clothes, inadequate hand or headset microphones, and other factors such as the use of social networks that might distract broadcasters while the game is live. Some sportscasters prefer headset microphones, and others prefer hand microphones because they produce a better voice sound.
- Voice effort to narrate important plays.
- Level of organization of interactions between sportscaster and commentator. The sportscaster describes what he or she sees in the game. The commenter makes comments according to the rules of the game and the skills of the team.

For the sports commentator, the approach is similar. The sports commentator may have a very high vocal demand during a long event, such as gymnastics. The commentator talks a lot more than the sportscaster does, describing the movements, the scores, and the history of the competition. However, the sports commentator uses much more conversation-like speech. The sports commentator does not have to use large vocal inflections, but it is important that the sports commentator's voice be healthy. Most commentators were players or head coaches before becoming commentators (Figure 5–1).

Training for Special Broadcaster Routines

For longer sporting events such as the Olympics and the World Cup, the sportscasters' and commentators' vocal preparation starts approximately 6 months in advance. Weekly speech therapy sessions are held, narration pilots of competitions with sportscasters and commentators in several events are held, and meetings are held with the staff members responsible for the broadcasts to be able to define all the details of the broadcast. Management must be aware of the speech potential of each professional and for how long the professionals can talk while safeguarding their health, thus ensuring vocal health throughout the entire competition.

It is the responsibility of the speech therapist, along with the technical staff, to choose the best microphone for each professional. It is relevant that each professional has his or her own microphone in order to avoid contamination of the team in case anyone gets sick.

The speech therapist conducts all the speech timing training for sportscasters, commentators, and on-field reporters. The training includes synchronizing the speech of each professional during the events. The profes-

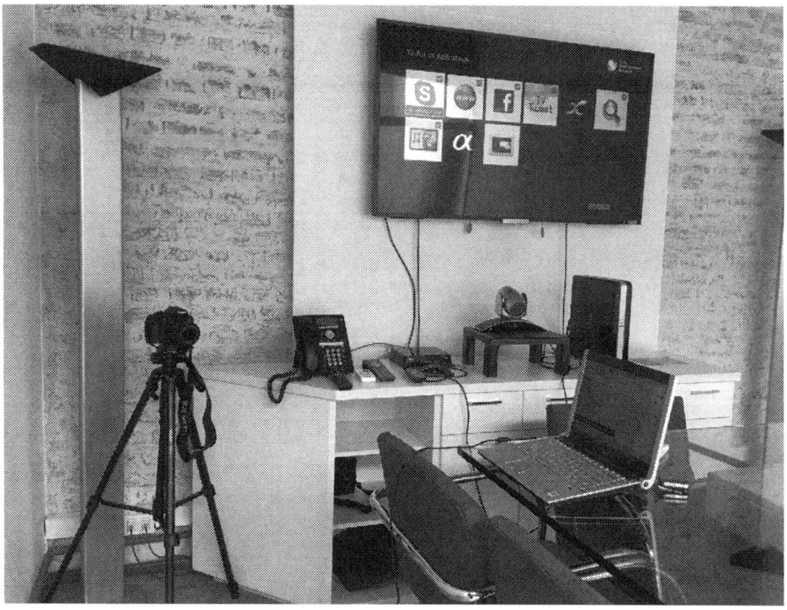

Figure 5–1. *SLP room in a sports network.*

sionals must learn to set the time to speak without interrupting each other sharply, and this moment must be denoted by a word that demonstrates that the speech space will be open, a body movement when the other wants to speak, or a different intonation.

The vocal warm-up and cool-down instructions are very important during this period. A sportscaster's voice must be flexible and adaptable to the different moments of a competition and must convey emotion, excitement, and confidence. Vocal inflections tend to be very quick during a match, and diction must be perfect, even when speaking quickly. Speed inflections are also frequent and follow the rhythm of the game. All these aspects are worked on during the speech therapy sessions. Even the "goal" yell style of the sportscaster is practiced so that the sportscaster can better explore narration style and signature.

Vocal Health

The greatest challenge video professionals face is constant upper airway inflammation. Rhinitis, sinusitis, colds, flu, laryngitis, and pharyngitis can cause hoarseness and affect work performance. Many professionals have to miss work for one or more days because of loss of voice. In these cases, the professionals receive orientation on the main voice care procedures and treatment and are sent to the network's physician or to an otolaryngologist who will provide the necessary prescriptions after examination (Gama, Kyrillos, & Feijó, 2005).

If the professional requires sick leave, he or she will receive instructions in order to care for his or her health and voice during this time. On returning, the professional will receive new instructions on voice care and exercises to help the voice recover back to normal.

In many cases, the broadcaster does not need to take time off work. In these cases, the speech therapist also intervenes to assist in voice quality maintenance and recovery.

The voice qualities normally expected for upper airway inflammatory diseases are hoarseness, breathiness, vocal instability, and medium to intense vocal breaks. Exercises may be done when there is an immediate need for vocal stabilization, but the results are not always positive. The exercises normally used in these cases are those for resonant voice technique (Lessac, 1997; Titze, 2001) and lax vox (Sihvo & Denizoglu, 2014).

Speech Therapy Assessment

Most professionals undergo a hiring evaluation with the speech therapist. The video stand-up of these professionals is analyzed, and a report is created on communicative performance.

The report describes the following: vocal quality, articulation quality and diction of the sounds, speech speed, organizational analysis of the speech (when recorded material was produced and written by the professional), resourcefulness in front of the camera, posture, hand gestures, and facial expressiveness according to the context of the story. The second part of the report contains the aspects that will be worked on and a time frame for results.

Speech therapy services are carried out on a priority basis. Treatment may begin for any of three reasons: a personal request by the professional, a request by the supervisors, or a request by the speech therapist.

Part of the speech therapist's job is to watch the news while on the air or through online recordings on the Internet. The objective of this analysis is to evaluate the professionals' performance within the news program's context and the dynamic between news stories.

The professional is also asked to answer a self-evaluation questionnaire about his or her on-camera performance (Appendix 5–1). This information is important to the speech therapist's work because it shows the awareness level and concern that this professional has toward the quality of his or her material (Pedrosa & Moreira-Ferreira, 2015). If the professional has vocal complaints, he or she is asked to fill out a voice-related quality of life form (Hogikyan & Sethuraman, 1999) to evaluate quality of life related to the voice disorder.

The evaluation protocol follows this open format to facilitate description of communication issues (Appendix 5–2) after the observation of conventional expressiveness patterns. The protocol consists of an auditory scene analysis of selected parameters (vocal quality, resonance, pitch, loudness, articulation, and pneumophonoarticulatory coordination), interpretation (rate, modulation, pauses, and emphasis), and psychodynamic factors (pleasantness, reliability, naturalness, and confidence). The psychodynamic evaluation refers to the social judgment expected from communication.

This form and all the questionnaires are available online to make it easier for the SLP to have access anywhere onsite or offsite. All the information is saved on the network's database, with an automatic backup. The protocol has an open format.

After asking for personal information, the SLP asks the professional to describe his or her activities because in television one job may have several different activities. Here, the focus is not only on vocal activities but also on what this professional's supervisors expect of his or her work. It is important to know how long the workday is in order to understand the physical and voice load. Origin or place of birth is important to profile the accent. Then, a brief medical history is obtained of complaints, personal and professional goals for the speech therapy, health problems, habits, other speech therapy treatment, main issues, hobbies, dental treatments, physical exercises, work history, and so on. The information about hobbies and other activities helps the SLP understand use of the voice outside of work. The SLP also asks about voice care habits the professional knows and uses.

The next step is understanding communication self-perception. The SLP needs to know what the professional thinks of his or her communication and what the professional would like to work on in order to correlate that with the professional's goals and time frame.

The evaluation begins with the observation of nonprofessional communication aspects. The description of these aspects in the protocol is done during the initial meeting. Because most professionals have two different voices, one professional and the other more natural, the SLP should avoid letting the professional know he or she is being evaluated, which makes assessing naturalness easier. At this point, speech and language characteristics are evaluated, including use of slang or informal language, answering with focus on the question, prolixity (tendency to speak or write in excess, verbiage), laconism (tendency to express oneself in few words, in a concise or brief manner), and spoken sentence structure.

Some professionals use inexpressive forms while reading scripts and do not bring out their own speech characteristics. In these cases, they randomly construct an artificial way of speaking using a specific modulation or musicality regardless of the subject (Stier, 2003).

From this point, the SLP starts working on evaluating the video material. The SLP needs to watch several videos produced by the professional in order to have a more accurate assessment of the professional's communication potential. Videos evaluated on the first day are saved in the professional's digital file, along with the evaluation questionnaire and the course of treatment.

During this first session, video records are made that simulate handoff (the moment that the reporter reads the text he or she wrote and presents the images of the story), links (the moment that the reporter appears during the news program talking live about a subject), and presentations with and without reading from a teleprompter.

The author uses a digital teleprompter, installed on a tablet or projected on a computer screen, and a professional digital video camera to simulate a presentation. Recordings are used for evaluation and training purposes. When a professional camera is not available, the author uses a cell phone camera. The evaluation form is filled out as the SLP and broadcaster watch or produce videos.

The professional's natural and professional voice styles are observed, additional audio recordings are made, and the differences are noted. The SLP should always ask the professional whether the difference between his or her professional voice and natural voice is desirable.

The SLP should help new professionals maintain this naturalness even during work so that they do not develop permanent and unwanted characteristics. With more experienced professionals who have established communication characteristics, the SLP may work on changing those habits only if it is their desire to do so.

During the first evaluation session, the SLP focuses on understanding the professional's communication profile and making him or her aware of it. By the end of the session, the professional should have a clear notion of his or her strengths and what can be developed further.

Diction and fluency articulation characteristics are evaluated in all the videos because it is easy to notice how they vary according to the subject, attention, and tiredness of the professional. The most observed articulation and fluency patterns in the Portuguese language are omission of last syllables and sentences, articulatory imprecision, tense articulation, and omission of /r/s and /s/s at the ends of words. For professionals with jobs in other languages, such as English and Spanish, the

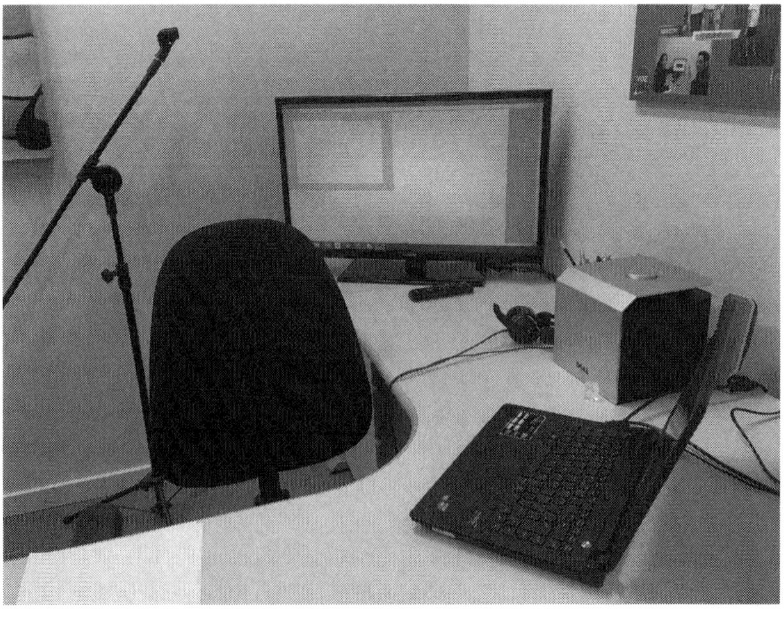

Figure 5–2. *SLP room in a network.*

SLP has to evaluate and work with the speech conditions for those languages (Figure 5–2).

Accent Training

Accent is a naturally special issue. Brazil is a large country, with different accents even within the same city. Therefore, for many years, television news attempted to standardize its reporters' and newscaster' accents. With the many changes that communication has undergone during the last 15 years, and even more in the last 10 years with the YouTube generation, accents are more tolerated. The philosophy of the network the author works for is to be more accepting of accents and change only a few characteristics when they are too prominent and may stand out more than the news story itself, especially in national news broadcasts. Therefore, my job is focused on changing small accent patterns, while keeping the main characteristics that localize the speaker. The accent protocol speech therapist Leonardo Lopes developed in his PhD research is our best reference. He also has experience with television news and was a speech therapist at this network's Manaus branch (Lopes et al., 2013).

Nonverbal Resources Training

The evaluation of nonverbal resources starts with two basic questions, the answers to which the author evaluates according to my personal experience and judgment and according to the results of the videos: Can I trust this person? Can I respect this person? (Cuddy, 2015). This judgment is what underpins the initial evaluation. The author also observes characteristics such as body posture and shoulder position and the movement of other body parts, such as the feet, legs, and hips, as well as head positions, types of hand gestures, looks, lip movements, cheeks, nostrils, and eyebrows.

Gestures can be repetitive, tense, inadequate, unrelated to the subject, adequate, associated with emphasis, or occurring before or after emphasis (Cotes, 2003). They must complement what is being said.

Gestural information associated with all of this other body information provides a wealth of detail about confidence, self-affirmation, truthfulness, and opinions on the subject. Almost all of the evaluations the viewer makes of the speaker are unconscious and contribute to the acceptance of the newscaster and consequently to ratings (Cotes, 2008; Cuddy, 2015).

After this, the author assesses the conditions of the phonoarticulatory structures, positioning, muscle tone, and movement during speech, mastication, and deglutition. The author evaluates the teeth and dental occlusion, the mandible and temporomandibular joint, the masseter muscle, the lips and tongue, and the hard and soft palates.

The evaluation is finalized by setting the main goals. Normally, the speech therapist's work with the television journalist can begin with aspects that the newscaster can easily identify and manipulate, such as body position and hand gestures, followed by voice quality and articulation, which are highly valued in more expressive narrations. The work on prosody is more complex in terms of voluntary control; it is more challenging and left for last (Penini, Padovan, & Vieira, 2011).

Expressiveness Training

Pleasantness, trustworthiness, naturalness, and confidence (Coelho, 2005) are evaluated as the end result of all aspects of communication. They are social perception judgments and correlated with the editorial profile of each show.

While trying to achieve naturalness, the SLP's goal is to make reading from the teleprompter not sound mechanical and as if the person is reading but rather as if the speaker were having a conversation with the viewer. The emphases and pauses, voice modulation, and sentence endings are evaluated, but they are only formally trained in a few cases.

The emphasis is the "bold" in the spoken word (Feijó & Kyrillos, 2004). The emphasis can be achieved by raising or lowering vocal pitch, loudness, or speech rate of one or more words in a sentence or by using more precise articulation (Feijó & Kyrillos, 2004). Emphasis can be moved around, when used with words that are not relevant to the main information, exaggerated sparingly or abundantly, or appropriately or inappropriately when unrelated to the main information. The emphasis is placed on the most important word or part of the sentence to help with comprehension. Every emphasis helps to highlight the most important information the speaker wishes to convey. The use of emphasis in spontaneous conversation occurs naturally. However, many speakers have difficulties expressing their ideas in this way. For example,

- **The** good news is that Mr. Paul won the tennis competition. (dislocated emphasis)
- The **good** news is that Mr. Paul won the tennis competition. (emphasis that highlights how good the news is)
- The **good news** is that **Mr. Paul won** the tennis **competition**. (exaggerated use of emphasis)

Pauses are important to speech because they allow time for the speaker to take a breath and for the listener to understand. They may be natural when they allow for good pneumophonoarticulatory coordination, but they may be either excessive or scarce in speech (Feijó & Kyrillos, 2004). During speech, the pause can be made at the grammatical pause or to highlight the information that will come next. When it is made solely for breathing, it may be dislocated in the speech:

1. The good news / is that Mr. Paul won the tennis competition. (emphatic pause)
2. The good news is that Mr. / Paul won the tennis competition. (dislocated pause)
3. The good news / is that Mr. Paul / won / the tennis competition. (exaggerated use of pauses)

Modulation is another speech characteristic that must be evaluated. It is the tonal speech variation, which may be classified as ascending, descending, or with variations. This modulation variation must be in relation to what is being said. The repetition of inadequate speech modulation causes the speech to be monotonous (Feijó & Kyrillos, 2004). It is very common for a reporter who did not have his or her natural communication stimulated to start reading offs or news headlines with an ascending or descending modulation. When the ending is ascending, it is out of context and conveys the feeling of lack of emotional control. When the ending is descending, it conveys a sense of tiredness or a lack of desire to communicate.

Speech rate is intimately linked to the importance and urgency of the news, the pace of the broadcast, and the presenter-reporter interaction. In terms of content and broadcast, it may be considered adequate, inadequate, fast, slow, varied, or constant. During the speech or recorded script, it is natural that speech not remain constant but that it have slight variations according to the intent and content of the message.

Speech rhythm is a very controversial classification in the literature. It is linked directly to modulation, emphasis (Feijó & Kyrillos, 2004), speech rate, and pauses. The author usually correlates rhythm with the concept of acceleration in physics: The result of acceleration is the variation of speed over time. In speech, the rhythm is like acceleration—that is, the variation of a few aspects such as speech rate, modulation, and emphasis strategy.

Voice naturalness classification is comparative. The author compares natural voice characteristics with professional voice characteristics and how much they differ from each other.

Voice projection is a classification similar to resonance, but it is important to point out that the newscaster speaks into a microphone in different situations. The newscaster may be in a studio, 6 feet away from the camera in a quiet environment. In this situation, it is not necessary to over-resonate or project the voice. When reporters are doing a story in an outdoor or noisy environment, the author suggests that they bring the microphone closer to the mouth to avoid shouting. When the environment is too loud, the author suggests reporters practice vocal projection with more intensity and no effort. Voice projection is closely linked to voice quality and resonance, as well as how far the journalist is from the camera. The camera is seen as the viewer, so there is no need to either shout at the viewer or talk too quietly, with no projection, making the voice difficult to hear.

When evaluating pitch, the author asks one question: Is this pitch appropriate to the physical type and professional activity of this individual? Pitch is adjusted only if necessary and with the professional's consent.

Long Take Training

The production process of a news program has changed throughout the years, and the broadcasting of a story is very fast, sometimes instantaneous. In the past, for a story to go on the air, it was necessary to wait for the news program to start so it could be broadcast in its entirety, or give brief bulletins that interrupted the regular programming. However, these bulletins were rare and hard to be inserted in the programming strategy. Today, many networks have enormous flexibility to cut in with news at any time, as needed. Large coverage of a story is done in real time and the regular programming is interrupted at any moment in order to give important news.

This flexibility was crucial for the networks to keep up with the updated information available on the Internet. Just like delivering the news first-hand to the viewers. This format requires more readiness to improvise good script organization, ability to narrate images, good command vocabulary, and knowledge of the place the event is happening and/or of the topic involved.

A lot of news pieces are broadcast without previously formatted scripts. Many facts are given using a technique called long take. A long take is a recording technique used in filmmaking. This recording technique has no cuts or edits. Contrary to the usual, the reporter does not previously write the script and then read it to overlay the images recorded. In this case, they record most of the story while showing what happened, where and how, while walking through the place where it took place. This strategy is practical with factual news stories, when time is short and when the place is rich in detail. In these cases, the reporter undergoes intense training, and their readiness to improvise is essential. This recording is always unedited.

The advantage of a long take is the opportunity of telling the story in a more realistic, more natural, and faster manner. The speech therapist's job in these cases is to assist the broadcaster or reporter to perfect his or her ability to organize the script and the story being told, to control his or her voice, and to use good orality to improvise while moving.

Exercises for Improving Improvised Communication

Improvising speech can be difficult and can put a lot of emotional pressure on the speaker.

Those who improvise on television show physical signs that occur before, during, and after the activity. Coelho (2005) conducted a study evaluating stress in live journalism, and the results revealed an increase in heart rate, cortisol levels, and vocal pitch. Today, most live segments are done without the reporter having done any prior script preparation. The report gathers the information and prepares to go live with a chance of being asked different questions from the presenter. Not memorizing the script before speaking allows the professional to speak more naturally. The professional assembles a script in advance, but not a memorized script.

In order to help the professional develop these improvisation, synthesis, information organization, and proper voice and speech skills, the training is wide ranging and involves several strategies such as narration of images on television with comments. In live news, the broadcasters describe the images and events they are seeing and experiencing, such as broadcasters involved in covering the tsunami in Japan or a road blockage on a main highway in Brazil. This coverage requires an in-depth knowledge of what is being talked about, reading and explaining scripts while timing themselves. It also involves command over verbal organization of the same topic in several different forms: chronological order, ordered from most to least important, reverse chronological order, and answering questions. Generally, training sessions are recorded, using either audio (voice recording on the computer) or video (using a professional camera), to monitor the body, voice, and speech production and to improve the professional's self-awareness. Professionals are also asked to take video selfies (using their cell phones) during training sessions because broadcast video selfies are used by some networks. This adds another level of awareness of their performance.

Case Study 1: Preparation of a Reporter

TDA, 26 years old. She came to the SLP for training for the first time when she was 24. She was prepared to be a television reporter. Her vocal quality evaluation scale was G0R0 B0A0S2 (G for grade of hoarseness, R for rough, B for breathy, A for asthenic, and S for strained) (Hirano, 1981). The otorhinolaryngologist evaluation results were normal.

Her pitch was high, and she had problems with articulation, diction, and interpretation of the text during loud reading. She spoke by using reserve air with an intense incoordination between speech and breath. Her high pitch, along with the uncoordinated breathing behavior during speech, ultimately infantilized her communication.

Training began with making her aware of her speech behavior and improving her use of reserve air. Even after each 30-minute training session and using different training strategies, she failed to notice the incoordination. Her body was constantly tense. Once training focused on reducing her pitch, good results were achieved. However, her communication remained sounding infantilized due to her speech-breath coordination.

After eight 30-minute sessions, she progressed very little regarding such communication skills as pitch, articulation, and reading interpretation of the text; the greatest challenge remained her inability to perceive her infantile communication behavior. Training then focused on auditory training and perception with auditory feedback. This included variation perception training with piano tonal variation, her own vocal tonal variation, and other people's voices, at different speech rates, with texts, poems, short stories, and improvised speech. Results were still inconsistent because she could not maintain the communication behavior she had learned. Once training included recording videos of herself and watching them at the end of the day, results started coming faster because she started to understand how to maintain the new communication behavior. She is currently a successful reporter who has worked for the network for 15 years doing other journalistic activities as editor video and text editor, and working for 4 years as a reporter.

Speech-Language Pathologist Services for Sportscasters

Vocal Preparation for Sportscasters

A sportscaster may have a degree in television journalism or radio or may have no college education at all. Sportscasters are generally very well-paid professionals. During the last 3 years, at the sports station where the author work, approximately 20 sportscasters, 28 to 75 years old, chose to invest in their careers by taking industry-related courses.

Vocal Preparation for Commentators

According to Wikipedia, "in sports broadcasting, a sports commentator (also known as sports announcer, sportscaster or play-by-play announcer . . . gives a running commentary of a game or event in real time, usually during a live broadcast, traditionally delivered in the historical present tense. The comments are normally a voiceover, with the sounds of the action and spectators also heard in the background. In the case of television commentary, the commentators are on screen rarely if at all during the event (although they may appear on camera at the start or near the end of the broadcast)."

The specialist who specializes in one or several sports is usually a professional who had no previous on-camera experience. He or she may have a journalistic background, with prior experience as a columnist for print journalism or specialized sports websites or may be a former athlete.

Their preparation from a communication standpoint involves all types of communication training, such as presentation of video communication styles; available resources, such as offs, narration, and teleprompter reading; personal interviews; synchronicity of their communication with the sportscaster's during sporting events; comment duration; and types of comments expected, depending on the audience and editorial perspective of the network. Other important topics are communication aspects such as voice care, diction improvement, fluency, speech speed, prosody, language organization, and on-camera body posture and body language.

Vocal Preparation for Large Sports Events

A large sporting event can last from 15 to 30 days. The SLP has to prepare the sportscasters and commentators in advance. Such events demand a more intense strategic and physical preparation from the professionals involved in the broadcast because of the higher workload, as well as all the added stressors they experience. They may have to speak for several hours straight, narrating different sporting events at all hours, even when they are outside of the country's time zone. They eat the food available to them at the venues, which is not part of their normal eating habits. The broadcast locations may not be ergonomically suitable to maintain a voice-friendly or comfortable body position for long periods. That is why vocal and physical training must be initiated well in advance so that the professional is adequately prepared for these demands.

Vocal Preparation for Covering the Olympic Games

The author has provided SLP services for broadcasters covering many international sporting events, such as the London Olympics in 2012, Rio Olympics in 2016, South Africa World Cup in 2010, and Brazil World Cup in 2014; three Pan American Games (Rio 2007, Guadalajara 2011, and Toronto 2015); and the Winter Olympic Games in Vancouver in 2010. The communication difficulties identified in these professionals were related to speech, voice, and language such as long sentences and unusual words. The primary evaluation revealed problems with diction; changes in-oral motor skills that affect speech; vocal projection; and voice problems such as asthenia, hoarseness, or voice breaks after speaking for short or long periods.

All the problems observed during the evaluation were worked on individually and then later in conjunction with other issues. For example, a hoarse voice is treated after an otolaryngologist diagnosis. As soon as an individual's voice reaches a better standard, narration work is started in order to assist in making this new vocal standard automatic during regular work activities.

For the Olympics, the work began 6 months ahead of time according to the following structure:

- A general meeting with all the reporters, sportscasters, commentators, and broadcasters was held to present the 6-month plan.
- We held weekly pilots for commentators who did not have experience as television sports commentators. They were all Olympic medal athletes or sports journalists without television experience. The pilots are a simulating transmission of the events. The sportscasters and commentators practice their activities as if it were the actual broadcast.
- We provided a weekly report distribution with brief voice and speech care instructions.
- The food served at the venues was researched in order to know what specific care each professional would have to take to avoid damaging their voice. For example, the food served in London would be sandwiches or would contain a lot of pepper. Both foods interfere with digestion, which can cause reflux and impair vocal quality.
- The local climate was taken into consideration at all of the events so that the professionals were prepared. Issues with temperature and humidity were discussed with the otolaryngologist. All professionals received the necessary information in case they had any voice health issues. When possible, local otolaryngologists were contacted in advance so that they could see the professionals in case of emergency.
- The SLP and the network's audio engineers selected the best microphone for each individual, addressing personal preferences as well. Having individual microphones was helpful in avoiding possible contamination in case anyone became ill and used someone else's equipment.
- Sportscasters and commentators received information about daily vocal rest, warming up, and cooling down.
- We held periodic meetings (every 15 days) with the sportscasters, commentators, reporters, broadcasters, and leadership to check the

progress of the work, the results, and any necessary planning changes.

- Whenever possible, sportscasters were able to choose the type of event they wished to cover. In these cases, the narration style was also taken into consideration to see whether it was a good fit with the narrated event.

Vocal Preparation for Reporters and Newscasters

Speech training attends to the needs of the news programs. Many newscasters are also reporters, meaning that the SLP works the same way with both groups, with the same skill sets, such as reading offs, doing links, reading a teleprompter, and so on. Interns and recently graduated journalists are taught to perform any journalistic video activity, such as presentation and reporting, and need to know how to read a teleprompter with the same interpretation as reading an off. In terms of technique, the reporter must have the following:

Head: The first sentence is almost always a headline, an affirmative sentence. The second explains the statement and introduces the subject.

Off: Text written by the reporter and based on the pictures provided by the reporting team.

Passage: The moment that the reporter appears in the matter. It gives credibility to what is being said. The passage can be used to describe something for which we have no image, to highlight one piece of information among others, to unite two situations, to highlight one interviewee, or to create a participatory passage.

The evaluation is initially done in order to map the personal and professional communication abilities of the journalist in several situations: reading off, teleprompter reading, improvisation, off-camera narration, and links. The initial evaluation includes the following:

- Self-assessment of recorded voice on camera, through listening to their video recordings, identifying different qualities and understanding how their voice would be perceived by their audience. This information helps plan exercises needed to improve vocal quality and vocal projection.
- Self-assessment of voice care practices, followed by ongoing education regarding vocal health practices.
- Evaluation of pronunciation of phonemes, fluency, rhythm, and speech speed. This helps the SLP plan speech enhancement exercises as needed.
- Evaluation of speech expressivity, the natural prosody used by the broadcaster to reflect the underlying intention and personal opinion about the script (mocking, disbelief, support, etc.).
- Offs reading style, which is the style of the reporter or broadcaster when narrating a script off screen. These narrations are edited into visual footage of televised stories. The SLP looks for the voice's ability to produce natural communication, clear articulation, engaging intonation, and authentic expressivity. Future training will target any aspects that need improvement.
- Teleprompter reading style, which involves the written display from which the broadcaster reads the news. This information is mostly prepared, but sometimes it is

improvised, such as with breaking live news. If the teleprompter is prepared, the broadcaster needs to identify fully with what he or she is reading, or it will sound fake to the audience (e.g., Michelle Obama's speech as she read it herself and then as it was read by Melania Trump). It should not look like reading, but rather as a form of self-expression. SLP training includes practicing to ensure understanding of the text and practicing different figures of speech and literary techniques while reading the text (e.g., metaphors, metonymy, euphemism, irony).

- Recounting skills. Broadcasters are asked to read a news story and then recount it without reading or teleprompter. The SLP evaluates their ability to organize ideas and facts; summarize; maintain clear and simple vocabulary; and avoid slang, corporate jargon, or seldom-used words. Training will target areas that need improvement.
- Body organization evaluation. The SLP evaluates the broadcaster's posture and hand and head gestures on television recordings. Training targets using body posture and gestures as second nature, this approach does not teach specific gestures. Broadcasters are made aware of their own posture and gestures by sitting them in front of a mirror and highlighting the effect of their gestures on the viewers (Vieira, 2005). Training aims for them to use these gestures as a natural resource of expressiveness rather than an extra movement that does not match with the content and acts as added noise.

Training Sessions

Training takes place during 30-minute sessions between the broadcaster and the speech therapist. The sessions take place at the network in the speech therapist's office or in a conference room.

One topic is chosen and practiced during each session. The professional receives voice, speech, or reading exercises to be practiced at home or during work. At the next session, the exercises are reviewed and an assessment of progress is made. Many topics require several training sessions. It is essential that the professional be self-aware of his or her speech and internalize what was learned.

The learning process varies for each aspect and for each individual. The process is determined by the complexity of each topic and the individual's ability to self-evaluate and self-monitor.

An experienced journalist already has many developed characteristics and does not need to work on a specific narration style. Therefore, the work is focused on constant performance evaluation, vocal exercises that help maintain voice and speech quality and facilitate voice projection, and warm-up and cool-down exercises.

Other experienced professionals seek speech therapy treatment to change speech or narration patterns in line with their work demands. They may be transitioning to a new broadcasting position, so they may need to work on some communication skills. The work is ongoing and tailored to individual and network needs.

Case Study: Preparation of a Sportscaster

TA, a 30-year-old motorsport commentator, referred to SLP services by his department to improve his communication. He used a non-projected nasal voice and had voice fatigue and a tight feeling in his throat during live coverage of sporting events.

The SLP assessment indicated normal vocal quality (G0R0B0A0S0) (G for grade of hoarseness, R for rough, B for breathy, A for asthenic, and S for strained) (Hirano, 1981), high pitch, reduced loudness, nasal sound, normal speech rate, strained voice, laryngo-pharyngeal voice (decreased oral resonance), moderate imprecise articulation, and use of reserve air during speech.

The first stage of training focused on improving communication and self-perception. Sessions included viewing the recordings of the sports events that he covered live. The evaluation protocol highlighted the following problems in communication: difficulty in pronouncing phonemes correctly or inaccuracy of speech, difficulty in maintaining voice volume until the end of a sentence, and noisy breathing during speech. These problems were treated by using speech amplification simultaneously during speech to improve the perception of speech pronunciation and speech volume. Respiratory noise is reduced with speech and breathing control exercises and use of respiratory support during speech. During the next sessions, the focus of training was on speech content, improvement of diction and articulation, and habituation of a speech rate that ensures precision of speech sounds. Training exercises included overarticulated speech, text reading, and spontaneous speech with auditory feedback.

The second step of training focused on voice health and care for the professional voice. It also introduced exercises to reduce pitch, loudness, and vocal fatigue; these included tongue vibrations, glottic firmness, and support sounds such as humming and sustained fricatives for lower pitch. The last step can be instant feedback provided during the recording or playback after the recording. Instant feedback training makes it easier to hear one's mistakes, correct them on the spot, and avoid them during the rest of the reading. Playback training allows time to analyse personal development better.

The last stage focused on the naturalness of speech during narration. Modulation concepts, emphasis, pauses, and finishing the sentences were presented but not taught. The sports commentator and the SLP focused on natural communication.

Throughout these 6 months, the commentator was preparing to assume more responsibilities during the broadcasting of sports events and competitions. After the 6 months, the network asked the SLP to prepare him to be a sportscaster. The training to be a sportscaster was a little different. He had already developed the communication aspects, but he needed to be able to talk for a long period. Training focused on impromptu speech concepts, analysis of images, and speech time because often it is not necessary for the sportscaster to describe what is going on in detail, and recognize that moment, as well as develop communication strategies for it is part of the training. The training sessions took place every 7 days, according to his schedule, for 1 year.

Speech Therapy Services for YouTubers

YouTube has more than one billion users who watch hours of video every day. The network display time has grown every year, and 80% of views are from outside the United States (YouTube information, 2016). YouTubers' communication patterns differ from those of traditional television, and it is important to understand this population and what they are doing.

The SLP service to YouTubers is a demand that has appeared more and more in the private office. YouTubers are gaining space, recognition, professionalism, and good remuneration. Many YouTubers produce their material in a homemade way; others are already linked to producers, and they produce periodic material with greater editorial quality.

Most YouTubers who seek speech therapy hope to work on their communication to make it more conscious and efficient without losing naturalness and spontaneity.

The communication pattern of the YouTubers differs from that of traditional television because most of the content is performed without a script, with intense use of the voice. The communication style is similar in most of the evaluated channels across countries. The language used by YouTubers is simple, according to the age of the speaker and the target audience.

Vocal Preparation for YouTubers

Vocal preparation is done in the traditional way. Evaluations include vocal quality, communicative performance, body language, and discourse analysis. However, in these cases, the work should greatly encourage the strengthening of the individual's natural speech patterns according to the purpose of the channel and its audience. A good example is the channels about games. In these channels, the speech rate is fast. There is no concern with the quality of the articulation of the sounds, and the author worked only on improving articulation in rare cases of moderate articulatory inaccuracy when the quality of the information was compromised. On television, any problem of articulation of speech sounds is worked out. The channels with the aim of teaching about some topic already consider the quality of the articulation of sounds and speech because they wish to demonstrate greater professionalism and the speaker wishes to appear credible.

Vocal quality is affected by several factors, such as health, prevention of future voice problems, and improvement of the speaker's self-image. A healthy voice also has greater acceptability and is more efficient when amplified by a microphone.

Case Study 3: Reparation of a YouTuber

MG, 30 years old, a YouTuber professional for 2 years. His speech style was teenage, and his vocal quality was classified as G2R2B1A1S0 (G for grade of hoarseness, R for rough, B for breathy, A for asthenic, and S for strained) (Hirano, 1981). His vocal projection was low and his pitch was high. The diagnosis was minor sulcus vocalis in the right vocal fold, glottal chink, and contralateral reaction. His speech rate was fast, he had moderate articulation inaccuracy impairing comprehension, and he had short breath during speech.

Discourse analysis showed simple vocabulary, long phrases, and some difficulties of objectively initiating the subject proposed in the video and concluding. Intense use of the vocative case was noted throughout his speech. He also addressed the viewer in the plural form, as if there were several viewers at the same time. The purpose of each of his videos was made apparent after approximately 1 minute.

His main complaints were related to his voice and his belief that the channel's audience is prejudiced because of it. When we looked at channel statistics, we noticed that viewers gave up watching the video after approximately 15 seconds. The beginning of the work focused on his vocal quality. A comprehensive voice rehabilitation program was suggested for 6 weeks (Behlau, Pontes, Pedrosa, Yamasaki, & Madazio, 2013; Pedrosa, Pontes, Pontes, Behlau, & Peccin, 2016). The program included articulatory exercises to improve articulation of speech sounds, speech amplification to increase perception of imprecision, as well as appreciation of positive results when the articulation improved. Video recording and speech audio features to aid the speaker's perception were explored extensively.

The language was analyzed, and the author proposed that he start the videos with direct language, without prolixity, and using only one vocative in the singular (e.g., "now," "pay attention," versus "attention all of you"). Language training was done through discourse reconstructions of taped videos and the impromptu training presented earlier in this chapter. As a result of this training, the audience increased, and the access time of each viewer increased.

In this way, he improved his vocal quality (G1R1B0A0S0) (G for grade of hoarseness, R for rough, B for breathy, A for asthenic, and S for strained) (Hirano, 1981), his pitch became slightly lower, his articulation improved, and his vocal projection improved. His language became more direct, without prolixity, and his improvised skills improved, which aided in its comic context.

Today, his YouTube channel is ranked among the largest Brazilian channels, with a very high level of access, and he broadened its audience, which previously had been teenagers. Today the target audience ranges from 15 to 45 years.

Vocal Preparation for Hosts During Merchandising on Television Programs

Merchandising during television shows is very common. For an advertisement to have positive results in sales, it is important that the advertisement focuses on the right audience and advertised product during the right program. The network understands that when the merchandising has good results, those good results are partly because of the form in which it is presented. These results clearly turn into more advertisements and greater financial returns. Similarly, today, advertisers clearly understand the benefit of having their product well represented.

The announcer who receives speech therapy services is usually a person who is accustomed to talking to the camera but may not be able to always lend a positive image to the advertised product. To avoid image conflicts during an advertisement, the author receives the merchandising texts 1 day before the recording.

The text is studied, and small changes in the text are suggested when necessary. Changes usually are related to the length of the sentences, the simplicity of the words, and how these combine with who is presenting the product.

Markings are made in the text as in musical scores to show the intent of each sentence or word. The end of each sentence is marked to show how to finish it according to the intention. These modifications represent the prosody of the speech so that it is as clear and attractive as possible. Merchandising may be for the retail market or it may not, and this difference requires clear differences in prosody. Retail, as with any television advertisement, demands faster speech, greater loudness, and intense melodic variation. In other cases, the communication varies according to the product and the text chosen. The tonic syllables of the words and the emphases represent the intention. The tonic syllables are also highlighted in the text to confirm the intonation of each word.

Before the recording is performed, the speaker warms up vocally and studies the text to be read before going to the teleprompter. This ensures achieving the desired final outcome of the recording.

References

American Speech-Language-Hearing Association (ASHA). (2010). *Professional issues in telepractice for speech-language pathologists* [Position statement]. Retrieved from http://www.asha.org/policy

Becker, B., & Teixeira, J. (2009). Narrativas jornalísticas audiovisuais: um estudo dos efeitos da convergência no JN e no UOL [Audiovisual journalistic narratives: A study on the effects of the convergence of JN and UOL]. *Rev Galáxia, 18*, 232–246.

Behlau, M., Feijó, D., Madazio, G., Rehder, M. I., Azevedo, R., & Ferreira, A. E. (2005). Voz profissional: Aspectos gerais e atuação fonoaudiológica [Professional voice: General aspects and speech therapy participation]. In M. Behlau (Ed.), *Voz: O livro do especialista* [Voice: The specialist's book] (pp. 296–332). São Paulo, Brazil: Revinter.

Behlau, M., Pontes, P., Pedrosa, V., Yamasaki, R., & Madazio, G. (2013). Presentation of the Comprehensive Vocal Rehabilitation Program for the treatment of behavioral dysphonia. *CoDAS, 25*(5), 492–496.

Castilho, M. S. (2015). A história do jornalismo Brasileiro [The history of Brazilian journalism]. *Observatório da Imprensa.* Retreived from http://observatoriodaimprensa.com.br/marcha-do-tempo/a-historia-do-jornalismo-brasileiro/

Coelho, M. A. (2005). O custo somático da expressividade—considerações sobre o stress no telejornalismo ao vivo [The somatic cost of expressiveness—stress considerations in live telejournalism]. In L. C. R. Kyrillos (Ed.), *Expressividade: da teoria à prática* (pp. 197–219). Rio de Janeiro, Brazil: Revinter.

Cotes, C. (2003). Avaliando o corpo [Evaluating the body]. In L. Kyrillos (Ed.), *Fonoaudiologia e Telejornalismo. Relatos de experiências na Rede Globo de Televisão* [Stories of experiences at Rede Globo Television Network] (pp. 19–31). Rio de Janeiro, Brazil: Revinter.

Cotes, C. (2008). *O estudo dos gestos vocais e corporais no telejornalismo brasileiro* [The study of vocal and bodily gestures in Brazilian television journalism]. São Paulo, Brazil: PUC-SP. Retrieved from http://www.pucsp.br/liaac/download/claudiacotes.pdf

Cuddy, A. (2015). *Presence.* New York, NY: Little Brown Company.

Feijó, D., & Kyrillos, L. (2004). *Fonoaudiologia e Telejornalismo* [Speech therapy and television news]. Rio de Janeiro, Brazil: Revinter.

Gama, A. C. C., Kyrillos, L., & Feijó, D. (2005). *Fonoaudiologia e Telejornalismo* [Speech therapy and television news]. Rio de Janeiro, Brazil: Revinter.

Hirano, M. (1981). *Clinical examination of the voice.* New York, NY: Springer-Verlag.

Hogikyan, N. D., & Sethuraman, G. (1999). Validation of an instrument to measure voice-related quality of life (V-RQOL). *Journal of Voice, 13*(4), 557–569.

Krotoski, A. (2011). What effect has the internet had on journalism? *The Guardian.* Retrieved from https://www.theguardian.com/technology/2011/feb/20/what-effect-internet-on-journalism

Kyrillos, L., & Cotes, C. (2008). A voz no telejornalismo [The voice in television news]. In I. B. Oliveira, A. A. F. Almeida, & T. Raize (Eds.), *Voz profissional* [Professional voice]. Produção científica da fonoaudiologia brasileira 2005–2007. São Paulo, Brazil: SBFa. Retrieved from http://www.sbfa.org.br/portal/voz_profissional/

Lessac, A. (1997). *The use and training of the human voice: A practical approach to speech and voice dynamics.* New York, NY: Drama Book Specialists.

Lopes, W. L., Lima, I. L. B., Silva, E. G., & Almeida, L. N. A. (2013). Sotaque e telejornalismo: evidências para a prática fonoaoudiológica [Accents and telejournalism: Evidence for speech therapy practice]. *CoDAS, 25*(5), 475–481.

Maia, A.S.C. (2011, August). *O telejornalismo no Brasil na atualidade: Em busca do telespectador* [TV journalism in Brazil currently: In search of the viewer]. Presented at Seminário Internacional—Análise de telejornalismo: desafios teórico-metodológicos. Retrieved from https://analisedetelejornalismo.files.wordpress.com/2011/08/maia_aline.pdf

Memória Globo. (2009). Retrieved from http://memoriaglobo.globo.com/perfis/talentos/glorinha-beuttenmuller.htm

Pedrosa, V., & Moreira-Ferreira, A. E. (2015). *Self perception protocols for professional speech voice.* Philadelphia, PA: The Voice Foundation.

Pedrosa, V., Pontes, A., Pontes, P., Behlau, M., & Peccin, S. M. (2016). The effectiveness of the comprehensive voice rehabilitation program compared with the vocal function exercises method in behavioral dysphonia: A randomized clinical trial. *Journal of Voice, 30*(3), 377.

Pennini, C., Padovani, M., & Vieira, V. (2011). *Características comunicativas na expressividade do telejornalismo* [Communication characteristics in telejournalism expressiveness]. Presented at 19º Congresso Brasileiro de Fonoaudiologia (19th Brazilian Speech Therapy Conference). 8º Congresso Internacional de Fonoaudiologia Comunicação Como um Direito de Todos (8th International Speech Therapy Conference Communication as a Right for All). São Paulo, Brazil: SBFa.

Porto, M. (2009). Novos apresentadores ou Novo Jornalismo? O Jornal Nacional antes e depois da saída de Cid Moreira [New presenters or New Journalism? National news before and after Cid Moreira left]. *Revista Comunicação e Espaço Público, Brasília*, 1–2.

Rezende, G. J. (2000). *Telejornalismo no Brasil: Um perfil editorial* [Television news in Brazil: An editorial profile]. São Paulo, Brazil: Summus.

Secchin, V. (2007). *Analisando os quatro principais telejornais da Globo à luz da análise do discurso crítica* [Analyzing the four main Globo news programs in the light of critical discourse analysis]. Viçosa: Universidade Federal de Viçosa. Retrieved from http://www.com.ufv.br/pdfs/tccs/2007/2007_vitorsecchin_in%C3%ADcio_analisejornaisdaglobo.pdf

Sihvo, M., & Denizoglu, I. (2014). *Lax Vox voice therapy technique.* Retrieved from http://www.laxvox.com/documents/LAXVOX%20handouts.pdf

Silva, E. C., & Penteado, R. Z. (2012). Mudanças no telejornalismo e as demandas de expressividade dos apresentadores [Changes in television news and the need for expressiveness by the presenters]. 10 Mostra acadêmica UNIMEP. Retrieved from http://www.unimep.br/phpg/mostraacademica/anais/10mostra/1/531.pdf

Sterling, C. H. (2009). *Encyclopedia of journalism.* Thousand Oaks, CA: Sage.

Stier, C. (2003). Oficina de narração [Narration Workshop]. In L. Kyrillos (Ed.), *Fonoaudiologia e Telejornalismo. Relatos de experiências na Rede Globo de Televisão* [Stories of experiences at Rede Globo Television Network] (pp. 19–31). Rio de Janeiro, Brazil: Revinter.

Temer, A. C. R. P. (2009). De tudo um pouco: o telejornalismo e a mistura dos gêneros [A little of everything: TV news and the mixture of genres]. *Anuário Unesco/Metodista de Comunicação Regional* (pp. 97–111). Retrieved from https://www.metodista.br/revistas/revistasims/index.php/AUM/article/viewFile/2194/2116

Titze, I. R. (2001). Acoustic interpretation of resonant voice. *Journal of Voice, 15*(4), 519–528.

UNESCO. (2016). United Nations Educational, Scientific and Cultural Organisation, *The News Manual.* Retrieved from http://www.thenewsmanual.net/Resources/glossary.html#N

Vieira, V. P. (2005). *O efeito da orientação fonoaudiológica na expressividade em estagiários do curso de jornalismo de emissora de televisão* [The effect of SLP intervention on expressivity in trainees of the television journalism course] [monografia de especialização em Voz]. São Paulo, Brazil: Centro de Estudos da Voz.

APPENDIX 5–1

Self-Evaluation Questionnaire of On-Video Communication

Name: ______________________ Date: __________

Profession ______________________ DOB: __________

Answer questions below considering your communication and how satisfied or not you are with any aspect. Consider numeric value of 1 as not satisfied at all and 6 very satisfied.

Question						
1. How adequate do you consider the quality of your voice for your professional performance?	1	2	3	4	5	6
2. How adequate do you consider your tone of voice for your professional performance?	1	2	3	4	5	6
3. How adequate do you consider your tone of voice for your physical type?	1	2	3	4	5	6
4. Can you make speed variations according to the content and the intention of the script you are narrating?	1	2	3	4	5	6
5. Can you make intonation variations according to the content and the intention of the script you are narrating?	1	2	3	4	5	6
6. How satisfied are you with your breath while reading the script?	1	2	3	4	5	6
7. How satisfied are you with your diction while working?	1	2	3	4	5	6
8. How satisfied are you with your pronunciation while working?	1	2	3	4	5	6
9. How satisfied are you with your accent?	1	2	3	4	5	6
10. Can you prioritize words and information from the script being read or improvised?	1	2	3	4	5	6
11. Can you take pauses while reading a script?	1	2	3	4	5	6
12. How easy is it for you to read an off or a teleprompter?	1	2	3	4	5	6
13. How easy is it for you to improvise script live?	1	2	3	4	5	6
14. How much difference does vocal warm-up make for your professional performance?	1	2	3	4	5	6
15. Do you make periodic self-evaluation of your videos?	1	2	3	4	5	6

APPENDIX 5–2

Evaluation Protocol

Evaluation Protocol Date: ____/____/____

Name ____

Age ________ BD ____/____/____/

Job description ____

E-mail ___________________________________ Cell phone ____________________

City of birth ____

Workload ____________________

History ____

____

____

____

Other work and voice activities

____

Self-perception of vocal quality

____

Natural voice and speech evaluation

Vocal quality		Vocal attack	
Pitch		Loudness	
Articulation		Diction	
Resonance		Rhythm	
Speech rate		Accent	
Natural vocal expression		Natural posture	
Natural facial expression		Natural gestures	
Pneumo-phono-articulatory coordination			
Profile/vices/organization			
Language			

Professional voice and speech resources on video

Record Video 1: reading an off about ______________________________

Fluency ______________________________

Emphasis ______________________________

Speech rate ______________________________

Speech naturality ______________________________

Voice projection ______________________________

Pitch ______________________________

Articulation/diction ______________________________

Nonverbal resources—body expressiveness

Facial expressions: describe patterns of eyebrow, eyes, chin, lips

____

Self-perception of the facial expression ______________________________

Body: describe patterns of posture, shoulders, movements, and gestures

____

____

____

Record Video 2: reading an off about ______________________________

Fluency ______________________________

Emphasis ______________________________

Speech rate ______________________________

Speech naturality ______________________________

Voice projection ______________________________

Pitch ______________________________

Articulation/diction ______________________________

Nonverbal resources—body expressiveness

Facial expressions: describe patterns of eyebrow, eyes, chin, lips

____

Self-perception of the facial expression ______________________________

Body: describe patterns of posture, shoulders, movements, and gestures

____

____

____

Record Video 3: performance in improvisation

Professional chooses a story to read and retell in an impromptu way

Fluency ______________________________

Organization of the story ______________________________

Language vices ______________________________

Emphasis ______________________________

Speech rate ______________________________

Speech naturality ______________________________

Voice projection ______________________________

Pitch ______________________________

Articulation/diction ______________________________

Nonverbal resources—body expressiveness

Facial expressions: describe patterns of eyebrow, eyes, chin, lips

____

Self-perception of the facial expression ______________________________________

Body: describe patterns of posture, shoulders, movements, and gestures

____

____

____

Phonoarticulatory organs: Chin, lips, tongue, nose, teeth

____

____

____

____

Conclusion ____

____

Main objectives/order/conduct/time

____

____

____

SLP. Vanessa Pedrosa

CHAPTER 6

Vocal Health Program for Teachers

Fabiana Zambon, Luiz Antonio Barbagli, and Mara Behlau

São Paulo Teachers Union—SinproSP

The São Paulo Teachers Union—SinproSP represents teachers from all levels and grades of private schools in the city of São Paulo, Brazil. Founded more than 60 years ago, the union has been responsible for increasing and guaranteeing the rights of teachers, serving as a leading example for similar institutions in other States of Brazil. Throughout the history of Brazilian education, private schools have had great social and political force, and have become an economic sector where, many times, the financial interests are priority. Accordingly, some employers tend not to respect the rights of teachers, and thus the union acts as the main source of support for these professionals.

SinproSP has over 25,000 affiliated teachers associated with it and is the most representative entity of this professional category in Brazil. The association to the union is optional, but recommended to all teachers. Affiliates have the right to use all the services provided by the union. Although the priority of its operation is to demand teachers rights and the political work, SinproSP offers many additional services and benefits, such as legal and social security–related advice, refresher professional education courses, summer camps for teachers' vacations or holidays, and medical care through agreements with many health professionals and companies from different backgrounds, in order to assist teachers, not only from the teaching perspective but also from the quality of life perspective. In addition, SinproSP is a pioneer in Brazil and in the world in developing its own reputable Vocal Health Program, which uses sound research methodology to support treatment and prevention of voice disorders in teachers.

Types of Schools in Brazil

In Brazil, schools are divided into public and private. The public schools are subdivided into state and municipal. In the city of São Paulo, about 62,603 teachers work in the private educational system (Ministry of Labor).

In general, public schools have unfavorable working conditions for voice usage, with an excessive amount of students per classroom, the classroom tends to be very noisy and teachers have no microphone available.

Some professionals teach in more than one private school, and others teach in both private and public schools concomitantly.

Working Conditions of Private School Teachers of São Paulo, Brazil

Private schools in the city of São Paulo, Brazil, present several different physical conditions. Most of them do not have classrooms acoustically prepared for vocal use, and the teachers have to compete with noise arising from the inside and the outside of the classroom. Few classes have air conditioning, and most have fans that are usually noisy.

Generally, teachers have an average number of students per class, which may vary from 10 to 40 students, according to the level of education. In higher education, classes usually have more students. Schools hardly ever offer microphones to teachers and, in most cases, when necessary, the teachers buy their own equipment.

Many schools still have blackboard and chalk—Some provide whiteboards or digital boards for their teachers.

Demographics of Teachers in Brazil

Behlau, Zambon, Guerrieri, and Roy (2012) conducted an epidemiological study of 3,265 individuals, representative of all the 27 States of Brazil, divided into two groups: 1,651 teachers and 1,614 nonteachers. All subjects answered a questionnaire that investigated the frequency and the adverse effects of voice disorders. The main result was that teachers reported higher frequency of vocal disorders during their professional life than nonteachers. Moreover, teachers referred a higher average of vocal signs and symptoms than the general population. They also reported more frequently the occurrence of limitations and restrictions in job activities, absences due to vocal problems in the year previous to the research, and 16,7% considered changing occupations in the future because of voice problems.

Demographics of Teachers Who Came to the Program

Choi-Cardim, Behlau, and Zambon (2010) studied the correlation between personal and professional demographics and vocal symptoms in 411 teachers, enrolled in the SinproSP Vocal Health Program. 256 needed voice treatment and 155 needed voice training sessions. Most of the teachers were females, 30 and 40 years old, teaching more than one grade, with an average of 30 students per classroom. Most of them reported excessive noise in the classroom, had some type of vocal care (e.g., hydration), used their voice excessively outside of their working environment (e.g., singing), and did not smoke or drink alcohol regularly. Teachers who needed treatment had the highest average of vocal symptoms.

Rodrigues, Zambon, Mathieson, and Behlau (2013) investigated vocal tract discomfort in 30 teachers with voice complaints enrolled in the SinproSP Vocal Health Program and 30 teachers with no voice complaints. The Vocal Tract Discomfort (VTD) Scale (Mathieson, Hirani, Epstein, Baken, Wood, & Rubin, 2009) was used for this purpose. Teachers with voice complaints present higher frequency and intensity of vocal tract discomfort symptoms. Discomfort sensation was related to some vocal signs and symptoms and with a worse self-perception of voice but was not correlated with vocal deviation.

Zambon, Moreti, and Behlau (2014) studied coping strategies identified in three groups: teachers with voice complaints who sought for treatment in the SinproSP Vocal Health Program, teachers with voice complaints who never looked for treatment, and teachers without vocal complaints. The main result was that teachers who sought voice treatment used more coping strategies focused on the problem—for example, I try to find as much information as possible about my voice problem (Epstein, Hirani, Stygall, & Newman, 2008). Although teachers usually get enrolled in the program with a high average of vocal signs and symptoms, this aspect was not correlated with coping. The greater feelings of limitation and restriction during vocal activities influenced greater coping with the problem.

Zambon, Moreti, Vargas, and Behlau (2015) used the ROC curve (Receiver Operating Characteristic curve) to analyze the efficiency characteristics and the cutoffs of the Voice Activity and Participation Profile (VAPP) protocol (Ricarte, Oliveira, & Behlau, 2013) that discriminate dysphonic from vocally healthy individuals, as well as teachers with and without dysphonia. The main result showed that the cutoff of the protocol was higher for teachers; however, the VAPP presented higher sensitivity and specificity for nonteachers.

Therapy Outcomes

Zambon, Ferraz, Oliveira, and Behlau (2011) investigated voice-related life activities impact and auditory-perceptual analysis in 23 teachers after 10 rehabilitation sessions within the Vocal Health Program and 10 teachers who did not receive any intervention. After treatment, teachers presented improvements on their vocal deviation and on almost all domains of the VAPP (Ricarte et al., 2013), except for the domain "effects on emotion," which demonstrated the need to include more strategies that address emotional health. Many teachers dropped out of treatment before completing the 10 sessions, which may indicate the need to shorten the program and re-assess teachers after eight sessions of treatment.

History of the Teachers' Vocal Health Program

The concern of SinproSP with the high occurrence of vocal problems in teachers began in 1993. They partnered with the PUC-SP Teachers Association (APROPUC) and their Voice Work Group (GT-VOZ PUC) to produce VHS film "What is good for me is good to the voice." Their aim was to educate teachers about vocal health care. At the same period, the union also began to offer courses and workshops on a regular basis about vocal care to their affiliated teachers in their head office. Given the great demand of teachers for these courses, the board of directors of the union saw the need to include more systematized actions to support the teachers in managing their voice problems and contribute to a more comprehensive resolution.

In 2001, the union hired a speech-language pathologist (first author) to initiate "The Teachers' Vocal Health Program." The program offered the teachers vocal assessment and counseling, in addition to lectures and onsite orientations in the schools. At this time, the actions of the program were exclusively preventive and did not include treatment. The teachers who needed rehabilitation were referred to accredited speech-language pathologists or otorhinolaryngologists affiliated with the union. As most teachers interested in the program already presented with vocal alterations, vocal training and treatment were included in the actions of the program in 2004. In the same year, a partnership was established with the "Centro de Estudos da Voz" (CEV), and the students of the graduate specialization program (Voice Specialization Course at "Centro de Estudos da Voz" —CECEV) of the institution started to receive their practical clinical training in the Vocal Health Program of the SinproSP (about

30 students per year). This resulted in clinical research that contributed to the advance of vocal science and the improvement of preventive, clinical, and vocal educational practices. This successful partnership is currently still thriving, and many studies have been conducted to understand the profile of teachers who look for clinical service, analyze their actions, and determine the best assessment and intervention instruments and techniques. The results of these studies have also contributed to updating the curriculum of the Graduate Specialization Program in Voice of the CEV–CECEV, in regard to teachers' voice production, problems, and management.

Structure of the Teachers' Vocal Health Program

The Teacher's Vocal Health Program offers specialized vocal health services to affiliated teachers, including vocal assessment, orientation, training, and treatment, with the aim to improve their voices and their communicative competence in teaching activities. These specialized vocal health services are conducted by the coordinator of the program and followed by graduate speech-language pathology students who are enrolled in the specialization course of the CEV–CECEV. This structure ensures that all the cases are thoroughly discussed, from diagnoses to treatment outcome. The coordinator works with the teachers 20 hours/week, 6 days a week (weekday afternoons plus Saturday mornings) averaging 3 to 4 hours/day. This ensures that teachers have a choice for receiving the needed voice care services either after their working hours during weekdays and/or on a weekend morning. Postgraduate students shadow the coordinator to get the needed voice management experience. Each student attends for 4 weeks, averaging 3 hours/day.

The teacher who seeks the specialized vocal health services is initially submitted to a detailed vocal assessment and referred to otorhinolaryngological evaluation through public medical services (free services) or through individual health care insurance. Depending on the diagnosis, teachers without vocal alterations are referred to vocal training sessions, while those with vocal alteration are referred to treatment sessions (see Vocal Treatment). All teachers receive information regarding vocal well-being, and are followed longitudinally, even after being discharged from treatment. In addition to these individualized interventions (vocal training and treatment), the SinproSP promotes workshops on communicative competence (in the Union) and offers lectures about voice and communicative competence to private schools (in the schools).

Vocal Assessment

Teachers attending the Vocal Health Program are submitted to a thorough vocal assessment, including personal and professional identification and characterization data, investigation of vocal signs and symptoms, auditory-perceptual and acoustic analysis of voice, and communicative competence.

Protocol of Personal and Professional Identification and Vocal Aspects

This protocol (Appendix 6–1) has the objective to investigate aspects of personal identification and work organization, and questions regarding habits and general health that may interfere with the teacher's voice, in addition to the vocal history of the family.

Personal identification and characterization data include name, address, gender, birthday, study discipline and level of education that the professional teaches, number of students per classroom, length of time in the teaching career, daily journey of work, and presence of noise in the working environment.

Regarding the habits that may interfere with the voice, the following issues are investigated: presence of vocal care habits; present and past smoking habits; alcohol consumption; excessive consumption of caffeine drinks; and excessive use of voice in activities other than work.

Questions about general health inquire about otorhinolaryngology appointments due to vocal problems, previous voice treatments, infection of upper and lower airways, general health problems, and use of medicines. The physicians managing the teachers are contacted when necessary in order to develop a multidisciplinary plan.

Finally, family history of voice problems is investigated, which helps in understanding if the vocal complaint of the teacher may have a congenital nature (e.g., vocal folds diaphragm or congenital cysts) or if it is only related to the professional use of voice. Although most teachers present problems related to vocal behavior, there are cases of organic dysphonia that must not be underestimated or inadvertently considered of functional nature.

During the evaluation, the teachers are asked to carefully describe their working environment, including aspects such as physical space of the classroom, type of board used (chalk or pen), presence of noise inside or outside the classroom, use of microphone, classroom communication strategies, and cleanliness and lighting of the classroom. They are also asked to record a video of themselves teaching, if possible. This is currently easier with the technology of smartphone and tablets. These videos are analyzed with each teacher, so they can develop the perception of voice use in their specific classroom environment, checking the intensity of speech, vocal quality, and/or speech rate. Environmental strategies that are easy to implement—such as reducing fan speed, shutting doors and windows, and getting closer to the students while speaking—are suggested.

Vocal Signs and Symptoms

The assessment protocol also investigates 14 signs and symptoms that may be related to voice problems. This list of signs and symptoms (LSS) was proposed by Roy, Merrill, Thibeaults, Parsa, Gray, and Smith (2004) in an American epidemiological study on teachers' voice. Later, Behlau, Zambon, Guerrieri, and Roy (2012) translated it into Brazilian Portuguese, and Zambon, Moreti, and Behlau (2014) found that teachers seeking voice care have an average of 8.6 voice symptoms. It might be interesting to highlight that a survey using this list, carried out on 3,265 individuals (1,651 teachers and 1,614 nonteachers)

Box 6–1

The LSS 14 signs and symptoms are as follows:

Symptoms that reflect phonatory aspects of voice: trouble speaking or singing softly, difficulty projecting voice, loss of singing range, discomfort while using voice, monotone voice (monopitch), effort to talk, a wobbly or shaky voice

Symptoms that reflect laryngopharyngeal problems: hoarseness, voice tires or changes quality after short use, chronic throat dryness, chronic throat soreness, frequent throat clearing

Symptoms that reflect pharyngoesophageal problems: bitter or acid taste, swallowing difficulties.

showed that Brazilian teachers present, on average, with 3.7 symptoms, while the general population presents with only 1.7 symptoms. The most common symptoms reported by teachers were: vocal fatigue and/or quality changes after short use of voice, effort to talk, and discomfort while using the voice.

Voice Recording

Teachers attending the Vocal Health Program have their voices registered in the voice laboratory of the institution using the Brazilian software Fono View (CTS Informática) and Vox Metria (CTS Informática). In the first assessment, the recording protocol includes sustained vowel /ε/, number counting from 1 to 10, sustained vowel /ε/ in weak and strong intensity, vowel /ε/ glissando up and down, and a testimony about the voice.

At the beginning and the end of all sessions of vocal training and treatment, the sustained vowel /ε/ and number counting from 1 to 10 are registered. This procedure has the aim to follow up the vocal evolution of the teacher in the aspects more related to the sound source (sustained vowel), as well as to the connected speech (number counting), in which speech rate (reduced, adequate, and fast rate), modulation (flat or rich), and pneumophonic coordination (coordination between breath and phonation or incoordination) are observed.

Orientation Regarding Vocal Well-Being

In all services provided by the Teacher's Vocal Health Program, teachers receive orientation about vocal well-being. This orientation includes questions related to their vocal hygiene practices, professional daily routine, working environment, as well as communicative competence in the classroom (see Communicative Competence Workshop). Three major aspects are covered: directly related to the voice, related to voice and body, and the impact of environment on the voice (See informational material developed in The Teacher's Vocal Health Program—Vocal Well-being Guide: A new perspective of voice care). Orientation is part both of vocal training interventions and in rehabilitation interventions, and it is always contextualized according to the teachers' vocal and working demands, thus the information provided makes more sense to the teacher and is easier to retain. Viable alternatives, such as talking closer to the students, a more modulated speech, or calling attention clapping hands, are offered for the teachers to validate the changes they need to make, avoiding a list of prohibitions that, many times, only alarm and concern the teachers. Strategies of co-responsibility, such as, "What can you do to change this?" (for example, "yelling in classroom"), are constantly used before offering a suggestion to solve the problem. This ensures that the teacher feels heard and supported and thus more open to change.

Vocal Training

Teachers without vocal problems are referred to vocal training sessions aiming to optimize the use of voice when teaching (better projection, less effort, more modulation, pneumophonic coordination), reduce signs and symptoms, reduce tension zones (laryngeal area, neck and cervical muscles), improve communication, and practice standardized voice warm-up and cool-down exercises. Although teachers are aware that improving their communicative competence contributes to the learning process of their students, the speech-language pathology traditional focus on the vocal aspects of teaching has led to the underestimation of the role of communication challenges in the development of their voice problems. During the assessment the communication competence aspects that need to be improved are identified. This may include articulation, projection, resonance, speech rate, modulation, loudness, pitch adjustments, and/or vocal control. Directed listening, turn-taking techniques, reduction of vocal aggressiveness, and appreciation of the students' questions are also implemented in these sessions. After the vocal training sessions, teachers are followed annually to control the voice quality and to maintain the vocal warm-up and cool-down exercises.

Vocal Treatment

Teachers with voice disorders are referred to voice treatment, which is planned according to each teacher's complaint, data from the SLP's vocal assessment, the patient's self-assessment (voice self-assessment protocols), and the results from otorhinolaryngological evaluation. The otorhinolaryngological assessment, with a defined conduct, is absolutely indispensable to start the treatment.

Rehabilitation is carried out in individual weekly sessions with duration of 30 minutes. The aim of these sessions is to develop strategies that, depending on the diagnosis and the teacher's needs, may include the following aspects: reducing vocal tract discomfort; improving vocal quality; increasing vocal resistance; improving vocal projection; in cases of larynx alterations, doing exercises with the aim to improve vocal folds vibration and/or glottal closure; decreasing the tension during phonation; improving the teacher's vocal–auditory perception; and optimizing the use of voice in the classroom. The main goal is to avoid removing the teacher from the classroom, working in parallel so as to improve the teacher's vocal condition day by day, and reach a performance more consistent with the process of good communication. In some cases, individual vocal amplification systems are suggested to avoid unnecessary tension during voice projection. Systems are implemented after specific training on their optimum use. This training includes loudness control, speed of speech, and speech articulation in the individual vocal amplification equipment.

Communicative Competence Workshop

With the aim to improve the communicative competence of teachers, workshops are held in groups of up to 10 teachers, in four weekly meetings of 2 hours and 30 minutes. They include voice and communication assessment (speech and listening aspects); strategies to improve communicative competence in the classroom and in different moments of teaching activities (meetings with parents and with the school board); orientation for vocal well-being, and conduction of vocal warm-up and cool-down exercises; and dynamics to improve the perception about teachers' own communication as well as that of the students. All the teachers are video-recorded in the first and the last meetings while speaking about a previously proposed topic, with the aim to improve communicative self-perception and evaluate the results reached in the four meetings. During the workshop verbal and nonverbal communicative aspects are addressed, such as objectivity of speech, vocal expression (voice changes according to the different emotions and classroom situations), speech rate, articulation, facial and body expression, gestures, the importance of active listening, among others.

Teachers with vocal alterations are referred to otorhinolaryngological evaluation and to a more detailed vocal assessment in the Teacher's Vocal Health Program. The communicative attitude as a whole—and not only the vocal aspects—is considered in this evaluation.

Case Study

A 38-year-old elementary school teacher has taught for 8 years, one daily period (4 hours a day) at a private school in the city of São Paulo.

She sought the Teacher's Vocal Health Program with the following complaint: "My voice has been hoarse for 4 years, previously with some improvement during holy days. Currently, hoarseness is constant; my voice does not improve on holidays and weekends anymore."

She has no history of smoking habits and alcohol compsuption, she does not make continuous use of medication, does not have any hearing complaint, does not present alterations in the upper and lower airways, and does not practice physical activity regularly. In addition, she does not use any vocal care procedures, does not have any excessive use of voice in activities other than work, and has no family history of voice disorders.

In the list of vocal signs and symptoms, she reports 10 symptoms: hoarseness, vocal tires or changes quality after short use, trouble speaking or singing softly, difficulty projecting voice, monotone voice (monopitch), effort to talk, chronic throat dryness, bitter or acid taste, swallowing difficulties, a wobbly or shaky voice.

The medical otorhinolaryngologic evaluation has shown a cyst in the right vocal fold, with contralateral reaction in the left vocal fold and spindle shaped glottic chink. It was prescribed reflux medication for gastroesophageal reflux (proton pump inhibitor). The management was vocal rehabilitation with eight speech therapy sessions followed by medical re-evaluation.

Speech-language pathologist assessment revealed a moderate rough, breathy, and tense voice, with frequency instability and voice breaks.

The teacher performed eight speech-therapy sessions, once a week, with 30 minutes duration. The main approach used was facilitating sounds to achieve a better source-filter interaction (Behlau & Pontes, 1990), with a particular emphasis in vibrating sounds (tongue and lip thrills) and nasal sounds. In addition, semi-occluded vocal tract exercises were performed (Simberg & Laine, 2007; Titze, 2000, 2006). The exercises were performed at the usual frequency and on ascending and descending musical scales. The patient was instructed to perform the exercise sequence every day, three times a day. During the treatment, she continued to teach.

During the process, the teacher was oriented on strategies for vocal well-being and on the use of voice and communication in the classroom, for example, expression (voice changes according to the different emotions and classroom situations), speech rate, articulation, facial and body expression, gestures, and the importance of active listening.

After eight speech therapy sessions, there was a considerable reduction of roughness and breathiness, with a more stable voice, without phonatorybreaks. In the otorhinolaryngological evaluation, it was observed: "Improvement of the mucosa wave in the direct vocal fold (where the cyst is located), with reduction of the reaction in the left vocal fold." After re-discussing the case with the speech-language pathologist, the otorhinolaryngologist has decided not to remove the cyst surgically, and it was defined that the teacher would receive medical and speech therapy monitoring every 6 months. She was instructed to maintain the vocal warm-up and cool-down exercises. Therefore, even if the lesion was not reabsorbed, the voice problem had a positive resolution.

Lectures in Schools

The main goal of the lecture is to sensitize the teachers to the importance of vocal care and to propagate the actions of the Teacher's Vocal Health Program. After the private school contacts the union, the speech-language pathologist responsible for the program goes to the school for a 1-hour lecture that covers the following content: risk aspects in the teacher's vocal use, signs and symptoms that suggest a voice problem, healthy and harmful aspects, and interference of the voice in teacher's communication. All teachers participating in the lecture receive a bottle to remind them to drink water, and a copy of the Vocal Well-being Guide. Specific actions are developed in celebration of the World Voice Day (April 16) or Week (Svec & Behlau, 2007), with support of the union, such as lectures in schools and dissemination of informational texts about the importance of voice for the teacher and vocal health care. Lectures may be offered by the union or requested by the schools during the school year, whether their teachers are part of the union or not.

Informational Material Developed in the Teacher's Vocal Health Program

During the 15 years of the Teacher's Vocal Health Program, Dr. Fabiana Zambon and Dr Mara Behlau (SinproSP and CEV partnership) developed operation materials to inform and educate teachers about the importance of their voice.

In 2006, the first edition of the "Vocal Well-being Guide: A new perspective of voice care" (Zambon & Behlau, 2006) was developed. This material is composed of 60 questions and answers about voice, divided into three chapters: aspects related to the voice, body, and environment. The material has been distributed in several private schools of São Paulo, Brazil, and is available at the SinproSP and the CEV websites with the aim to inform the teachers about the main aspects of vocal care. The guide had wide national reach, and its reproduction is authorized by the union, provided that the source is cited. In 2011, the second edition of the guide was released. Currently, the material is in its third edition, and has been the main reference on the topic of voice care in Brazil (available in Portuguese and English at the website http://www.sinprosp.org.br). Thirty five thousand copies have been printed and distributed, and the electronic file is available in the SinproSP and the CEV websites with free authorization for reproduction. It is estimated that the material has received thousands of accesses and sharing (Figure 6–1).

In 2010, the booklet "The Teacher's Voice: Aspects of the Professional Vocal Suffering" was issued to share the results of an important Brazilian epidemiological study of teachers' voice, conducted by the SinproSP and the CEV in partnership with the University of Utah (Zambon & Behlau, 2010) (Figure 6–2).

In 2012, also in partnership with the CEV, the SinproSP released the film "My Voice, My Life," with the objective of educating and sensitizing teachers about the importance of taking care of their vocal health. The film is available at the website http://www.sinprosp.org.br, with legends in English. The teachers' testimonies touched the authors and members of the union: teachers felt represented in their pain and identified in the difficult reality of teaching. The film had important international repercussion, confirming what the science already knows, that the teacher's voice is a worldwide problem (Figure 6–3).

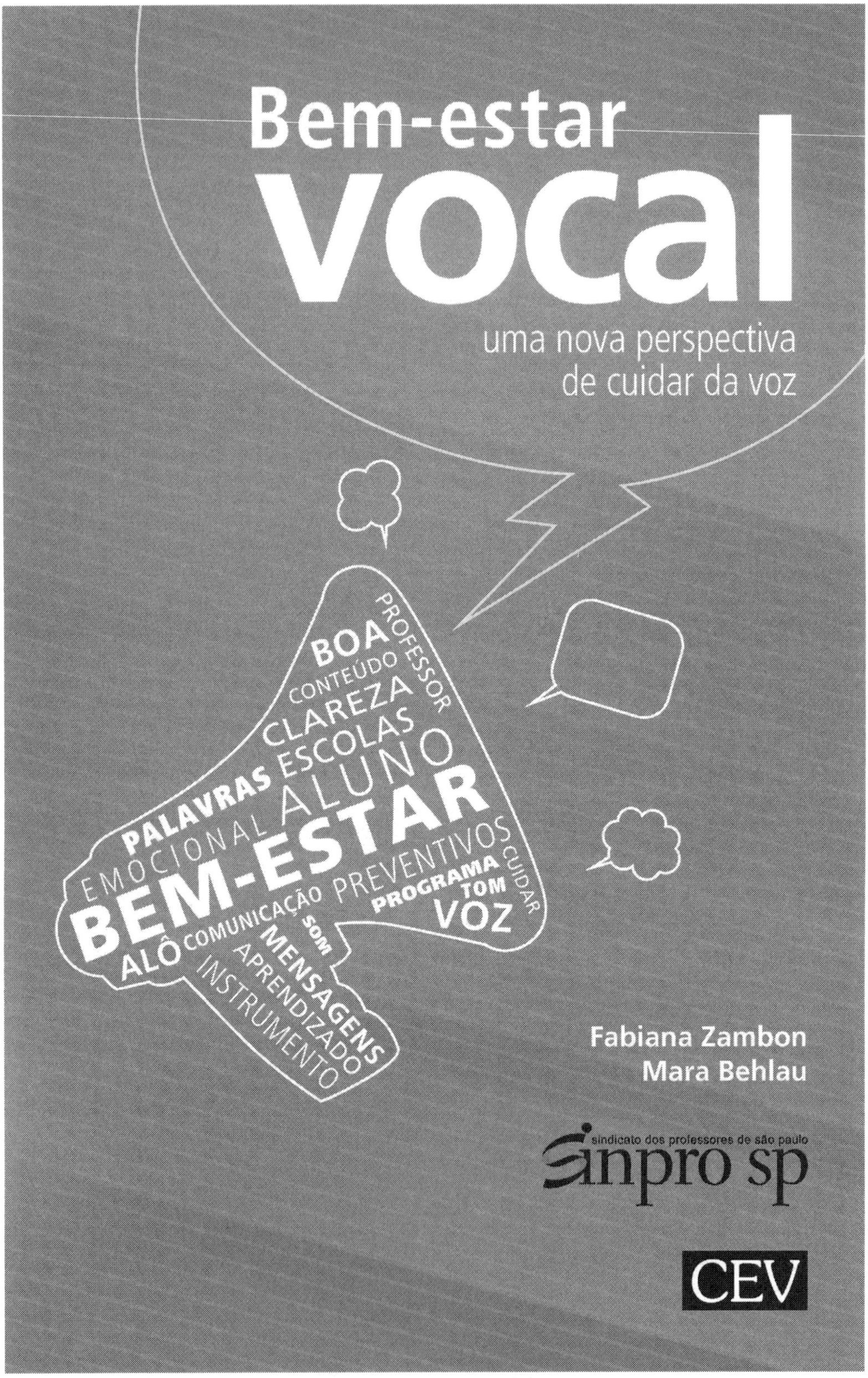

Figure 6–1. *Vocal Well-being Guide: A new perspective of voice care (Third edition).*

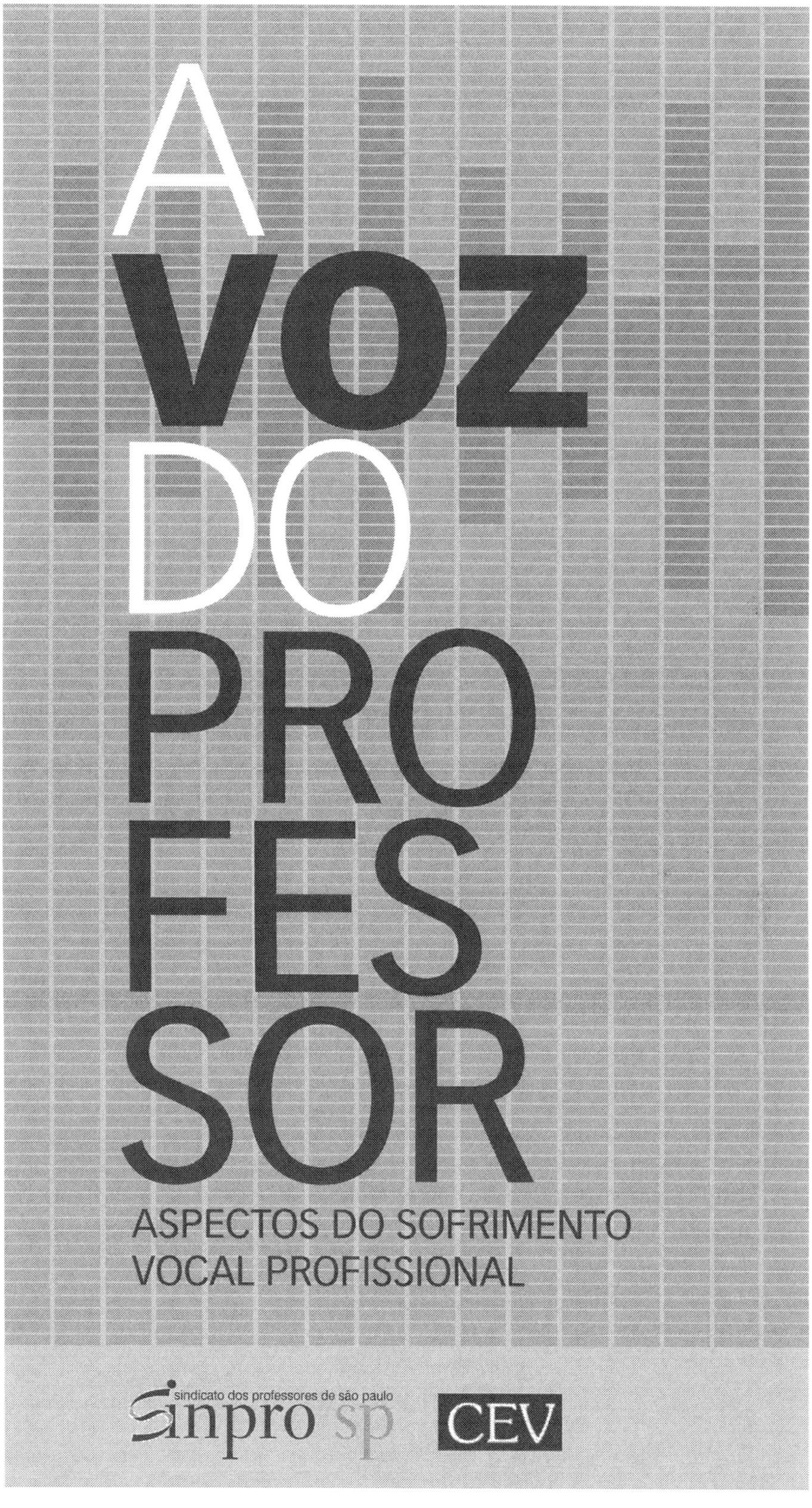

Figure 6–2. *The teacher's voice: Aspects of the professional vocal suffering.*

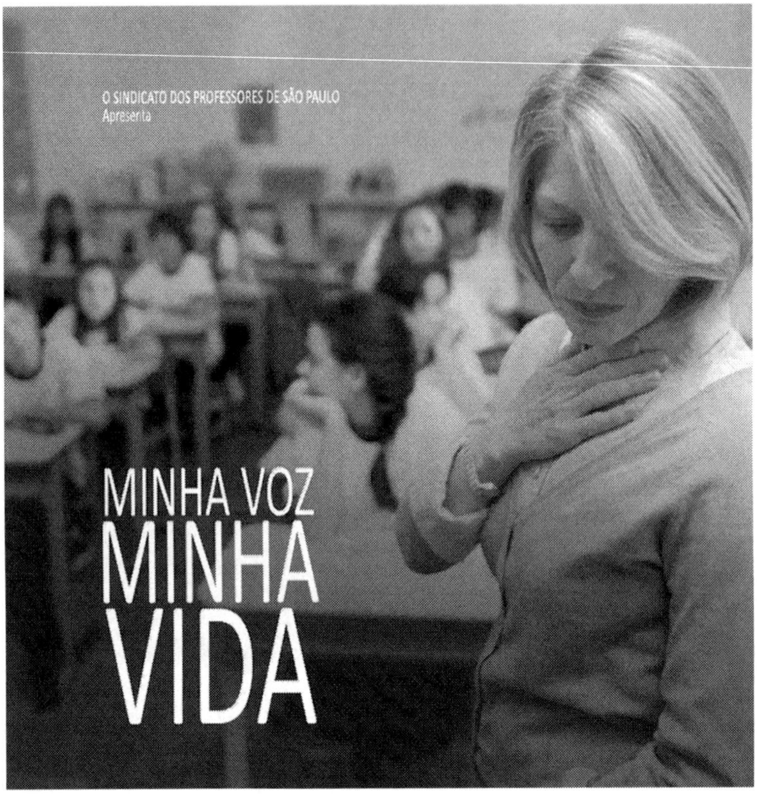

Figure 6–3. *Film* My Voice, My Life.

Future Actions

It is predicted that several interventions with private schools teachers will be expanded through the following actions:

- Self-assessment of voice and communicative competence as soon as the teacher associates to the union
- Small texts and educational material, with quizzes to verify the knowledge on voice
- Dissemination of good practices for voice and communication
- The making of authorized videos with parts of the trainings and testimonies from the participant teachers available, in order to stimulate greater adherence to the program
- Publicity partnership with the directors of private schools to support the teachers in the required changes
- Insistent referral of the alarming results from the studies developed in the program to the competent government organs, in order to conquer improvements in public policies

References

Behlau, M., & Pontes, P. (1990). ***Princípios da reabilitação vocal nas disfonias*** [Principles of vocal rehabilitation in dysphonia]. EPPM.

Behlau, M., Zambon, F., Guerrieri, A. C., & Roy, N. (2012). Epidemiology of voice disorders in teachers and nonteachers in Brazil: Prevalence and adverse effects. *Journal of Voice, 26*(5), 665.e9–e18.

Choi-Cardim, K., Behlau, M., & Zambon, F. (2010). Sintomas vocais e perfil de professores em um programa de saúde vocal [Vocal symptoms and teacher profile in a vocal health program]. *Revista CEFAC, 12*(5), 811–819.

Epstein, R., Hirani, S. P., Stygall, J., & Newman, P. (2008). How do individuals cope with voice disorders? Introducing the Voice Disability Coping Questionnaire. *Journal of Voice, 23*, 209–217.

Mathieson, L., Hirani, S. P., Epstein, R., Baken, R. J., Wood, G., & Rubin, J. S. (2009). Laryngeal manual therapy: A preliminary study to examine its treatment effects in the management of muscle tension dysphonia. *Journal of Voice, 23*(3), 253–266.

Ministério do Trabalho. Retrieved from http://trabalho.gov.br/rais

Ricarte, A., Oliveira, G., & Behlau, M. (2013). Validação do Protocolo Perfil de Participação e Atividades Vocais no Brasil [Validation of the Protocol Profile of Participation and Vocal Activities in Brazil]. *CoDAS, 25*(3), 242–249.

Rodrigues, G., Zambon, F., Mathieson, L., & Behlau, M. (2013). Vocal tract discomfort in teachers: Its relationship to self-reported voice disorders. *Journal of Voice, 27*(4), 473–480.

Roy, N., Merrill, R. M., Thibeaults, S., Parsa, R., Gray, S. D., & Smith, E. M. (2004). Prevalence of voice disorders in teachers in the general population. *Journal of Speech, Language, and Hearing Research, 47*, 281–293.

Simberg, S., & Laine, A. (2007). The resonance tube method in voice therapy: Description and practical implementation. *Logopedics, Phoniatrics, Vocology, 32*(4), 165–170.

Svec, J. G., & Behlau, M. (2007). April 16th: The World Voice Day. *Folia Phoniatrica et Logopaedica, 59*(2), 53–54.

Titze, I. (2000). Phonation into a straw as a voice building exercise, *Journal of Singing, 57*(1), 27–28.

Titze, I. (2006). Voice training and therapy with a semi-occluded vocal tract: Rationale and scientific underpinnings. *Journal of Speech, Language, and Hearing Research, 49*, 448–459.

Zambon, F., & Behlau, M. (2006). *Bem-estar vocal: Uma nova perspectiva de cuidar da voz* [Vocal well-being: A new perspective of taking care of the voice]. SinproSP, CEV. Retrieved from http://www.sinprosp.org.br

Zambon, F., & Behlau, M. (2010). *A voz do professor: Aspectos do sofrimento vocal profissional* [The voice of the teacher: Aspects of professional vocal suffering]. SinproSP, CEV. Retrieved from http://www.sinprosp.org.br

Zambon, F., Ferraz, P., Oliveira, G., & Behlau, M. (2011). Voice rehabilitation effect on teachers' voice-related life activities and perceptual analysis. *Flemish Journal Logopedie, 24*, 155–160.

Zambon, F., Moreti, F., & Behlau, M. (2014). Coping strategies in teachers with vocal complaint. *Journal of Voice, 28*(3), 341–348.

Zambon, F., Moreti, F., Vargas, A. C. T., & Behlau, M. (2015). Efficiency and cutoff values of the Voice Activity and Participation Profile for nonteachers and teachers. *CoDAS, 27*(6), 598–603.

APPENDIX 6–1

Protocol of Personal and Professional Identification and Vocal Aspects

Name: ______________________________

Address: ______________________________

Date of Birth: ______________________________

Subject: ______________________________

Grade of education that you teach: ______________________________

Number of students per classroom: ______________________________

Length of time in the teaching career: ______________________________

Teaching periods per day:
( ) 1 period—4 hours/day ( ) 2 periods—8 hours/day ( ) 4 periods—12 hours/day

Presence of noise in the working environment: ( ) Yes ( ) No

Describe: ______________________________

Previous otorhinolaryngology evaluation due to vocal problems: ( ) Yes ( ) No

Describe: ______________________________

Previous voice treatments: ( ) Yes ( ) No

Describe: ______________________________

Do you use any vocal care procedures? ( ) Yes ( ) No

Describe: ______________________________

Do you use any medicine regularly? ( ) Yes ( ) No

Describe: ______________________________

Do you have any excessive use of voice in activities other than work? ( ) Yes ( ) No

Describe: ______________________________

Do you smoke? ( ) Yes ( ) No

Do you drink alcohol? ( ) Yes ( ) No ( ) Sometimes

Do you have: ( ) Sinus ( ) Allergic Rhinitis ( ) Bronchitis ( ) Asthma ( ) Frequent Colds
( ) Tonsillitis or Pharyngitis

Do you have hearing difficulty? ( ) Yes ( ) No

Describe: ____

Do you have family history of voice problems? ( ) Yes ( ) No

Describe: ____

CHAPTER 7

Vocal Health and Communication Training of Telemarketers in Brazil

Ana Elisa Moreira-Ferreira

Growth of Teleservices Job Market in Brazil

In Brazil, the telemarketing sector represents a great market share of economy and employability, especially for young people with no experience in corporate environments.

Reports of the first teleservice centers in Brazil date back from the 1950s, when a company named "Yellow Pages" created a sellers team to commercialize classified ads by phone. During the following 20 years, the centers continued to use this channel, more focused in selling their products and services. The first telemarketing campaign was released in the 1970s by the Ford Motor Company. However, it was in the 1980s that telephone operating companies, credit card companies, and major publishers spread the culture of phone contact between companies and clients with objectives other than selling (ABT, 2011).

By this time, the term *telemarketing* was used to refer to all phone actions that would bring clients closer to the companies. The great growth of this segment came after the 1990s, especially after the creation of the "Consumer Protection Code," which established and guaranteed the clients's rights. There was an expansion and privatization of telecommunication companies, technological advances, and improvement of the purchasing power of the population in general. This led to an increase in the competition and search for consumers. With these advances, by the end of the century the market constituted great "Call Centers" (Brazil used the same English name). The definition of telemarketing got differentiated from *teleservices*: the first is used exclusively for sales actions, and the second, for all other customer relationship services by telephone. Almost 53% of all call centers are outsourced by other service providers and 47% are owned by the operating companies (Carrochano, 2007).

In 2011, the sector of services, which included teleservices, reached its apex, representing 69% of the gross domestic product (GDP) (IBGE, 2011). The sector increased 235% between 2010 and 2012, with more than 1.2 million of working professionals—that is, almost 1% of the Brazilian population, working directly in teleservices (ABT, 2011).

Currently, this segment is respected for its economic representation and its professional associations of employers and employees. The ease it has brought to the lives of consumers in big cities and remote areas has made teleservice a crucial part of the current job market in Brazil.

Telemarketing Operators' Profile

The 2006 study conducted by Brazilian Association of Teleservices showed that 60% of the telemarketing operators were 25 years old or younger and 57% were female (ABT, 2011).

Because previous experience is not required in most call centers, the work shift is 6 hours a day (which allows to reconcile study and job), and the salary is low (minimum wage floor), the job attracts a pre-university public or young adults attending higher education, and it is mainly seen as a transient job that pays for one's bills and studies. However, due to the increase and the strong organizational structure of this sector for over 40 years, many entry-level telemarketers have ended up attaining a professional career in this area; many began as operators and later on became supervisors, managers, directors, and even owners of big companies, encouraging young people to follow their path and even pursue undergraduate and graduate degrees in call center management.

Furthermore, there are specialized centers that already offer much higher salaries when the jobs require specific college graduation (pharmaceutical companies, special bank sectors, specialized technical sales, among others) or bilingual skills.

History of Speech Pathology Services for Teleservices

Brazilian labor law for teleservices is very strong, with active professional associations and regulatory rules that determine working hours, breaks and periods of rest, workplace aspects, conditions of equipment and furniture, among others (Brazil, 2007). The current labor law also addresses workers' health, determining guidelines for operators' mental, body, good for auditory, vocal, and visual health (Brazil, 2007). This legislation has supported providing several speech-language services for teleoperators, such as periodic exams and orientations on promotion of vocal health and prevention of vocal problems.

The growing realization that taking care of operators' vocal health is a way of preventing vocal alterations, offering welfare, increasing the quality of communication with clients and thus increasing revenue, has made companies adopt and expand on the implementation of vocal health programs (VHPs) and programs that target improvement of communicative competence programs (ICCPs) for teleservices operators.

Brazilian speech-language pathology services followed this growth. In the 1980s, the teleservice companies' biggest concern was limited to the aspects related to operators' vocal health and well-being. Accordingly, initial services focused on the prevention of work-related dysphonia and providing isolated lectures about healthy habits (Ferreira & Migliorini, 2002; Ferreira & Moreira-Ferreira, 2014). Later on, these activities were organized into comprehensive and long-term VHPs that were offered by occupational speech-language pathologists (Moreira-Ferreira, 2011), a new subspecialization recognized by the professional council (CFFa, 2014).

The next stage of speech-language pathology services emphasized vocal expressiveness. Researchers became aware that the voice and the words of the operator on the phone were responsible for the construction of a mental image (Gélinas-Chebat & Chebat, 1996; Gélinas-Chebat, Chebat, & Boivin, 1999) and, the more positive the image created in the client's mind of the operator, the better the relationship between both parties (Moreira-Ferreira, 2007). Thus, by the end of the 1990s, SLPs started to work with the psychodynamic of the voice through improving the expressiveness of the operator's voice, guiding the operator on different aspects of prosody in order to communicate positive attitudes, such as cordiality and safety.

Soon the SLPs' services expanded beyond the voice, because the operators needed to be turned into professional communicators. At the beginning, Brazilian SLPs followed the procedure guidelines originally created in the United States (the pioneer country in teleservices), communication followed exactly what was in the scripts and internal manuals of service. However, it was noticed that Brazilian clients wanted more than an efficient service, they wanted a close relationship with the company and its representative—the teleoperator. The teleservice professional would need to go beyond the scripts and beyond demonstrating technical knowledge, into creating a more personal, not intimate, conversation atmosphere. This characteristic may come from the Brazilian culture, which is highly communicative, colloquial even in professional relationships. A large part of the population also rejects orientations exclusively guided by rules, needing clear arguments posed with care and politeness.The work shows that consumers not only want a solution to their problems, but they also want to be treated with respect and cordiality, and made to feel like a unique client. This information brought a revolution to the operator's profile, from the selection of the applicants to the training methods. Following scripts was no more enough; it became necessary for the teleoperator to communicate really well. The training targeting communicative competence in the relationship with clients started to be called organizational speech-language pathology services (Moreira-Ferreira, 2011; Moreira-Ferreira, Oliveira, & Algodoal, 2011).

Teleservice operators has been one of the most studied populations among voice professionals by SLPs in Brazil, due to our broad performance and interest in this area (Oliveira et al. 2008).

Development of Organizational Speech-Language Pathology Services

In the 1990s. individual SLPs worked with teleoperators as freelance SLPs. By 1998 the Univoz was created with the aim to professionalize and structure the SLP services provided to telemarketers. Their director is also their consultant SLP (the primary author), who delivers communicative competence and vocal health programs as well as professional training and supervision for other SLPs. In the past 19 years, more than 60 SLPs have worked at Univoz, in projects of different dimensions. In one of its more recent projects, 24 professionals specialized in voice were all involved at the same time.

When new SLPs enter the Univoz team, they receive training on occupational and organizational speech-language pathology, depending on the project in which they will be involved. This initial theoretical and practical training takes at least 32 hours; it also includes the observation of activities while being implemented and providing feedback.

The Univoz team of SLPs acts directly at the teleservice centers and, periodically, holds work meetings for the discussion of activities and updates on research, at the Univoz head office.

The consultant SLP services are very diverse; they include, but are not limited to, giving lectures, training clients, and training and managing the team of SLPs.

Univoz provides service for several companies in Brazil, especially in the State of São Paulo (Southeast region of the country). It creates a tailored database for each company.

Some of their call center clients own their own companies (i.e., they hire their own teleoperators), and others are outsourcers, who are not involved in the hiring. The number of teleoperators hired varies from 20 to 8,000. In the past 19 years, they provided training programs for more than 50 companies, attending to the needs of about 30,000 teleoperators.

Vocal Health Program (VHP)

The complete VHP is not required by law at the companies. For this reason, the only companies that implement it completely and longitudinally are the ones that recognize its benefits to the employees and the results in quality, productivity, and reduction of costs with labor liabilities related to occupational health.

The actions can be implemented in isolation, but it should be understood that improvement actions are part of a mutual support scenario and cannot be seen as part of a "coffee shop menu" (Taylor, Baldry, Bain, & Ellis, 2011) from which the company chooses individual actions or actions that are easier to implement and manage. The National Institute for Occupational Safety and Health recommends, in the document Total Worker Health (NIOSH, 2012), that any approach in occupational health should always be implemented comprehensively and integrally.

When we are hired to manage a VHP, the method used by UNIVOZ is as follows: implementing all the necessary and effective actions to reduce the risk factors for work-related voice disorders (CFFa, 2006) and to protect the voice of the professional (teacher, teleservices operator, seller, lecturer, trainer, among others) longitudinally, interrelated and integrated to the policies of organizational and occupational health and involving all instances, from the professional and his or her managers to the occupational health team and the executives of the companies. Figure 7–1 describes all the actions that we have implemented in companies by type. However, the choice to implement the program longitudinally and completely belongs to the company, and many of them start with isolated stages or are restricted to a single activity.

Our goals in the VHP include the health and well-being of the operator, providing comfort for working. Regarding the companies, we are committed to act for the reduction of the following indicators related to vocal problems:

- presenteeism—reducing the loss of work hours or productivity;
- absenteeism rate—reducing the absense of the employee;
- number of leaves due to voice-related alterations;
- withdrawal rates due to voice problems; and
- reduction of health events—costs with actions involving health issues.

We describe below all the actions from the VHP, and to each one, we present different cases describing the actions and the obtained results in several of the companies where we have performed.

Vocoergonomics Assessment

The publications from the group of Dr. Erkki Vilkman since 2000 (Lehto, Alku, Bäckström, & Vilkman, 2005; Lehto, Rantala, Vilkman, Alku, & Backstrom, 2003; Vilkman, 2000, 2004) have brought many reflections to our work at Univoz. We already worked with the analysis of voice-related ergonomics, but based on these studies, we started to call vocoergonomics all the care with extrinsic and intrinsic factors that might expose the professional to the risk of developing dysphonia.

The voice problems of the operator affect the operator's productivity and quality of life, and are related to several factors. For a broad view of occupational voice disorders, the comprehension of all risk factors must be included to make it possible to avoid, modify, or control them.

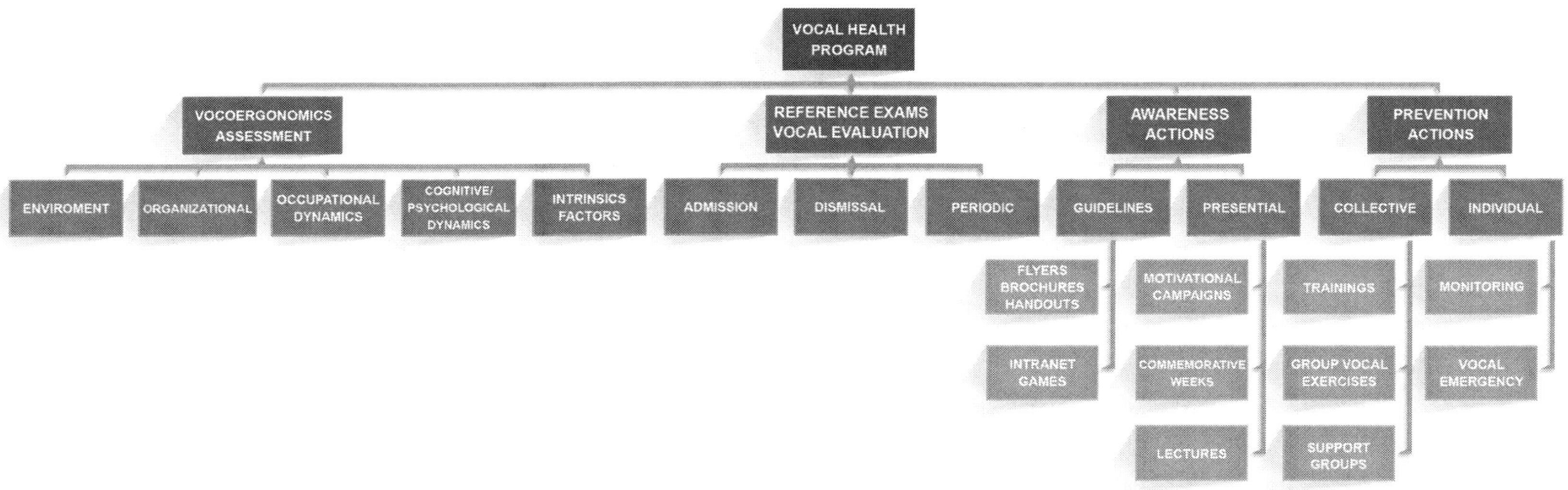

Figure 7–1. *Description of the complete Vocal Health Program (VHP) implemented by Univoz in teleservice centers.*

In teleservices, it is not enough to have reduced occupational voice working hours (6 hours/day); it is necessary to act in all health determinants and focus the efforts on the changeable factors (Jones, Sigmon, Hock, Nelson, Sullivan, & Ogren, 2002).

When a VHP is implemented, the first action is the vocoergonomics assessment, which allows the identification of potential occupational risks for voice problems. Risk is the evaluated potential of harmful consequences that might result in a threat to vocal health. The probability of occurrence of a vocal problem when the professional is exposed to specific risk situations is assessed.

As the voice is multifactorial and concausal, we evaluate several factors within vocal ergonomics.

Since voice is multifactorial and concausal, several factors are assessed within vocoergonomics. The aim of this analysis is to observe what still should be improved before or during the VHP. We understand that the professional should not be the only one responsible for his or her vocal care. The actions must have the company's support, contributing to a healthy environment. For example, it is not effective if the speech-language pathologist emphasizes the need for professionals to drink water and water is not easily available, or if the operators are asked to maintain good posture and the available chairs are not proper. The intervention in occupational vocal health starts with the whole company being made aware that favorable ergonomic conditions must be provided to improve professional performance, reducing health risks. Thus, we distribute brochures and vocal health manuals, and give lectures to the managers so they can understand their responsibility regarding their employees' vocal health.

So, within the concept of vocoergonomics (Figure 7–2), we map the following:

a. Extrinsic factors
   i. Environment (physical ergonomic factor)
      - Environmental noise and sound competition
      - Temperature and care with the air conditioning
      - Individual headset use
      - Furniture according to the ergonomic rules
      - Possibility to keep the water in the work station
   ii. Organizational
      - Style: active or receptive operation
      - Characteristics of the communication with the client
      - Working routines

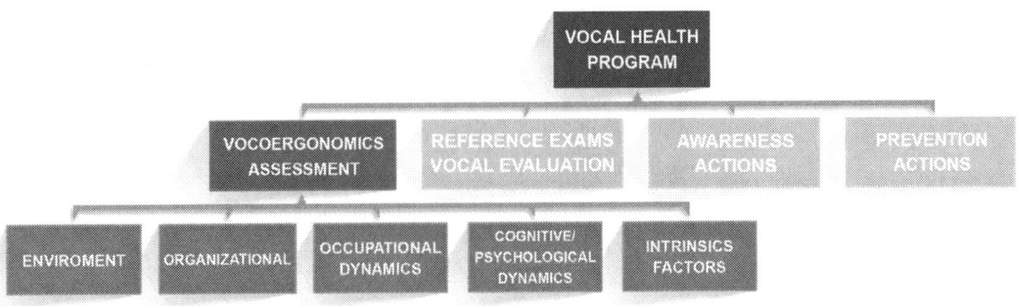

Figure 7–2. *Description of the actions in Vocoergonomics Assessment implemented by Univoz in teleservice centers.*

- Working goals
- Health actions available
- Occupational health policies

iii. Occupational dynamics
- Number of calls
- Control of average service time
- Work breaks
- Daily hours

iv. Cognitive and psychological dynamics
- Complexity of the work method
- Need of script reading
- Exposure to large amounts of information
- Occupational pressures by the dynamics of work

To collect these data, the SLP performs observations of the environment; studies internal documents, regulations, and manuals; carries out meetings with the managers of occupational health; interviews the leaders for data collection; and applies online questionnaires that include the voice professional.

b. Intrinsic factors
Using self-evaluation questionnaires, we map vocal health and habits of the entire population of operators.

An important index of vocal health in call centers is the occurence and the incidence of vocal alteration complaints and self-reported signs and symptoms. A study from Hazlett, Moorhead, and Duffy (2009) have shown that one in every four teleservice operator reports symptoms of vocal alterations. The most common complaints are from sensations of vocal discomfort, such as pressure, dryness, laryngeal globus, fatigue, and the presence of rough voice quality, without vocal projection, frequently with the presence of sound breaks and loss of vocal flexibility (Hazlett et al., 2009).

In our practice we used validated protocols, such as the Vocal Tract Discomfort Scale (VTDS) (Mathieson, Hirani, Epstein, Baken, Wood, & Rubin, 2009). Moreover, we use the Talkativeness and Vocal Loudness Test, published in English (Bastian & Thomas, 2016) and translated into Portuguese (Behlau & Pontes, 2009). This test was also applied to a population of teleservice operators (Padilha et al., 2012), showing that they report speaking more and stronger in work situations, and that women working in this profession tend to speak more than men in professional and social situations (Padilha et al., 2012).

Due to the specificities of this population, we have also developed other protocols, such as the Vocal Profile in Teleservices Questionnaire (VPTQ®) (Appendix 7–1) with questions regarding broad issues. The questionnaire is available on the Internet, intranet, or in printed protocol. In Brazil, the legislation for ergonomics in teleservices (Brazil, 2007) recommends that operators are not required to participate in health actions; therefore, they are invited to fill in the questionnaire. Thus, before that, engagement actions are necessary so a greater number of professionals volunteer to participate, making it possible to draw a more accurate profile of the center's vocal health.

As soon as all the data in vocoergonomics are mapped, we elaborate a report to the company that includes recommendations of actions according to the need of promotion and prevention in occupational or extra-occupational vocal health.

Case 1 (Box 7–1) shows the importance of being alert not only to characteristics of the voice professional, but to the entire environment and the occupational risks to which he or she is exposed.

Box 7–1

Case 1

We were hired to implement a VHP for 3,000 operators from a call center of the financial segment in 2005. Before taking any action, we performed a vocoergonomics analysis to identify which risk factors for vocal health were present and made recommendations for each one of them.

We found a very favorable environment regarding the items "ii" to "iv" of the Vocoergonomics Analysis. However, analyzing the item "b"—Intrinsic Factors:

- through the self-perception questionnaire, which was answerd by 62% of the operators (Appendix 7–1), we noticed frequent complaints of tension on shoulders, neck, nape, and jaw, which are risk factors for vocal health, besides pain in the arms and the back;
- by observing the operators while working, it was identified inadequate posture, with hyperextension of the head and lifting of shoulders.

When applying the item "i" of Vocoergonomics—Environment, analyzing the adequacy of the furniture to the ergonomic rules, we could notice that the computer tower was under the monitor. This was causing inadequate posture of the operators with the lifting of shoulders and hyperextension of the head to maintain alignment with the monitor.

In the vocoergonomics report, we recommended changing the position of equipment to realign the posture of operators. The recommendation was readly accepted and the position of the tower was changed, with immediate reduction of body tension complaints in spontaneous reports from the operators.

After this intervention, the VHP was implemented, already with effective reduction of body tension from the first action in vocoergonomics.

Reference Exams

Admission, dismissal, and periodic vocal exams (Figure 7–3) are reference evaluations conducted by most centers, providing documents for following up the professionals and identifying dysphonia.

The teleoperator will be acting essentially with his or her voice, and hiring the teleoperator with any kind of alteration is a risk for the company. It is known how much voice disorders adversely impact job performance and attendance. An epidemiologic study of the prevalence and risk factors of voice disorders in general adult population showed occupational consequences and effects (Roy, Merrill, Gray, & Smith, 2005). Participants indicated that their voice had limited or rendered them unable to do certain tasks in their current job, and they reported that they had been absent from work for 1 to 4 days in the past year due to voice problems (Roy et al., 2005).

It is a duty of the company not to submit a dysphonic individual to the risk of worsening his or her vocal condition due to risk factors related to the professional use of voice. Therefore, in our projects, three types of vocal evaluation are performed in teleservice centers (see Figure 7–3):

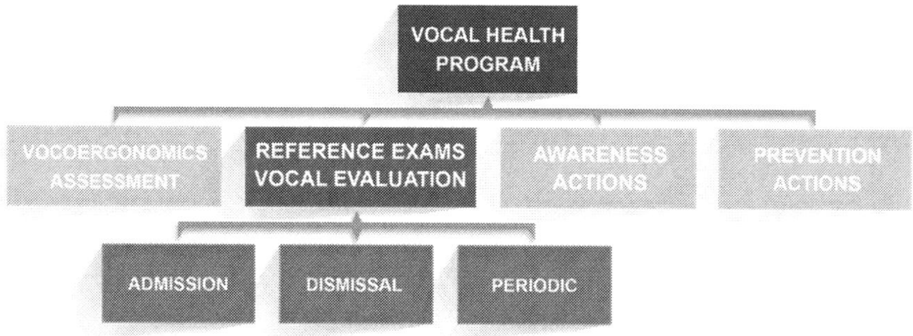

***Figure 7–3.** Description of the actions of Reference Exams implemented by Univoz in teleservice centers.*

a. Vocal assessment upon admission
   Carried out upon the operator's admission with the aims to

   i. identify if the applicant presents previously existing dysphonia or risk of worsening vocal conditions that may impair, complicate, or prevent professional practice, contributing to the decision of the company about hiring him or not;
   ii. identify the presence of evident or imminent risk for vocal alterations that might be, in the future, characterized as work-related dysphonia.

   Laryngoscopy is a relatively expensive exam in Brazil to be used for all the applicants in the hiring period. Before the operator is considered a regular employee in the company, there is no coverage of corporate health insurance. Hence, only the clinical speech-language vocal assessment is performed.

   However, since there is no direct acoustic, auditory, and visual correlate to identify dysphonia, some of our clients request complementary exams when the Admissional Vocal Assessment shows any level of dysphonia. Thus, the applicant is submitted to evaluation by an otorhinolaryngologist, nasofibroscopy and/or telaryngoscopy, and stroboscopy in order to confirm whether the auditory alteration diagnosed by the SLP is accompanied by lesion of the vocal folds or not, and what is the risk level in hiring him or her. All exams are analyzed by the occupational physician, who provides the certificate of occupational health, classifying the applicant as able or unable to work in teleservices.

   When the exams are carried out at the doctor's office in the company, there is greater transdisciplinary integration, and the SLPs are able to work very closely with the occupational physician, discussing each case and making together the decision on the risk level of hiring the applicant.

b. Periodic vocal assessment
   Periodically (usually anually), the speech-language evaluation is repeated in order to observe the evolution in vocal quality, signs and symptoms, and complaints related to the voice.

   If any alteration or complaint is identified, in case the company has implemented the VHP, this operator receives special attention from our team of SLPs (we discuss this topic in items 4 and 5). In the companies where we are hired only to perform the Reference Exams, the operator is referred to an otorhinolaryngologist and to a SLP from the corporate health insurance that, by law, every company must provide, and follows the treatment independently from the company. Periodic reports must then be sent to the medical control and occupational health program (MCOHP) of the company (also required by law) that verifies if the employee is under treatment and follow-up. The role of the SLP from our team, at this moment, is to participate on this follow-up and assist the occupational physician in the decision of whether the operator

i. will be kept in the position with or without speech-language follow-up;
ii. needs a temporary layoff (medical leave); or
iii. presents a vocal health condition that prevents him or her from taking calls and needs to be "readapted"—that is, must be reallocated to a function that requires less from the voice.

In our experience, this last case is rare in companies with implemented VHP, since our work is comprehensively directed toward preventing the worsening of vocal alterations.

c. Dismissal vocal assessment
The vocal assessment is also repeated at the dismissal evaluation to verify and document if the operator maintained a healthy voice when dismissed from this call center.

All the evaluations are filed, generating documentation to protect the company and the employee. In Brazil, there are already lawsuits filed by operators against companies claiming to have developed dysphonia due to their work in teleservices. These documents legally support both sides, employer and employee.

The evaluations are always performed by a SLP expert in voice. The assessment takes 30 minutes and is conducted at Univoz or within the structures of the company.

An important indicator of the operator's vocal health is the presence of self-reported signs and symptoms of alterations, since studies have shown prevalence or high incidence of them in operators, when compared with the average of the population (Dassie-Leite, Lourenço & Behlau, 2011; Hazlett et al., 2009; Piwowarczyk, Oliveira, Lourenço, & Behlau, 2012). The following protocols are applied:

a. Self-assessment protocols:
   i. Vocal Profile in Teleservices Questionnaire (VPTQ®) (see Appendix 7–1)—has the aim to get information on self-reported signs and symptoms, presence of voice-related habits, vocal use in social situations, professional use of voice in previous and current activities, past history of vocal health, general health data. It is the same protocol described in item 1 (Vocoergonomics Analysis), allowing a longitudinal comparison of the results.
   ii. Vocal Tract Discomfort (VTD) Scale (Mathieson et al., 2009; Rodrigues, Zambon, Mathieson, & Behlau, 2013)—has the aim to map the self-perception of frequency and intensity of sensations/symptoms of dysphonia. Applied in the periodic evaluations, it allows the follow-up of worsenings after the exposure period to teleservice work, or reductions after any intervention.
   iii. Specific protocols—We also apply protocols such as Voice Activity and Participation Profile (VAPP), Voice-related Quality of Life (V-RQOL), or VTD for vocal health issues. How-

ever, during our performance, we have identified the need to develop customized protocols, with more specific questions regarding the professional practice of each employee. Hence, we have developed the Self-perception of Voice Impact on the Quality of Life and Performance in Call Centers® (Appendix 7–2), presented at The Voice Foundation's 44th Symposium (Pedrosa & Moreira-Ferreira, 2015). The protocol has the aim to map the consciousness of the operator on the aspects of his or her voice that might interfere in his or her professional performance and quality of life.

b. Vocal Assessment in Teleservices—The auditory-perceptual evaluation is carried out using phonatory tasks such as vowels [ε] (sustained, gliding up and down, weak and strong intensity), numbers counting from 1 to 10, a sustained /s/ and /z/, text reading, and answer the question, "What do you think about your voice?," and others, in order to obtain data regarding vocal quality, maximum phonation time, breathing and pneumophonic coordination, articulation, fluency and speech rate, resonance, pitch and loudness, resistance, and flexibility. In some cases, complementary acoustic analysis are also conducted. This protocol has specific teleservice tasks, such as the simulation of greeting phrases and other parts to examine the operator's vocal expressiveness.

The periodic and dismissal assessments use the same instruments of the Admissional Vocal Assessment, added by questions that allow comparison of the self-perception of the current vocal health condition with the one from the first Reference Evaluation (Admissional Vocal Assessment). We have noticed that the operators present more signs and symptoms of voice alterations and vocal quality alterations in the periodic assessment than in the admissional assessment. The profession of teleservice operator put them at risk for presenting dysphonia; therefore, the annual reassessment is indispensable.

It is also important to investigate the presence of distal and proximal pain to the larynx, since they are prevalent in teleoperators (Constancio, Moreti, Guerrieri, & Behlau, 2012), and therefore we also added, to the evaluation, questions that map these complaints (see Appendix 7–1). Hereafter, we discuss a case (Box 7–2) of application and follow-up of reference exams in a call center.

Box 7–2

Case 2

For one of our clients, we performed admissional exams for hiring new operators for the expansion of the central service or for substituting those who were dismissed. The vocal assessment was performed in a second stage, only with those who presented professional competence for the position. The company was a center of help desk receptive service to answer questions about software, with about 45 operators between 21 and 30 years of age.

We performed 224 admissional vocal assessments from 2009 to 2015. In this evaluation, we identified the presence of dysphonia or the imminent risk of developing it by the presence of signs and symptoms and data from the vocal quality evaluation of the applicants. The reports were sent to the occupational physician, who was responsible for the decision of hiring or not, providing the occupational health certificate (OHC).

Previous to the admissional exams, we performed an ergonomic study to evaluate the level of exposure risk to the occupational use of voice. In this study we noticed that the center represented low risk for triggering dysphonia, since the vocoergonomics factors were under control, such as:

- *Physical ergonomy*—good environmental conditions (regulated and clean air conditioning, offer of water during the working period, balanced temperature);
- *Organizational ergonomy*—absence of pressure regarding the average time of calls;
- *Occupational dynamics*—presence of three rest breaks during the 6-hour shift and a special room for resting; number of calls per day that allows for small breaks between calls;
- *Cognitive and psychological dynamics*—low levels of stress in the relationship with the client on the phone; and
- *Offer of promotion and prevention actions* (periodic vocal assessment and lecture with our team of SLPs).

Because it was a low-risk center, we established with the MCOHP that operators with mild dysphonia and/or with up to three self-reported symptoms could be hired, and would be followed up to watch the evolution of the alteration.

In this period, from the 224 evaluations performed (Table 7–1), 10.2% were not hired for being out of this profile. Moderate or severe dysphonia represented a risk for the company and for the applicant. All other applicants were hired.

During these 5 years, only six (2.7%) operators presented important complaints of worsening of the vocal condition in the periodic reassessment (Table 7–2), which was considered a low occurrence of vocal alterations in teleservices when compared to other centers where we have worked. These subjects were referred to medical treatment and speech-language follow-up with a professional from the corporate health insurance, with good response to treatment. Only one operator (diagnosed with unilateral vocal fold cyst, see Table 7–2) had an

Table 7–1. Distribution of Admissional Vocal Assessment Results in Case 2

Results of Admissional Vocal Assessments	N	%
Neutral or adapted voice	142	63.4
Mild dysphonia	59	26.4
Moderate to severe dysphonia	23	10.2
Total	224	100

Table 7–2. *Comparison of Admissional and Periodic Evaluation With Otorhinolaryngological Exam of Operators Who Presented Worsening of Vocal Condition, Case 2*

Vocal Assessment			
Admissional	**Periodic**	**N**	**%**
Neutral	Mild dysphonia Otorhinolaryngological exam—bilateral thickening of vocal folds	2	33.2
Mild dysphonia	Mild dysphonia/increase in signs and symptoms Otorhinolaryngological exam—Signs of gastroesophageal reflux and infection of the upper airways	3	50
Severe dysphonia	Intense dysphonia/increase in signs and symptoms Otorhinolaryngological exam—unilateral vocal fold cyst	1	16.8

extended medical leave and was included in the Career Plan to apply for another position in the company that would not need the professional use of voice very frequently.

It may be noticed that the Admissional Vocal Assessment does not eliminate an applicant but may reduce the risk of hiring operators who will develop dysphonia throughout their career. Besides, it is not enough to evaluate only in the admission; it is necessary to follow up and provide orientation to the operator for that risk to be effectively reduced. Therefore, the importance of vocal health lectures, campaigns, and actions that will be discussed next.

Actions of Vocal Health Promotion—Awareness Actions

The objective of promotion actions is to raise awareness for the need to change the behavior of operators regarding their lifestyle, their actions and habits toward voice, seeking better conditions for professional vocal use.

In the great centers it is necessary to quickly disseminate the orientations to make sure that everybody will get the basic information on health-related issues. One way to reach a large population in a short period of time is by promoting Awareness Actions (Figure 7–4) that are implemented punctually, collectively, and interactively to get the attention of professionals to voice-related aspects.

Therefore, such actions are designed to sensitize the operators regarding:

- their role as voice professional;
- the risk factors for dysphonia;
- ways to avoid dysphonia, either work-related or not; and
- conscious expressiveness as a way to approach the client.

The more motivational and interactive are such actions, the better the result engaging the professionals and the better the learning

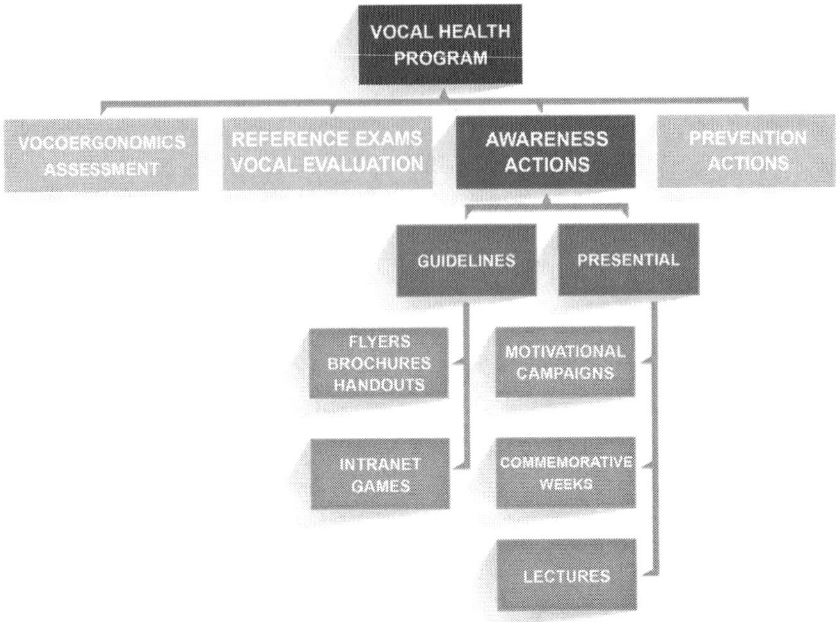

***Figure 7–4.** Description of Vocal Health Promotion Actions for Awareness, implemented by Univoz in teleservice centers.*

and effective use of the information provided. Therefore, in Univoz we implement Awareness Actions in several ways:

a. Guidelines—orientations regarding vocal health and well-being in flyers, handouts, or brochures with easy tips for daily routine, distributed to all operators. The guidelines are also placed on intranet programs with warnings on the screens on voice healthy habits or voice exercises or in an Internet games format;
b. Motivational campaigns—collective actions including games (e.g., as in Figure 7–5, a game to recognize familiar voices), plays, contests, competitions, theater (e.g., as in Figure 7–6, a vocal health and expressiveness theater acted by teleservices operators), choral singing, and others. Because it is a young population, these actions are very well received and have high adherence.
c. Commemorative weeks—in Brazil there are commemorative weeks, such as the Quality of Life Week and the Internal Work-related Accidents Prevention Week, when we include the voice theme as an integrated part of general health care. In April, due to the World Voice Day (April 16th), many companies have already included in their activities calendar actions for the awareness of vocal health and expressiveness with different activities and gifts (Figure 7–7), as an apple to remember the importance of good alimentation habits, or notepad and cards with guidance on vocal health habits and expressiveness.
d. Lectures—with 1 to 2 hours duration, they have interactive and creative methodology. Despite the short time, we propose dynamics to sensitize more effectively for the voice theme (Figure 7–8). In the lectures we also include topics related to the operators'

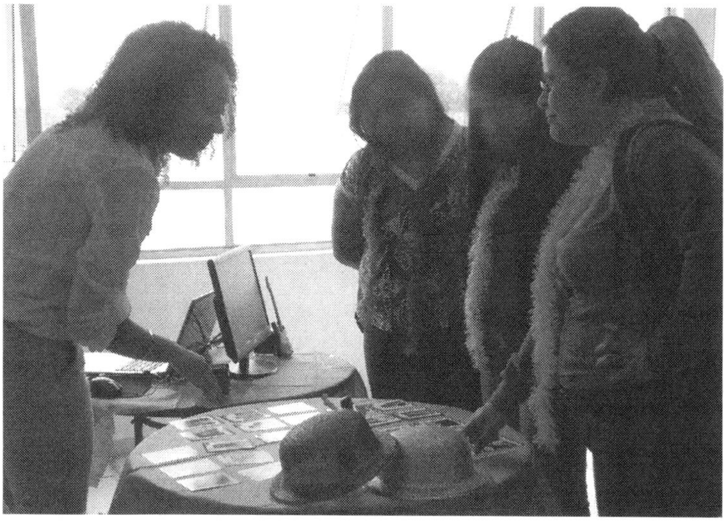

Figure 7–5. *Motivational campaigns with a game to recognize familiar voices with Adriana Pio, SLP in Univoz.*

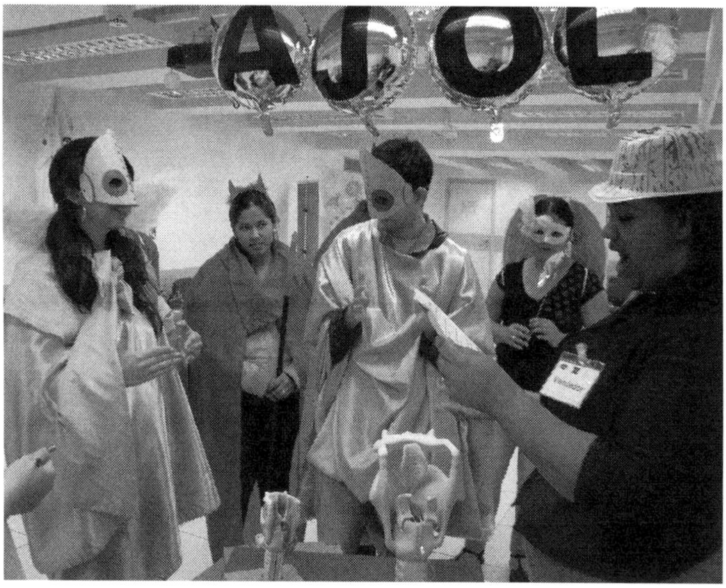

Figure 7–6. *Vocal health and expressiveness theater acted by teleoperator in a motivational campaign.*

auditory health, such as the correct use of headphones and protection from noise exposure inside and outside the call centers (Trompette & Chatillon, 2012). The Regulation (Brazil, 2007) of the Ministry of Health, already mentioned in this chapter,

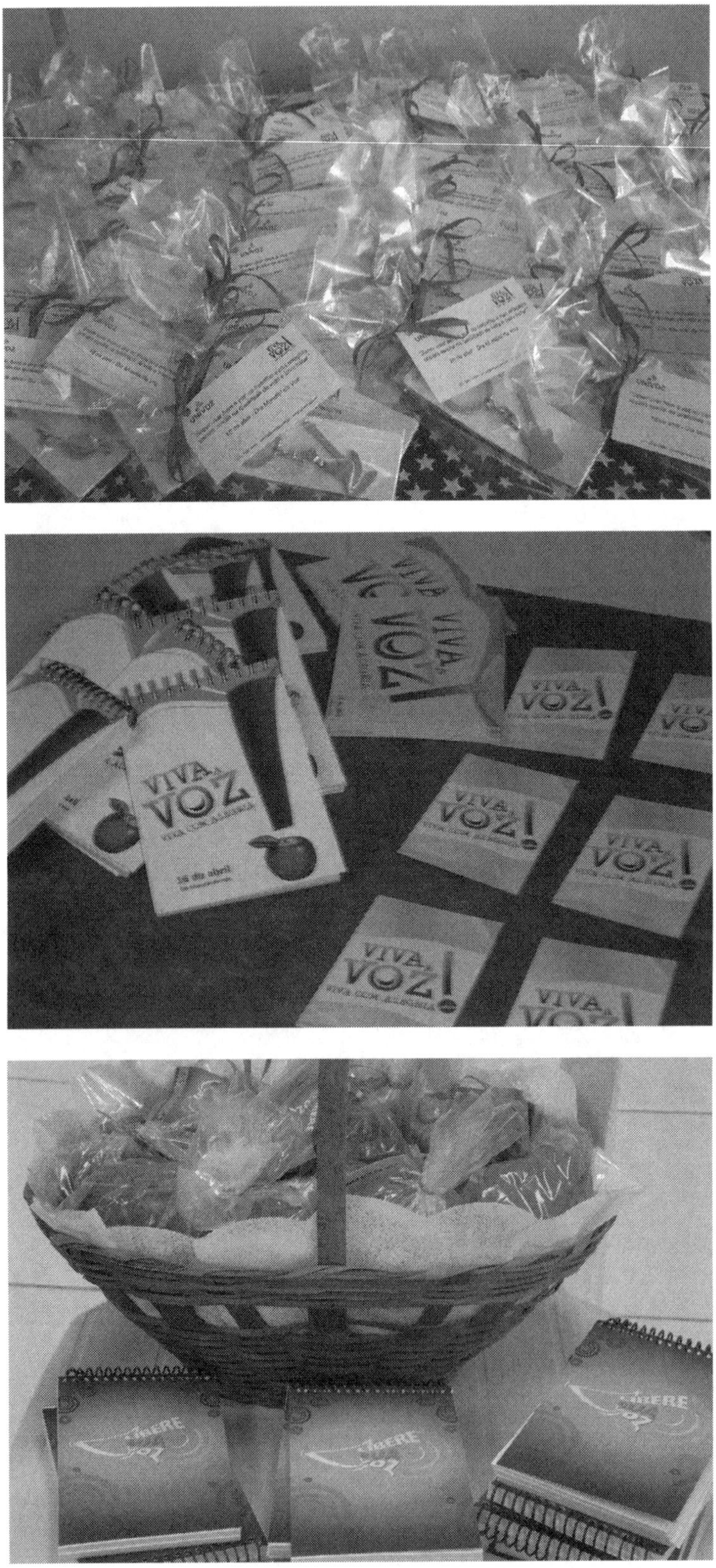

Figure 7–7. *Different types of gifts delivered on World Voice Day.*

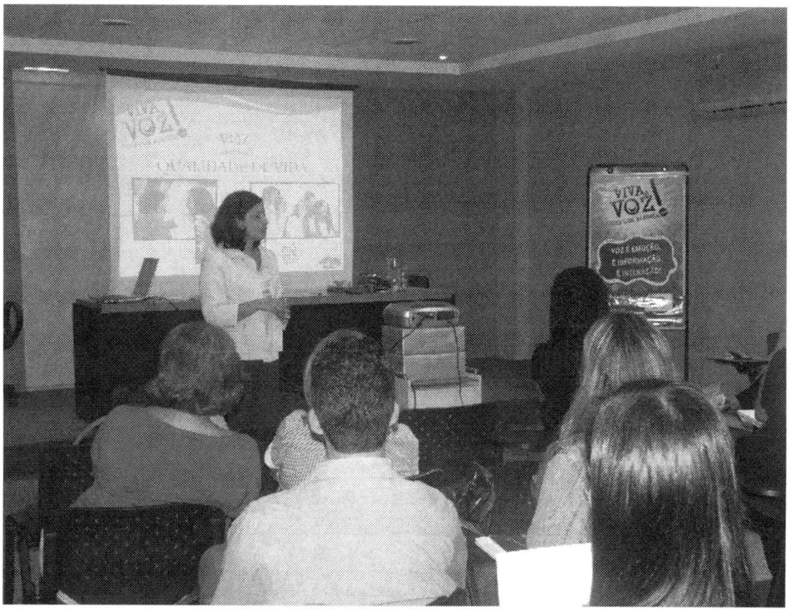

A

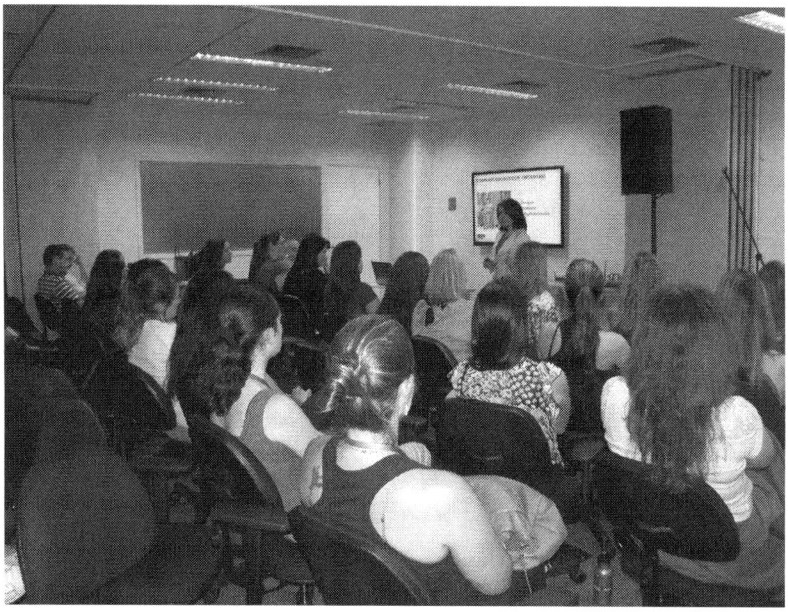

B

Figure 7–8. ***A.*** *Lecture on vocal health for teleservices operators by Ana Elisa Moreira-Ferreira, SLP in Univoz.* ***B.*** *Lecture on expressiveness for teleservices operators by Ana Elisa Moreira-Ferreira, SLP in Univoz.*

demands that the companies offer an initial lecture on the aspects of health. Therefore, every year, Univoz gives a 1-hour lecture on vocal health and expressiveness for the newly hired of a big call center in the city of São Paulo, Brazil, with more than 5,000 operators, including an update on the theme for employees who have participated in previous years. The operators are divided into groups of 100 to 200 participants, and the lectures are offered at different times during 2 weeks in the beginning of each year.

Box 7–3

Case 3

Since 2008, Univoz conducts a voice campaign in a responsive call center in the city of São Paulo, Brazil, in celebration of the World Voice Day. Since this center with 62 employees has a low turnover, each year we need to create a new topic and format so the campaign will arouse interest.

Here we present the data from the 2013 Voice Campaign. The theme was "FREE YOUR VOICE®," and it included a singing workshop, providing an experience of vocal warm-up exercises, its effect on singing and spoken voice, guidance on vocal well-being, and the benefits of singing to the voice.

In order to obtain success in the campaigns, it is necessary to engage the entire company. To obtain 100% of adhesion, the managers changed the schedules of the operators, interrupting their work for 1 hour and releasing groups of up to six operators to participate on the proposed activity. Posters were distributed around the entire company and call center, inviting everybody for the action and disclosing the agenda.

A room was specially prepared for the activity with thematic party decoration, banners, and props of the proposed theme music to sing at the end of the activity (Figure 7–9)—in this case, a "Baião," typical and very popular Brazilian music. The activity consisted of the following stages:

- First stage—Questionnaire in a Program (Figure 7–10)—computer terminals were installed with a questionnaire to get information regarding habits, present signs and symptoms, and knowledge on voice. The operators filled it when they entered the room, while waiting for the rest of the group.
- Second stage—Presentation of the activity by the voice specialist speech-language pathologist—in the first 15 minutes, we explained the proposal, the importance of voice to the operator, and the issues about vocal health care; we then introduced the importance of warming up for the professional use of voice and its effects on the operator's voice, making an analogy to the warmup performed by singers.
- Third stage—Vocal warmup (see Figure 7–9A)—we performed basic and universal warm-up exercises in group, and then some introductory vocalizations to singing, to provide the vocal experience.
- Fourth stage—Singing activity (see Figure 7–9B)—we proposed singing the theme song of the Campaign

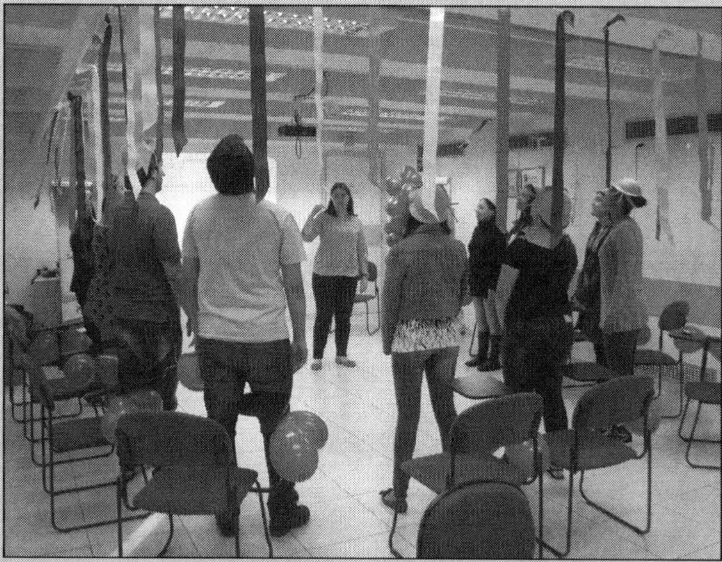

A

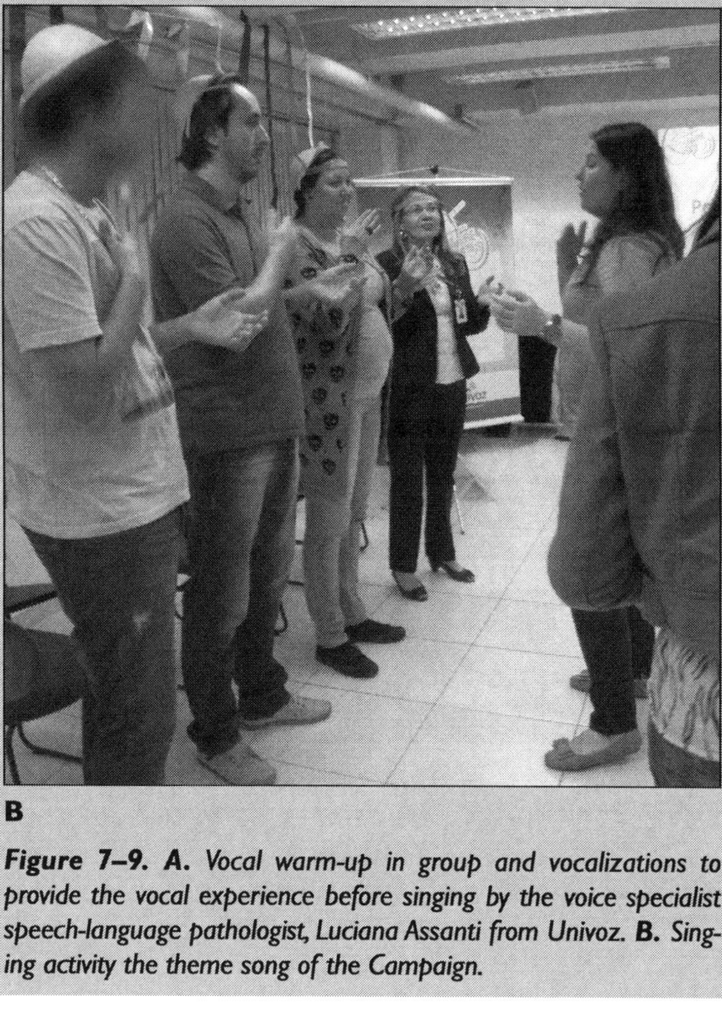

B

Figure 7–9. A. *Vocal warm-up in group and vocalizations to provide the vocal experience before singing by the voice specialist speech-language pathologist, Luciana Assanti from Univoz.* ***B.*** *Singing activity the theme song of the Campaign.*

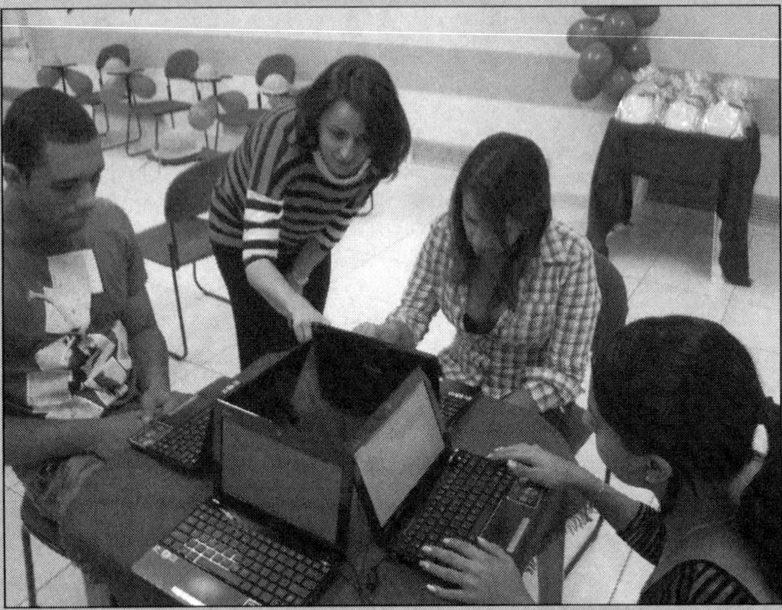

***Figure 7–10.** Computer terminals with Survey Monkey Questionnaire.*

while talking about rhythm, melody, and other aspects. At the end, everybody sang the song and gave testimony of the effects of the exercises in singing. We emphasized that the importance of vocal care is not only for vocal elite professionals, but operators also benefit from it.

- Fifth stage—Gifts—at the end, everybody got a brochure with orientations about voice, a ticket to see a musical play about "Baião," and a key ring with musical notes for participation in the activity (Figure 7–11).

To understand if the action brought any changes, we applied a satisfaction and adherence assessment 30 days after the activity. The results were very positive, with 100% of the subjects satisfied or very satisfied with the activity and its benefits (Table 7–3). We also wanted to know what kinds of benefits were noticed, and we asked an open question: "Which benefits have you noticed in your voice or your professional performance?" (Table 7–4). The answers were classified by semantic similarity into four types: general awareness, habits, voice quality, and vocal performance. The employees who answered this question (55 participants, 89%) reported up to three benefits. "General awareness" answers were the most mentioned, and finally, 16.1% reported feeling impacts on vocal quality (see Table 7–4). This confirms that punctual actions do not promote effective changes in phonatory adjustments and vocal quality, and do not guarantee changes in vocal habits, but are effective in increasing interest for the topic and general awareness for vocal care.

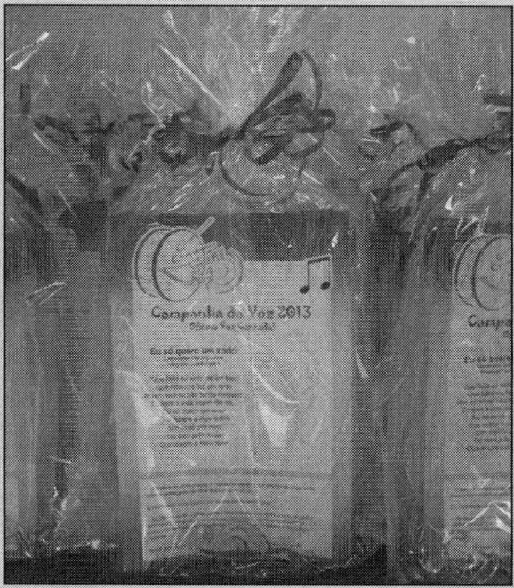

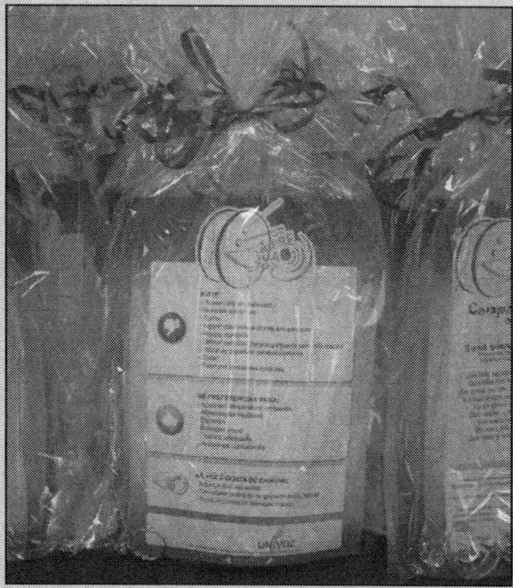

Figure 7–11. *Gifts—brochure with orientations about voice, a ticket to see a musical play about "Baião," and a key ring with musical notes for participation in the activity.*

Table 7–3. *Demonstration of the Satisfaction Level With the Benefits Brought by the Voice Campaign to the Voice or Professional Performance*

Satisfaction With the Benefits From Actions	N	%
Very satisfied	57	91.9
Satisfied	05	8.1
Somewhat satisfied	—	—
Total	62	100

Table 7–4. *Responses to the Question, "What Benefits Have You Noticed in Your Voice or Professional Performance With the Voice Campaign?" (N = 62)*

Benefits			
Type	**Examples**	**N**	**%**
General awareness	"Greater attention when I speak," "Greater concern to use the voice inside and outside of work"	32	51.6
Habits	"I drink more water," "I do some exercises before working," "More voice rest"	19	30.6
Professional performance	"Better use of voice with the customer," "I put more emotion to the voice on the phone"	16	25.8
Voice quality	"I feel more comfortable speaking," "I avoid speaking without breathing," "My voice is less shouted"	10	16.1

The Case 3, (Box 7–3) presented also contributes to the reflection on the importance of all the actions implemented in the companies having tools to measure the results, helping the team of SLPs to understand the impact of our actions. Therefore, Univoz has several ways of measuring these results in order to improve the approaches, get to know better the population we work with and what sensitizes them, as well as show the companies the effects and benefits offered.

We also highlight that, despite providing awareness, there is no guarantee that the changes in vocal behavior will have a lasting maintenance. For the actions to bring deep engagement with change, they must be long term and include closer follow-up to the voice professional. Therefore, these Awareness Actions are usually introductory to the implementation of the follow-up actions of a comprehensive VHP.

Collective Prevention Actions—Training and Exercises

We define prevention as educational measures that provide effective changes on vocal behavior and healthy voice production, reducing the risk for dysphonia and/or increasing the resistance of the voice professional to be exposed to these occupational risk factors. The actions in the work environment and organization are also preventive; therefore, they are implemented in the very beginning of the projects, as described in item 1, Vocoergonomics Assessment.

But for the changes to be effective, it is important that the operators experience the voice production, the exercises, the healthy vocal adjustments, and notice their benefits to their voice. Although we still need more research to generate conclusive evidence that voice training improves vocal efficiency of voice professionals (Hazlett, Duffy, & Moorhead, 2011), we know how much trainings increase the knowledge about voice, the awareness of the risks and how to avoid them, and the voice quality (Hazlett et al., 2011), and that the practice of exercises contributes to the well-being of the teleservice operator and to the reduction of signs and symptoms related to voice problems (Lehto et al., 2005).

Therefore, in a comprehensive VHP, these are the most important actions to actually change vocal behavior and prevent alterations. These actions are permanently, frequently, and interrelatedly implemented.

In the VHP managed by Univoz, as soon as the operators are hired, still in the training and integration period, they participate on the lecture (mentioned in the previous item) with basic information. However, as soon as they start working, the Collective Prevention Actions are initiated (Figure 7–12):

a. Training—4 to 8 hours in duration, depending on the company, they may be divided into several shorter weekly, biweekly, or monthly meetings. These trainings are held right after admission, but also annually, to reinforce and renew the knowledge. Between 10 and 20 operators participate each time, and it is held in a classroom with support of didactic material, such as PowerPoint, handouts, dynamics, and other resources for the conduction of specific exercises. It is a playful activity, with practical actions that include contents regarding

   - voice production;
   - breathing, projection, and resonance;
   - knowledge of usual pitch and loudness;
   - improving articulation and diction;
   - speech rate;
   - intonation and prosody;
   - comfortable vocal phonation; and
   - warm-up and cool-down exercises.

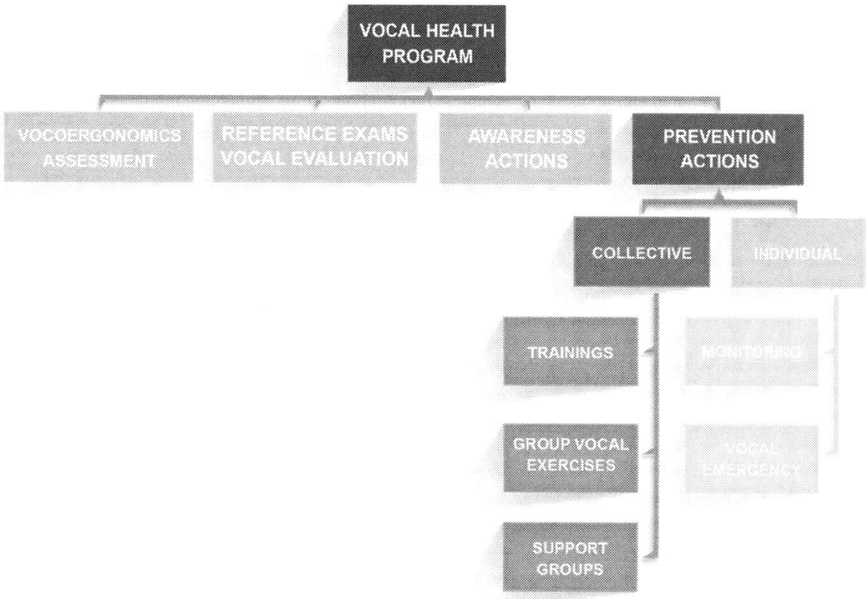

Figure 7–12. *Description of the Collective Prevention Actions implemented by Univoz in teleservices centers.*

Even when implemented punctually or shortly, the trainings are very important to help the operator to reduce signs and symptoms and to find a more comfortable phonation during professional practice and, why not, also out of work. In a research with a group of operators after a short training, 60% of the participants reported improvement in vocal habits, and none reported anything negative about the effects of this action on their voices (Lehto et al., 2003). At Univoz, the same effects have been noticed after these actions.

b. Group vocal exercises—After going through training, the operators are ready to attend the groups of Vocal Exercises. Short breaks are scheduled along the work shift in the very system—"Univoz break" or "voice break"—and the operator may be away from his or her position to perform vocal exercises in groups. There are many challenges in this activity:

- offering the right exercise for each moment, since they are not necessarily having their breaks in the beginning of the shift (for vocal warm-up), or at the end of it (so we can help the cool-down);
- offering the adequate amount and time of exercises not to cause vocal fatigue;
- offering universal exercises that help everybody in the group, without differentiating them by demand, profile, complaint, vocal alteration, among others; and
- making sufficient break time for the proper performance of the exercise.

Usually, the leader offers between 5 and 15 minutes of break in groups of three to five operators at a time. These groups have been proven to be very effective, since the trainings do not guarantee that operators do the exercises regurlarly, nor that they have time for doing it or feel comfortable doing it by themselves. The practice conducted by the SLP reduces the embarassment and guarantees that they do it more frequently and correctly.

In our experience we observe that the improvements in the operators' vocal health are easily noticed by them, as they report, in pre- and post-intervention self-evaluations, reduction of signs and symptoms, improvements in phonatory comfort, and better voice expressiveness. However, the benefits are not exclusive to the employees: the companies also have gains when the number of absences for voice problems decrease, the leaves are almost absent, and the professional performance improves, as shown in Case 4 (Box 7–4).

c. Support groups—Sometimes the groups cannot be carried out with all the operators due to the elevated number of professionals, the work shifts, or the workplace with little space, preventing us from gathering people around the work stations. We cannot forget that the performance of vocal exercises produces noise that might interfere with the attention of the operators that are working and the interaction with clients on the phone. Thus, in some centers, Univoz implements support groups in which only the operators with more complaints of vocal alteration and/or with diagnosed dysphonia participate. In these cases, this activity is a support to the operator in treatment with a SLP outside of the workplace. These operators also have special breaks, in addition to those determined by law, so the SLP may invite them to participate on the activity at the designated time.

In the group, the operator can express his annoyance with dysphonia, ask questions about the healthy production of voice, and even perform specific warm-up and cool-down exercises according to the operator's problem, other than the universal exercises carried out in the action of

Box 7–4

Case 4

In 2005, we presented the results of a project conducted in a hybrid call center (receptive and active) regarding the contribution of the VHP to the professional performance of telemarketing operators in the XIII Brazilian Speech-Language Pathology and Audiology Congress (Moreira-Ferreira, 2005). It is known that voice alterations hinder communication (Vilkman, 2000) and, therefore, may also hinder the operator's professional performance and relationship with the client. In our experience, we noticed that operators who went through voice programs reported improvements at work, and not only in signs and symptoms or vocal quality.

At the time, we implemented a Vocal Conservation Program (VCP) for 20 operators (55% male; 45% female) between 19 and 43 years of age (average of 25 years). The VCP consisted of (a) diagnosis of the company—voco-ergonomics analysis; (b) vocal evaluation with auditory-perceptual analysis, vocal profile questionnaire, and professional performance evaluation (classification based on the supervisor's monitoring sheet, considering the days of presence, lateness, and leaves, number of calls per day, average time of calls, as well as the quality of interaction with the client—attitude and communication); (c) trainings (8 hours talking about health and professional use of voice); and (d) program of exercises (15 daily minutes in groups with five participants each, once a week conducted by the SLP in a room close to the center, and four times a week followed by the leader of the team who had been trained weekly on the exercises of that period).

We were interested in analyzing if the VCP implemented contributed to the professional performance of the telemarketing operators. After 6 months of VCP, the item 2—vocal assessment—was conducted again. In this period, the center was not submitted to any other intervention in training, and the data collected pre- and post-VCP were compared.

Before the VCP we had the following population profile:

- 25% (five operators) did not present dysphonia, 50% (10 operators) presented mild, 20% (four operators) moderate, and 5% (one operator) severe dysphonia;
- 76% of the operators reported more than three signs and symptoms of alterations; and
- compared to the center's performance sheet, all operators with moderate to severe dysphonia presented low professional performance, obtaining, pre-VCP, the classifications 10th, 12th (two operators), 15th, and 18th in the ranking of relationship with clients.

After the VCP interventions the vocal assessment showed that

- 75% improved on the level of dysphonia, going from severe to moderate and from moderate to mild; one operator with dysphonia (who held the 12th place on the performance evaluation) was dismissed due to organizational issues.
- There was a decrease in the number of operators with more than three symptoms (first week: 76%; last week: 47%), reducing mainly the complaints of fatigue, volume/tone alteration, effort, throat clearing, and dryness. The symptom "sore throat" did not present reduction, probably for being associated with nonfunctional alterations, and therefore not being impacted by exercises.
- In correlating dysphonia with the performance evaluation registered by the center, it was noticed that all the four dysphonic operators (not considering the one dismissed) obtained better performance, going to first, seventh, fifth, and second places.
- Moreover, it was noticed that when the voice specialist conducted the exercises, 100% of the operators participated in the activity. In the other days, when the exercise was conducted by the leader, the adhesion was 80%.

The Vocal Conservation Program (VCP) proved to be efficient for the improvement of operators' vocal quality and presence of signs and symptoms, and may have positively influenced their professional performance.

item "b." The SLP makes an interface so there is no conflict between the exercises. The groups are gathered according to some criteria, such as level and type of dysphonia, presence or absence of lesion. At Univoz, we have assumed as a criterion to accept no more than four participants in each group, since it requires more specific work.

Individual Prevention Actions

The health programs established in companies usually have a collective character, attending employees globally and in groups. However, Brazilian VCPs also assume a closer character, due to the high risk of vocal alterations to which these employees are exposed. There are several activities considered as Individual Prevention Actions (Figure 7–13). In the projects implemented by Univoz we perform the following:

a. Monitoring—Periodic follow-up of the operator by telephone recording. This might be offered to all the operators of the center or only to the ones with moderate or severe alterations, and the periodicity may vary depending on the vocal alteration:

- monthly to the ones with no complaints; or
- weekly or biweekly to the ones already in the risk group, with complaints or vocal alterations of mild or worse levels.

The operator may be approached in person, which we call "*In loco* or online monitoring," when the voice specialist goes to the work station. This offers the possibility to connect the headset to the equipment to listen to the interaction between client and operator in real time. One call is listened to, and at the end, the operator takes an approximate 5-minute break so

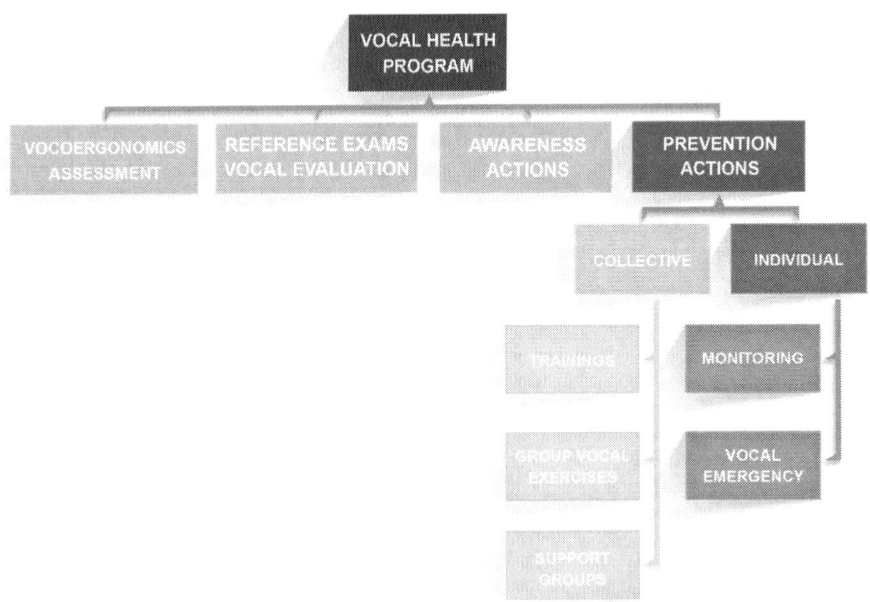

Figure 7–13. *Description of Individual Prevention Actions implemented by Univoz in teleservice centers.*

the SLP may answer his or her questions and provide orientation on the observed issues, such as

- noticed signs and symptoms;
- vocal quality alterations;
- need for expressiveness adjustments; and
- even other aspects of speech and language, if the project includes these topics (as we see in item II of this chapter).

Another type of follow-up is using wiretapping software in a "Quality call monitoring" process—that is, using the system, the voice specialist listens offline to some calls between operator and client and then schedules an approximatey 15-minute meeting for feedback. Quality Call Monitoring is a simple and easy process and, with the feedback, produces significant results in the development of vocal awareness and the information provided to each operator, according to his or her particular vocal characteristics. Identifying a vocal problem when it starts is also an efficient process, because it does not depend on the operator to notice the problem and have the initiative to seek the speech-language pathology team or to go to the doctor's office at the company.

b. Vocal emergency care—(Case 5, Box 7–3). When projects are applied to call centers with a large number of operators (generally more than 500), one or more voice specialists work full time with the client to perform the VCP activities. Since our presence is constant, we can also implement the vocal emergency care. At any moment, the operator may search for the voice specialist's help, in case he or she feels any alterations in vocal quality or worsening of signs and symptoms that may be difficult, limiting, or preventing his professional performance.

At this moment, the SLP immediately receives the teleoperator in person, keeping a focused process of listening to the vocal complaints and specifically guiding him or her, working quickly in cases of acute dysphonia and the presence of related signs and symptoms (Moreira-Ferreira & Dragone, 2008). Our goal in this action is

- to retake a healthy and comfortable vocal condition;
- to keep the operator working, provided that he or she is in condition for that without risking his vocal health; and
- to reduce the absenteeism due to voice-related problems that tend to get worse when there is no quick intervention.

The voice specialist usually is located at the doctor's office, where he is able to work in partnership with the occupational physicians and nurses. During 20 to 30 minutes, we conduct a brief anamnesis, gathering information about the operator's history on the program, the results of his or her vocal screening and therapeutical tasks, in order to observe whether the reported complaint is related to the professional use of voice or to other situations of use, or if there is any evidence of a condition related to other causes (upper respiratory tract infection, gastroesophageal reflux disease, and others). In this last case, the voice specialist provides orientation regarding vocal care and refers the subject to the company's occupational physician. When implemented, the emergency care presupposes that we have data from previous VCP monitoring for a better understanding of the dysphonic condition. These data are available on the computerized systems that Univoz implements with the clients. The case must then be followed up for a few days, observing the evolution and considering the need for other conducts.

Box 7–5

Case 5

We have worked in a hybrid negotiation call center, with VCP implemented for more than 2 years, with all the registered data from each operator, and with emergency room implemented. During 2 years, we registered 556 attendances (Table 7–5). From the operators who have attended emergency care, almost 64% (Table 7–6) were kept working in the center, without the need to lose hours or days of work, 5.2% remained in the center while in relative rest (resting 15 minutes for each hour of work), and about 30% were referred to the doctor's office for presenting signs of associated organic conditions.

Table 7–5. *Number of Emergency Care Performed Between 2007 and 2008*

Period	N	%
2007	68	12.3
2008	488	87.7
Total	556	100

Table 7–6. *Conduct After Emergency Care (%)*

Conduct	N	%
Stayed working at the center	357	64.2
Stayed at the center in relative rest	29	5.2
Referred to the occupational physician	170	30.6
Total	556	100

However, we were concerned about whether keeping them taking calls was the right conduct. The immediate intervention with only one vocal screening and without the support of a medical diagnosis left some doubts.

Thus, we conducted a retrospective analysis of the records. We analyzed the complaint and history, the vocal quality, and the vocal signs and symptoms self-reported when the emergency care was performed and after a few days. We also compared the immediate result of the intervention, the conduct facing the condition diagnosed by the SLP (keep working, vocal reduction/rest, and/or referral to the occupational physician), and the follow-up after this intervention—all subjects were reassessed between the first and seventh days after the event.

From the 357 employees who were maintained at the center, 94% reported improvement of the condition and comfortable professional performance after the intervention, indicating that the conduct actually helped improve the voice (Table 7–7). All subjects among the 6% that reported the same complaint or

Table 7–7. *Report About Vocal Quality and/or Signs and Symptoms Among the Operators That Kept Working at the Center, at Follow-Up (1 to 7 days after the Emergency Care)*

Report	N	%
Improvement	335	94
Same or worse	22	6
Total	357	100

worsening of the condition were referred to the occupational physician.

Data showed that the emergency care was sensitive for the correct identification of dysphonia in most cases and for guiding the necessary approach facing this condition. For the voice professional, having the support of the SLP in vocal emergencies may contribute to a quicker recovery in cases of dysphonia caused by the occupational use of voice, avoiding the risk of more serious harm to vocal health, and providing the adequate orientation on the other cases. For the company, the emergency care helps keep the operator working comfortably, avoiding losses by absenteism.

Improvement of Communicative Competence Program (ICCP)

The teleservice operator is not only a voice professional, but also a language professional (Moreira-Ferreira, 2007). At the beginning of teleservices, prescribed scripts were provided, and the operator only read the orientations to the clients, in order to avoid mistakes in the procedures. Slowly, with the changes observed in the consumer's profile and the understanding of the need to better serve the clients, the scripts were extinguished, demanding greater skills, from the operator, to interact professionally and explain to the clients the procedures and rules of the company.

With this change, the communication of teleoperators needed to be improved to gain more expressiveness from the vocal point of view, with prosody and intonational variations that translate his attitude and transmit the adequate intention, such as politeness, security, interest, and calm. We know how much voice is a convincing resource in telephone communication (Gélinas-Chebat & Chebat, 1996; Gélinas-Chebat et al., 1999). The operator must comprehend that even small intensity, rate, or melodic variations may transmit more positive or negative clues about his or her attitude and interest in serving the client (Moreira-Ferreira, 2007; Moreira-Ferreira et al. 2014).

The operator also needed to develop his or her verbal and nonverbal communicative abilities to provide correct, clear, and convincing explanations, with arguments that make the client understand the internal procedures of the company and that help the client in his or her needs and decision making. Thus, besides the voice, linguistic-discursive resources also contribute for the client to make an image of the teleservice professional (Moreira-Ferreira, 2007), which has a direct influence on the satisfaction rates of the client with this relationship.

The operator, then, must develop communicative competence, which is understood as the ability to mobilize his or her cognitive skills to establish, by verbal and nonverbal resources, an interaction that includes understanding and being understood, influencing the interlocutor's behavior, and thus generating positive responses.

Since 1998, Univoz works taking actions for training teleoperators in their communicative profile. These actions, initially more focused in vocal expressiveness, vocabulary, and grammar by courses within the company, started to gain a broader dimension, being structured into Improvement of Communicative Competence Program (ICCP).

During these years, we have worked with call centers for sales and post-sales, trading, orientation, services, compliance with customer complaints, among others, and we have always been concerned about developing specific communication styles. We know there is a vocal style (Behlau, Feijó, Madazio, Rehder, Azevero, & Moreira-Ferreira, 2005) for each voice professional, but there is also a language and a communicative behavior that is more suitable to each client profile and that represents more appropriately the company's profile. Therefore, in teleservices, there are several communication styles. For example,

- an active sales center needs an operator with fluency, positive expression facing the client's negative response, a voice that expresses motivation with the product represented, and great ability to identify the client's needs and to base his arguments on them;
- an emergency service center (health, public safety, fire, and others), on the other hand, requires an operator able to provide direct questions and objective explanations, with a higher speech rate, showing readiness and agility without losing intelligibility not to demonstrate haste or lack of interest, and a vocal psychodynamic that transmits security and, at the same time, shelters the person in a situation of risk.

Teleservice companies understand the need to develop the voice, speech, language, listening abilities, and communicative attitude of their agents. As good as the selection process is, the operators always need to be trained. Each professional has been through different previous experiences, in centers more or less demanding with regard to professional communication. It is the company's responsibility to line up the operation style of his or her performance. With this purpose, it seeks teaching and learning strategies that promote effective changes in communicative competence.

Our SLPs, qualified to understand vocal psychodynamics, language structure, discourse analysis, and communicative attitude, as well as how to improve them for better interaction, help to develop this competence within the corporative environment, for all positions and functions. In Brazil, this area is known as "Organizational or Corporate Speech-Language Pathology" (Moreira-Ferreira, 2011; Moreira-Ferreira, Oliveira, & Algodoal, 2011), the exact translation from English (Christensen, 2006; Feinstein-Whittaker, Wilner, & Sikorski, 2012; Schwartz, 1995). Because it is a relatively new area, there is still no deep approach to it in undergraduate school.

Working with teleoperators includes several aspects of communicative competence, such as vocal expressiveness, grammar components, semantic aspects, among others, as described in Table 7–8.

CURIOSITY

An interesting example of working with language rules refers to the use of the gerund. In Brazilian Portuguese, the suffix "-ndo" corresponds to "-ing" in English. However, in Portuguese, the use of gerund is specific, transmitting the idea of a current ongoing action that will continue, and it is not used, as in English, to express actions in the present. For example, the sentence, "*Eu estou te enviando um e-mail*" ("I am sending you an e-mail"):

- should not be used in the gerund "estou enviando" ("am sending," literally) because it would give the impression that the action is beginning and might take some time;
- the correct use is, "Eu enviei para você um e-mail"—"I just sent you an e-mail"; or even
- "Eu enviarei para você um e-mail"—"I will send you an e-mail."

What happens is that the teleservice scripts, when they got to Brazil, were translated literally from English to Portuguese, and this

Table 7–8. *Aspects Approached With the Operators Regarding Communicative Competence*

Aspects of voice expressiveness in communication	
1. Vocal psychodynamic	The voice is specific for each context and may be adapted to the client's profile, the characteristics of the represented product or service, and even to each situation of communication on the phone. Train the expressiveness of the voice so it transmits the necessary and adequate attitude to the type of center the employee represents and to the intention of each sentence during the interaction.
2. Mitigate regionalisms	Brazil presents about 15 different accents, with intonational variations of phonemic production. We train the operators to mitigate their accents, making communication clearer despite the origin of the client.
Grammatical aspects of communication	
3. Brazilian Portuguese rules	Basic review of grammar rules, in order to avoid common mistakes of verbal and nominal conjugation, and others.
Vocabulary and semantic aspects of communication	
4. Language etiquette	Depending on the client, the product, the service, or the company's profile, more or less formality in communication is required. In this item, the operator is introduced to language etiquette, which includes, for example, forms of treatment more or less personal, expected phraseology, greeting or closing phrases, and others.
5. Professional language	Training to reduce language support, informal words, slang, idiomatic expressions, and others that suggest lack of professionalism.
6. Technical vocabulary	Every company has its own technical vocabulary that is not necessarily known by the client. The operators are guided on how to clearly explain each procedure.
7. Cordiality expressions	They are guided on which words express more cordiality and which are appropriate for each moment of interaction with the client.
8. Impact expressions	Words and expressions that help transmit certain attitudes such as security, service agility, interest, and others are trained. In the sentences below, it is noticeable the difference between them, with sentence number 2 expressing more agility: 1. "I will look for it" 2. "Sir, please wait while I look for it *right now*. It is *very quick*."
Aspects of communication structure	
9. Clear and objective language	Training on how to give information and complex orientations clearly, cohesively, and objectively, without losing time in the call.

continues

Table 7–8. *continued*

Aspects of discourse in communication	
10. Negotiation	In this aspect, approaches may vary according to the style of teleservices, but they always need orientation on how to highlight advantages, flexible benefits, and others.
11. Argumentation	The clients know their rights and demand clear explanations from companies. Training argumentation is essential for the client to feel satisfied and accept the orientation.
12. Survey and direction of the call	Relevant questions for understanding the scenario/problem presented by the client: ordering of questions, types of questions, best structure to ask without exposing, offending, or doubting the client.
13. Active listening	How to listen paying total attention, to retain, memorize, understand, and search for solutions to the client.
14. Humanization of service	The expression "humanization" has been used in Brazil to define a more interactive and conversational approach between the operator and his client. Without losing the characteristic of a professional communication, closer expressions are introduced, making the conversation fluid.
Aspects of intention in communication	
15. Communicative attitude	We understand as communicative attitude aspects related to "wanting" to communicate and "understanding" the need to adjust communication to the listener. This ability of interaction is related to multiple factors, such as personality aspects of the speaker, his or her emotion and feelings during interaction, his or her emotional intelligence to deal with the other on a phone conversation, among others.

verb tense began to be used incorrectly, passing the idea of an action that will happen in the future, when the operator is actually referring to something he or she just did. Thus, it is necessary to include this kind of guideline in the training.

The most basic structure of a ICCP has four actions, as follows.

Corporate Communication Diagnosis

The previous stage to any action in communication for a call center (Moreira-Ferreira, 2003), the corporate communication diagnosis aims to identify the communicative profile of the working operators and the desired profile to satisfy the needs of the client. It can be performed by

a. Individual interviews—evaluate the spontaneous oral communication abilities of the operator;
b. Evaluation in real work situation—evaluate the vocal expressiveness and the linguistic-discursive resources in the interaction with the client;
c. "Self-Perception of Teleservice Communication (SPTC®) protocol—this protocol developed by Univoz and published as part of a book in Brazil (in press), has the aim to survey the perception of the operator regarding his or her communication in

specific professional situations in teleservices (Appendix 7–3).

Based on the aspects evaluated on this stage, it is possible to draw the communicative profile of the operator and understand how outdated he or she is from the expected for the teleservice market, helping to define the actions that should be implemented to improve communication.

Selection Process by Communicative Profile

This process is to select among the applicants those who meet the communicative profile of the company. The selection criteria include communication characteristics listed in Table 7–8, aligned with the profile of the company. For the selection, we perform individual interviews, tests regarding knowledge in Portuguese and other aspects of communication, group dynamics, and simulated calls.

Monitoring the Quality of Communicative Competence

The monitoring process of communicative competence quality is implemented with weekly, biweekly, or monthly periodicity, contemplating

a. listening to calls to assess the client-operator communication;
b. fulfilling the monitoring sheet that contemplates all the items that must be evaluated, oriented, and improved; and
c. individual feedback—15- to 30-minute meetings to provide orientation regarding the issues that need improvement.

It is a continuous action to improve the operator's professional performance. At this point, specific orientations and exercises are offered, along with complementary materials aimed at developing the communicative abilities, promoting effective behavioral changes. It is usually performed by a professional called a quality monitor, who does not always provide effective guidelines to promote voice, speech, language, listening, and attitudes, due to his or her lack of specific graduation in communication. The corporate SLP has the ability to perform this task with greater efficacy. In many companies, this monitoring is part of the operator's professional performance protocol, recognizing him or her when excellence levels of communication are reached in the interaction with the client.

Communicative Competence Trainings

This is a scheduled and planned moment (Moreira-Ferreira, Oliveira, & Algodoal, 2011), using topics and methods that allow the development of the operators' communication abilities. These professionals must improve the aspects of voice, speech, language, listening, discourse, communication attitude, and emotional control, using them effectively in practice. Therefore, following the guidelines for the teaching and learning of adults, corporate training must be very practical, using a facilitating didacts for learning. Simulations and experiences, dynamics, exercises, corporate games, plays, and other activities are used with this purpose.

These trainings have different hours and frequency formats, according to the center and the project. They may be applied punctually (only one training on a predetermined theme, usually with 6-hour duration) or longitudinally (involving several meetings with varied hours and long-term application, named "Learning Trail"). In our practice, the latter has the best results in improving communication. The themes chosen are aligned with the diagnosis and the needs for customer relationship. The most common are related in Table 7–8.

Box 7–6

Case 6

Since 2005 we have worked in a Customer Assistance Support (CAS) department of a chain of stores with over 50 selling points in Brazil. This call center performs post-sale receptive service, providing information about delivery deadlines for purchased merchandise, exchange policies, substitution of damaged products, and other issues regarding the post-sale.

Univoz was hired due to the need to improve the quality of assistance perceived by the client (a satisfaction survey showed less than 80% of satisfaction with the assistance received). Our aim was to improve the performance in the oral professional communication of the 20 teleoperators (at the time) so it reached levels above 90% of excellence and none of them was below 80% (which was their mean range before the project).

As in other call centers, operators had 6-hour shifts with regulated breaks and went through technical training, according to the company's rules, products, and services. However, they were not submitted to the "Quality Call Monitoring." Thus, we implemented the following:

1. diagnosis of the call center, determining the communicative profile of the operators, which showed the need to improve items 1, 3 to 7, 9, 11 to 13, and 15 of Table 7–8;
2. the technical procedure monitoring process, which started to be carried out by the company, in order to verify if the clients were receiving correct and comprehensive information;
3. communicative competence monitoring—weekly listening of calls to fulfill the monitoring sheet, and 28 meetings for feedback, conducted by the corporate SLPs from Univoz with the aim to improve the operator's communication (first monitoring was carried out before any training actions); and
4. the cycle of trainings in competence communication—monthly communication workshop (eight 2-hour meetings; up to 10 operators per group).

In the first monitoring, the sheet showed that 65% of the operators (Table 7–9) had important communication deficits, with scores lower than 80 points; only 5% received scores over

Table 7–9. *Distribution of Operators by Score Range Received in the First and Last Monitoring of Communicative Competence*

	First Monitoring		Last Monitoring	
Monitoring Score Ranges	**N**	**%**	**N**	**%**
0 ↔ 80	13	65	3	15
80.01 ↔ 90	6	30	13	65
90.01 ↔ 100	1	5	4	20

90%. Difficulties were diagnosed in all the assessed levels, especially in vocal psychodynamics, in the ability to listen and understand the client, in using polite and professional expressions, and in argumentation.

After feedback and workshops, the monitoring evaluations showed improvements on the aspects emphasized in 80% of the operators (Table 7–10). The mean score on the monitoring sheet increased from 69.42 to 79.78%, and the evolution of scores (Figure 7–14) shows that the number of operators with scores between 80.01 and 90% went from 6 (30%) to 13 (65%), and the number of scores over 90% went from 1 (5%) to 4 operators (20%). However, not all subjects improved: 1 (5) operator kept the same score, and 3 (15%) obtained lower scores when compared to the first monitoring, showing that the learning of communication is not linear and also depends on the commitment and the motivation of the speaker.

We are currently still consultants in this company. We are always updating and modifying the project in order to adjust to the market needs and the operation profile, and training newly hired operators to keep the quality level we have conquered. Today, the company has over 70 employees and the excellence levels have been kept over 95%. This case was described in detail on a chapter of a book published in Brazil (Moreira-Ferreira & Moraes, 2014).

Table 7–10. *Comparison Between Operators' Scores Received in the First and the Last Monitoring of Communicative Competence*

Scores of the Last Monitoring Compared to the First	N	%
Higher	16	80
Equal	1	5
Lower	3	15

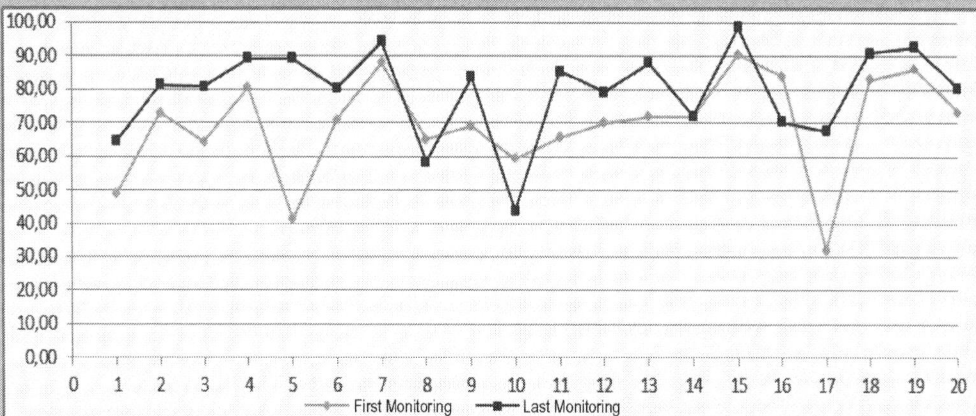

Figure 7–14. *Comparison of the operators' scores in the first and the last monitoring after the implementation of the project.*

Conclusion

Implementing longitudinal projects in teleservice centers is very challenging. The companies are more and more interested in hiring punctual actions with lower costs, that promote fantastic results in the short term. However, modifying aspects of voice, speech, language, and communicative attitudes means altering communication habits, which is only conquered with daily orientations and practices in real situations of professional communication.

In Brazil, this is a consolidated and still promising area for speech-language pathology. A new advance regarding occupational vocal health is a document, in the approval phase, about dysphonia in voice professionals, which is known as work-related voice disorder (CFFa, 2006). In the future, this document may favor health actions.

The creativity of Brazilian SLPs, allied with the space and the importance provided by the companies, have made the Vocal Health Program (VHS) and the Improvement of Communicative Competence Program (ICCP) an important working niche for our professional performance and for science in Brazil. This has allowed that some studies with populations of teleservice operators were published with great access in open Brazilian and international journals (Oliveira et al., 2008).

The advantage of being executed by SLPs —specifically by voice specialists, in the case of VHS, and corporate SLPs, in the case of ICCP—lies on our expertise in evaluating voice and communication and in finding strategies for exercises, dynamics, and specific orientations to promote vocal quality, the improvement of vocal expressiveness, and the linguistic resources of teleservice professionals.

For me and my company, working in this area is a privilege, because we notice several advantages with our approaches:

- for the operator, who has his or her vocal health preserved and communication improved, with positive consequences for well-being and professional performance within the company and along his or her career;
- for the company, which reduces health care costs, increases the well-being of their employees, improves the interpersonal relationship with the clients, and as a consequence, harvests motivated and productive operators, and improves the company's image in front of the public;
- for the public service, which reduces the investment on citizens on medical leave for occupational conditions and also has a more capable and prepared population for the job market, with more communicative professionals; and
- for the client, who will be assisted by a healthy, motivated, and competent professional, able to offer him or her the support he or she needs.

For speech-language pathology, the gains are equally evident. Teleservices have allowed us to put our actions into practice with great populations of voice professionals, and to broaden our work to an important area for comprehensive health: communicative competence.

References

Associação Brasileira de Telesserviços (ABT). (2011). *O que é telemarketing?* Retrieved from http://www.abt.org.br/telemarketing.asp

Bastian, R. W., & Thomas, J. P. (2016). Talkativeness and vocal loudness: Do they correlate with laryngeal pathology? A study of the vocal overdoer/underdoer continuum. *Journal of Voice, 30*, 557–562.

Behlau, M., Feijó, D., Madazio, G., Rehder, M. I.., Azevedo, R., & Ferreira, A. E. (2005). Voz profissional: aspectos gerais e atuação fonoaudiológica. In Behlau, M. (Ed.), *Voz: O livro do especialista* (pp. 296–332). Rio de Janeiro, Brazil: Revinter.

Behlau, M., & Pontes, P. (2009). *Higiene vocal – cuidando da voz* (4th ed.). Rio de Janeiro, Brazil: Revinter.

Brazil. (2007). Anexo II da NR-17. Portaria SIT n.º 09, 30 de março de 2007, 07, Trabalho em Teleatendimento/Telemarketing. Ministério do Trabalho e Emprego. Retrieved from http://portal.mte.gov.br/data/files/FF8080812BE914E6012BEFBDACD94B74/nr_17_anexo2.pdf

Carrochano, M. C. (2007). *Jovens, Sindicato e Trabalho no Setor de Telesserviço.* Retrieved from http://www.ibase.br/userimages/telemarketing_final.pdf

Christensen, B. (2006). Corporate speech-language pathology: Is it right for you? *The ASHA Leader, 11*, 14–25. Retrieved from http://leader.pubs.asha.org/article.aspx?articleid=2278238

CFFa. Conselho Federal de Fonoaudiologia (2006). *Distúrbio de Voz Relacionado ao Trabalho—DVRT. Ministério da Saúde, Secretaria de Vigilância em Saúde.* Retrieved from http://www.fonoaudiologia.org.br/paginas_internas/noticiasIntegra.asp?id=319

CFFa. Conselho Federal de Fonoaudiologia. (2014). Res. CFFa nº 453/2014. *Diário Oficial da União.* Retrieved from http://www.fonoaudiologia.org.br/cffa/wp-content/uploads/2013/07/res-453-2014-novas-especialidades.pdf

Constancio, S., Moreti, F., Guerrieri, A. C., & Behlau, M. (2012). Dores corporais em teleoperadores e sua relação com o uso da voz em atividades laborais. *Rev. Soc. Bras. Fonoaudiol, 17*, 4, 377–384.

Dassie-Leite, A. P., Lourenco, L., & Behlau, M. (2011). Relação entre dados ocupacionais, sintomas e avaliação vocal de operadores de telesserviços. *Rev. Soc. Bras. Fonoaudiol, 6*, 1, 59–63.

Feinstein-Whittaker, M., Wilner, L. K., & Sikorski, L. D. (2012). A growing niche in corporate America. *The ASHA Leader, 17*, 28–31. Retrieved from http://www.asha.org/Publications/leader/2012/120313/A-Growing-Niche-in-Corporate-America.htm

Ferreira, L. P., & Migliorini, D. R. (2002). Fonoaudiologia e Telemarketing: como tudo começou. In R. G. Alloza & R. B. W. Salsztein (Ed.), *Fonoaudiologia na empresa: Atuação em call center* (pp. 1–8). Rio de Janeiro, Brazil: Revinter.

Ferreira, L. P., & Moreira-Ferreira, A. E. (2014). Fonoaudiologia nas empresas de telesserviços. In L. P. Ferreira, M. A. Andrada e Silva, & S. P. Pinto Giannini (Ed.), *Distúrbio de voz relacionado ao trabalho: Práticas fonoaudiológicas.* São Paulo, Brazil: Ed. Roca

Gélinas-Chebat, C., & Chebat, J. C. (1996). Voice and advertising: Effects of intonation and intensity of voice on source credibility, attitudes toward the advertised service and the intent to buy. *Perceptual and Motor Skills, 83*, 243–262.

Gélinas-Chebat, C., Chebat, J. C., & Boivin, R. (1999). Impact of male and female voice cues on consumers' attitudes. In *Int. Congress Phonetic Sciences - ICPHS*, Telemarketing. San Francisco, CA, 2nd ed., pp. 1577–1580.

Hazlett, D. E., Duffy, O. M., & Moorhead, S. A. (2011). Review of the impact of voice training on the vocal quality of professional voice users: Implications for vocal health and recommendations for further research. *Journal of Voice, 25*(2), 181–191.

Hazlett, D. E., Moorhead, S. A., & Duffy, O. M. (2009). Occupational voice demands and their impact on the call-centre industry. *BMC Public Health, 9*, 108. Retrieved from http://www.biomedcentral.com/1471-2458/9/108

Hazlett, D. E., Moorhead, S. A., & Duffy, O. M. (2011). Working voices. An epidemiological study of occupational voice demands and their impact on the call center industry—IOSH Research Committee. *IOSH*, University of Ulster, England. Retrieved from https://www.iosh.co.uk/~/media/Documents/Books%20and%20resources/Published%20research/Working_voices.ashx

IBGE - Pesquisa Mensal de Emprego do Instituto Brasileiro de Geografia e Estatística. (2011). Retrieved from http://www.ibge.gov.br/home/estatistica/pesquisas/pesquisa_resultados.php?id_pesquisa=38

Jones, K., Sigmon, J., Hock, L., Nelson, E., Sullivan, M., & Ogren, F. (2002). Prevalence and risk factors for voice problems among telemarketers. *Archives of Otolaryngology-Head and Neck Surgery, 128*(5), 571–577.

Lehto, L., Alku, P., Bäckström, T., & Vilkman, E. (2005). Voice symptoms of call-centre customer service advisers experienced during a work-day and effects of a short vocal training course. *Logopedics, Phoniatrics, Vocology, 30*(1), 14–27.

Lehto, L., Rantala, L., Vilkman, E., Alku, P., & Backstrom, T. (2003). Experiences of a short vocal training course for call-centre customer service advisors. *Folia Phoniatrica et Logopaedica, 55*, 163–176.

Mathieson, L., Hirani, S. P., Epstein, R., Baken, R. J., Wood, G., & Rubin, J. S. (2009). Laryngeal manual therapy: A preliminary study to examine its treatment effects in the management of muscle tension dysphonia. *Journal of Voice, 23*, 353–366.

Moreira-Ferreira, A. E. (2003). Diagnóstico empresarial fonoaudiológico em Call center: essencial para o sucesso de nossas atuações. In R. B. W. Salzstein & R. G. Alloza (Ed.), *Conhecimentos Essenciais para Atuar Bem em Empresas - Call Center*. São Paulo, Brazil: Pulso.

Moreira-Ferreira, A. E. (2005). Contribuição do programa de conservação vocal no desempenho profissional do operador de telemarketing. *XIII Congresso Brasileiro de Fonoaudiologia*. Santos, São Paulo, Brazil.

Moreira-Ferreira, A. E. (2007). *Recursos de expressividade oral e linguístico-discursivos de operadores de telemarketing: Relação com a sensação gerada em prováveis clientes e o desempenho profissional.* Pontifícia Universidade Católica. Retrieved from http://www.sapientia.pucsp.br/tde_busca/arquivo.php?codArquivo=4364

Moreira-Ferreira, A. E. (2011). *Fonoaudiologia do Trabalho e Fonoaudiologia Organizacional: Diferenças e similaridades das áreas de atuação em empresas.* Sociedade Brasileira de Fonoaudiologia (SBFa.). Retrieved from http://www.sbfa.org.br/CursoDepartamento%20/22011.htm

Moreira-Ferreira, A. E., & Dragone, M. L. S. (2008). Pronto atendimento em voz – efeitos no desempenho profissional e na saúde vocal de teleoperadores. In *Anais do 16º Congresso Brasileiro de Fonoaudiologia, Soc. Bras. Fonoaudiol.* São Paulo, Brazil.

Moreira-Ferreira, A. E., & Moraes, M. (2014). Programa de monitoria para aprimoramento do desempenho em comunicação oral profissional em serviços de atendimento ao cliente. In L. P. Ferreira, M. A. Andrada e Silva, & S. P. Pinto Giannini (Eds.), *Distúrbio de Voz Relacionado ao Trabalho: Práticas Fonoaudiológicas* (pp. 203–212). São Paulo, Brazil: Roca

Moreira-Ferreira, A. E., Oliveira, S., & Algodoal, J. (2011). A voz no telesserviços. In I. B. Oliveira, A. A. F. Almeida, T. Raize, & M. Behlau (Eds.), *A atuação fonoaudiológica em Voz Profissional* (pp. 21–55). São Paulo, Brazil: SBFa, Roca.

Moreira-Ferreira, A. E. M., Spina, S. L., Algodoal, J., & Barrichelo, V. (2014). Atuação Fonoaudiológica nos telesserviços—Saúde e Aprimoramento. In I. Marchesan, H. J. Silva, & M. C. Tomé (Eds.), *Tratado das Especialidades em fonoaudiologia—SBFa* (pp. 230–239). São Paulo, Brazil: Guanagara Koogan.

National Institute for Occupational Safety and Health (NIOSH). (2012). *The Research Compendium: The NIOSH Total Worker Health™ Program: Seminal Research Papers* 2012, DHHS (NIOSH) Publication, 146, May 2012. Retrieved from http://www.cdc.gov/niosh/docs/2012-146/default.html

Oliveira, S., Raize, T., Algodoal, J., Moreira-Ferreira, A. E., & Marchiori, M. Q. (2008). A voz no telesserviço. In I. B. Oliveira, A. A. F. Almeida, & T. Raize (Eds.), *Voz profissional—produção científica da fonoaudiologia brasileira.* São Paulo, Brazil: Sociedade Brasileira de Fonoaudiologia. Retrieved from http://www.sbfa.org.br/portal/voz_profissional/

Padilha, M. P., Moreti, F., Raize, T., Sauda, C., Lourenço, L., Oliveira, G., & Behlau, M. (2012). Grau de quantidade de fala e intensidade vocal de teleoperadores em ambiente laboral e extralaboral. *Rev. Soc. Bras. Fonoaudiol., 17*(4), 385–390.

Pedrosa,V., & Moreira-Ferreira, A. E. (2015). *Proposed self-assessment protocols for professional speaking voice.* Presented at the Voice Foundation 44th Annual Symposium: Care of the Professional Voice, Philadelphia, PA.

Piwowarczyk, T. C., Oliveira, G., Lourenço, L., & Behlau, M. (2012). Vocal symptoms, voice activity, and participation profile and professional performance of call center operators. *Journal of Voice, 26,* 194–200.

Rodrigues, G., Zambon, F., Mathieson, L., & Behlau, M. (2013). Vocal tract discomfort in teachers: Its relationship to self-reported voice disorders. *Journal of Voice, 27*(4), 473–480.

Roy, N., Merrill, R. M., Gray, S. D., & Smith, E. M. (2005). Voice disorders in the general population: Prevalence, risk factors, and occupational impact. *Laryngoscope, 115,* 1988–1995.

Schwartz, K. (1995). From clinic to conference room. *American Speech-Language-Hearing Association.* Retrieved from http://www.asha.org/uploadedFiles/0695ashamag.pdf

Taylor, P., Baldry, C., Bain, P., & Ellis, V. (2011). A unique working environment: Health, sickness and absence management in UK call centres, *Work, Employment and Society, 17*(3), 435–458.

Trompette, N., & Chatillon, J. (2012). Survey of noise exposure and background noise in call centers using headphones. *Journal of Occupational and Environmental Hygiene, 9*(6), 381–386.

Vilkman, E. (2000). Voice problems at work: A challenge for occupational safety and health arrangement. *Folia Phoniatrica et Logopaedica, 52,* 120–125.

Vilkman, E. (2004). Occupational safety and health aspects of voice and speech professions. *Folia Phoniatrica et Logopaedica, 56,* 220–253.

APPENDIX 7–1

Vocal Profile in Teleservices Questionnaire (VPTQ®)

Developed by Ana Elisa Moreira-Ferreira from Univoz

UNIVOZ **VOCAL PROFILE IN TELESERVICES QUESTIONNAIRE - VPTQ®** page 1

The data entered by you will be in complete secrecy, serving only as a source of data for the Health Program Vocal and scientific research. Therefore, we kindly ask that this protocol is filled with sincerity. If you have doubts on any question, leave it blank so that we can guide you later. The UNIVOZ, thanks for your attention and time dedicated.

Date: ___/___/___ **Company:** ________ **Identification number:** ________

Complete name: ________________

Date of birth: ___/___/___ **Age:** ________ **Male ( )** **Female ( )**

SENSATIONS AND SYMPTOMS

01. The following are sensations or symptoms that you may feel. Please indicate the frequency with which they occur in general and by week, and if it related with work or not.

ALTERNATIVES	Never	Rarely	Often	Always	Which frequency per week?	It happens before (B), during (D) or after (A)
Aching throat	( )N	( )R	( )O	( )A	( )2 ( )3 or 4 ( )5 or +	( )B ( )D ( ) A
Burning	( )N	( )R	( )O	( )A	( )2 ( )3 or 4 ( )5 or +	( )B ( )D ( ) A
Dry throat	( )N	( )R	( )O	( )A	( )2 ( )3 or 4 ( )5 or +	( )B ( )D ( ) A
Dry mouth	( )N	( )R	( )O	( )A	( )2 ( )3 or 4 ( )5 or +	( )B ( )D ( ) A
Irritable	( )N	( )R	( )O	( )A	( )2 ( )3 or 4 ( )5 or +	( )B ( )D ( ) A
Tightening of the throat	( )N	( )R	( )O	( )A	( )2 ( )3 or 4 ( )5 or +	( )B ( )D ( ) A
Lumb of the throat	( )N	( )R	( )O	( )A	( )2 ( )3 or 4 ( )5 or +	( )B ( )D ( ) A
Difficulty swallowing	( )N	( )R	( )O	( )A	( )2 ( )3 or 4 ( )5 or +	( )B ( )D ( ) A
Breathlessness	( )N	( )R	( )O	( )A	( )2 ( )3 or 4 ( )5 or +	( )B ( )D ( ) A
Dry throat clearing	( )N	( )R	( )O	( )A	( )2 ( )3 or 4 ( )5 or +	( )B ( )D ( ) A
Produtive throat clearing	( )N	( )R	( )O	( )A	( )2 ( )3 or 4 ( )5 or +	( )B ( )D ( ) A
Discomfort in the throat	( )N	( )R	( )O	( )A	( )2 ( )3 or 4 ( )5 or +	( )B ( )D ( ) A
Cough	( )N	( )R	( )O	( )A	( )2 ( )3 or 4 ( )5 or +	( )B ( )D ( ) A
Vocal fatigue	( )N	( )R	( )O	( )A	( )2 ( )3 or 4 ( )5 or +	( )B ( )D ( ) A
Effort	( )N	( )R	( )O	( )A	( )2 ( )3 or 4 ( )5 or +	( )B ( )D ( ) A
Hoarseness	( )N	( )R	( )O	( )A	( )2 ( )3 or 4 ( )5 or +	( )B ( )D ( ) A
Voice breaks or failure	( )N	( )R	( )O	( )A	( )2 ( )3 or 4 ( )5 or +	( )B ( )D ( ) A
Aphonia per hours	( )N	( )R	( )O	( )A	( )2 ( )3 or 4 ( )5 or +	( )B ( )D ( ) A
Aphonia per 1 or more days	( )N	( )R	( )O	( )A	( )2 ( )3 or 4 ( )5 or +	( )B ( )D ( ) A
Weak voice	( )N	( )R	( )O	( )A	( )2 ( )3 or 4 ( )5 or +	( )B ( )D ( ) A
Deeper voice	( )N	( )R	( )O	( )A	( )2 ( )3 or 4 ( )5 or +	( )B ( )D ( ) A
Higher voice	( )N	( )R	( )O	( )A	( )2 ( )3 or 4 ( )5 or +	( )B ( )D ( ) A
Voice worse in the morning	( )N	( )R	( )O	( )A	( )2 ( )3 or 4 ( )5 or +	
Voice worse at night	( )N	( )R	( )O	( )A	( )2 ( )3 or 4 ( )5 or +	

UNIVOZ

VOCAL PROFILE IN TELESERVICES QUESTIONNAIRE - VPTQ® -

WORK AND TRAINING

02. About your previous jobs:

Function	How many years?	Did you use the voice at work ?		Explain
1. ____	____	No ( )	Yes ( )	____
2. ____	____	No ( )	Yes ( )	____
3. ____	____	No ( )	Yes ( )	____

03. Do you work in another activity that requires the use of voice? How many hours per day??

Classes	( )	____ Hours/day	Theater	( )	____	Hours/day
Sing	( )	____ Hours/day	Others	____		

04. Do you have attended any of these vocal works, courses or training? When?

Voice	( )	Speech Therapy	( )	Sing or Theatre	( )	
Oratory	( )	Communication	( )	Others	( )	____

DATA ABOUT YOUR VOCAL BEHAVIOR

05. Do you think you have the habit of talking: (you may mark more than one option)

Fast	( )	or	Slow	( )
Excessive	( )	or	Few	( )
Strong	( )	or	Weak	( )
High	( )	or	Low	( )

06. Check the aspects of verbal communication that you believe have difficulties?

Voice	( )	Pronunciation	( )	Speed of speech	( )	Vocabulary	( )
Entonationn.	( )	Articulation	( )	Grammar rules	( )	Slangs	( )

07. Do you think your voice is appropriate to its: (you may mark more than one option)

Job ( ) Physical structure ( ) Personality ( )

08. Do you have any voice complaint?

No ( ) Yes ( ) Describe: ____

How long? ____

09. If you answer "yes" to the previous question, how was the beginning of the voice change?

Slow ( ) Sudden ( ) Floating ( ) Do not know

UNIVOZ

WORK AND TRAINING

10. Have you ever stopped working for problems in his voice?

No ( ) Yes ( ) How many times? ____________

How long? ____________

11. Have you had voice problems previously?

No ( ) Yes ( ) Which professional was consulted? ____________

What treatment was carried? ____________

12. What do you do or use to improve your voice? ____________

13. Which of the following interfere with your voice or the sensations in the throat? What causes?

		Describe what you feel
Air conditioning	( )	____________
Speaking in noisy environment	( )	____________
State of stress or nervous	( )	____________
Using much the voice (talking too much)	( )	____________
Flus, colds, or allergies	( )	____________
Sudden change in temperature	( )	____________
Smoke, dust, or strong smells	( )	____________
Relationship difficulties in the company	( )	____________
Relationship difficulties with the customers	( )	____________
Stressfull calls	( )	____________
Others	( )	____________

ABOUT YOUR HEALTH DATAS

14. As you consider your health?

Very good ( ) Good ( ) Regular ( ) Bad ( )

15. Do you use to have any of these health changes?

Rhinitis, allergies, and sinusitis	( )	Laryngitis, pharyngitis, and tonsillitis	( )
Frequent cold or flu	( )	Stomach burn, heartburn, reflux (return from stomach)	( )

Hormonal ( ) Digestive ( ) Neurologic ( ) Emotional ( )

16. Do you use any of these medicines?

No	( )	Yes	( )	Which one?			
Hormones	( )	Diuretics	( )	For high pressure	( )	Anti-allergy	( )

17. Do you follow any other treatment for health?? Qual? ____________

No ( ) Yes ( ) Which one? ____________

STRESS DATA

18. Usually experience pain and / or tension:

Head	( )	Neck	( )	Throat	( )	During chewing	( )
Nape	( )	Back	( )	Mandibule	( )	When open mouth	( )
Shoulders	( )	Arms	( )	Body	( )	When swallows	( )

19. When do you feel these feelings?

At work ( ) Off work ( ) Constantly ( )

20. Do you considered yourself as a tense person?

No ( ) Yes ( ) What do you do when you are tense? ____________

21. Do you practice some physical activity?

No ( ) Yes ( ) Which and how often? ____________

22. Do you considered yourself as person with tendency to:

Frustration	( )	Anxiety	( )	Depression	( )	Oscillation of humor	( )
Affliction	( )	Anguish	( )	Concern	( )	____________	( )

23. Some of these feelings above are connected/related to your voice?

No ( ) Yes ( ) Which? ____________

24. Do you feel stressed with some of these factors listed below? (you may tick more than one)

		How are you affected?
Customer relationship	( )	____________
Relationships in business	( )	____________
Internal charges / goals	( )	____________
Health problems	( )	____________
Problems with voice	( )	____________

UNIVOZ

25. Do you practice any of these habits listed below? (you may tick more than one)

		Describe when, how often/many/much
Resting the voice	( )	______
Exercises for voice	( )	______
Shout out	( )	______
Speaking in noisy environment	( )	______
Consume water at work	( )	______
Consuming water out of work	( )	______
Consuming ice water	( )	______
Consuming coffee	( )	______
Consuming alcoholic beverage	( )	______
Bad eating habits	( )	______
Smoking	( )	How many/day? ______ How long? ______

Use this space for other comments that you think is important about the subjects of this questionnaire

______

______

DATA ___/___/______ Signature ______

Thank you for your attention and dedication in completing this questionnaire.

Protocol developed by SLP.Ms.Ana Elisa Moreira-Ferreira at Univoz, according to the structure of VHI. To use this questionnaire for work purposes or research is necessary permission of the author. Our contacts are in the page footer for those interested in. Thank you

APPENDIX 7–2

Self-Perception of Voice Impact on the Quality of Life and Performance in Call Centers®

Developed by Ana Elisa Moreira-Ferreira from Univoz

UNIVOZ

Self-Perception of Voice Impact on the Quality of Life and Performance in Call Centers®

Name:____Date:_____/______/_______

Considering that communication and voice are used as work tolls in call center, analyze the statements below and put a line around the frequency of your behavior, assigning the following value:

0 = Never
1 = Almost never
2 = Sometimes
3 = Almost always
4 = Always

1	I feel that I can't control myself and the tension while I speak to the client	0 1 2 3 4
2	The client notices that I'm nervous by the tone of my voice and the way I speak	0 1 2 3 4
3	I find it difficult to argue when the client is nervous	0 1 2 3 4
4	Selling situations or difficult waiting affect my voice	0 1 2 3 4
5	I feel tension in my voice when the client complaints	0 1 2 3 4
6	Professional goals affect my voice	0 1 2 3 4
7	I have to clear throat from the throat in difficult situations while I speak to the client	0 1 2 3 4
8	I feel my throat narrowing when communication becomes tenser	0 1 2 3 4
9	Uneasy feelings in my voice or throat arise during the waiting	0 1 2 3 4
10	My voice becomes rough at the end of difficult callings	0 1 2 3 4
11	My voice changes or I feel tired of speaking at the end of the day	0 1 2 3 4
12	The voice changes refrain or damage my work	0 1 2 3 4
13	My communication problem raises objections while dealing with the client	0 1 2 3 4
14	My communication problem restrains my performance	0 1 2 3 4
15	My communication problem causes me economic loss	0 1 2 3 4
16	I feel that I'm in disadvantage at work due to the way I talk	0 1 2 3 4
17	I think the clients notice my communication problem	0 1 2 3 4
18	Clients complain that they can't hear me or that they can't understand what I say	0 1 2 3 4
19	I grow angry or upset when clients or supervisors say something about my voice	0 1 2 3 4
20	I get feedbacks from monitoring to better express emotion in my voice	0 1 2 3 4
21	I recognize that I lack "smiling" in my voice	0 1 2 3 4
22	My voice doesn't express the required emotion/attitude to deal with the client	0 1 2 3 4

Is there any further information you'd like to report about your voice and communication skills?

____

____

APPENDIX 7–3

Self-Perception of Teleservice Communication (SPTC®)

Developed by Ana Elisa Moreira-Ferreira from Univoz

UNIVOZ

Self-Perception of Teleservice Communication – SPTC®

Name:____________________________________Date:____/_____/______

Answer the questions bellow considering your perceptions about in teleservice communication. Consider "0" for "totally disagree" and "5" for "totally agree".

1. My voice combines with the company I represent	0 1 2 3 4 5
2. My voice combines with the product and service that represented	0 1 2 3 4 5
3. My voice well represents my personality	0 1 2 3 4 5
4 My voice is related to my physical structure	0 1 2 3 4 5
5 My voice is suitable for customer relationship	0 1 2 3 4 5
6 I can convey the appropriate emotion for the moment by my voice	0 1 2 3 4 5
7 Through my voice, I can convince the customer	0 1 2 3 4 5
8 I use my voice to calm the customer	0 1 2 3 4 5
9 I convey credibility and security when I speak in attendance	0 1 2 3 4 5
10 I convey calm and patience when I talk to the customer	0 1 2 3 4 5
11 I am able to control my voice when I'm nervous about the customer	0 1 2 3 4 5
12 I speak clearly and articulating all sounds	0 1 2 3 4 5
13 The speed of my speech is adequate to the calls	0 1 2 3 4 5
14 The client can fully understand what I say	0 1 2 3 4 5
15 The intensity of my voice is suited to phone	0 1 2 3 4 5
16 I have adequate vocabulary for service	0 1 2 3 4 5
17 I pay attention to language support/informal words and try to avoid them	0 1 2 3 4 5
18 I formulate objectively sentences and clear to guide the client	0 1 2 3 4 5
19 My explanations about the products and services are convincing	0 1 2 3 4 5
20 I have strong arguments to guide the customer	0 1 2 3 4 5
21 I think I have an expressiveness communication	0 1 2 3 4 5

Is there any further information you'd like to report about your voice and communication skills?

____

____

Protocol developed by SLP.Ms.Ana Elisa Moreira-Ferreira at Univoz, according to the structure of VHI.
To use this questionnaire for work purposes or research is necessary permission of the author.
Our contacts are in the page footer for those interested in. Thank you.

UNIVOZ – Organizational and Occupational Speech-Language Pathology Company

(55 11) 3262-2009 - ana.elisa@univoz.com.br - www.univoz.com.br

SECTION V

Practices and Outcomes of an Expert From North America

CHAPTER 8

Speaking From the Soul: Theatre Voice and Text Work for Clergy

Kate Burke

Introduction

Clergy of any denomination must be excellent communicators. Conventional public speaking training and seminary homiletics courses do not provide the targeted training that creates powerful preachers. Theatre voice and text training, rather, provide professional training that prepares clergy for their work, in the same way that it equips actors to tell stories with power and imagination, cultivate effortless, clear, resonant, flowing voices that fill large spaces, and reach listeners with a compelling message. Clergy need these gifts as much or more than actors on the stage, if their aim is to proclaim God's Word and speak from the soul.

Clergy Population Served

This chapter is written from the Christian perspective, which dominates in the United States. Catholicism/Christianity, Islam, and Hinduism constitute the three leading faith denominations worldwide. While excellent communication skills are required of clergy regardless of church affiliation, such skills are also crucial for all who minister to a congregation, including deacons, lectors, leaders of scripture study, religious educators of young people, choir directors, and community liaisons.

"The United States has a greater number of religious groups than any other country in the world" ("U.S. religious groups," n.d., para. 2). A quick demographic sketch of the Baptist and Episcopal denominations bears this out. The 2009 U.S. Religious Landscape survey found that Baptists represent the largest denominational family in the United States, making up about one-sixth (17%) of the total U.S. adult population. (Survey conducted by the Pew Trust, www.pewforum.org). The Baptist World Alliance reports that 235 "member bodies" exist in 122 countries spanning Africa, the Asia Pacific, the Caribbean, Central America, Europe, North America and South America. (http://www.bwanet.org). The Episcopal church is also an international one, with 7,000 churches worldwide, 11 seminaries ("Episcopal Church," n.d.), and over 131 institutions of higher learning which are registered members of Colleges and Universities of the Anglican Communion ("CUAC," n.d., para. 2). The author has worked with clergy from the following traditions: Baptist, Episcopal, Catholic, Presbyterian, Methodist, and

Church of Christ. Rabbis and "presidents" of Latter Day Saints churches (called "stakes") have also participated, as have atheists engaged in contemplative practice.

What Clergy Do

The Reverend Mary Jo Smiley heard a young Reverend Martin Luther King, Jr. speak at the Dexter Avenue Baptist Church. " . . . there's a difference between a preacher [and] a minster . . . ML had a control of words . . . you sat there awed. You understood every word . . . And you felt as if he was speaking directly to you" (Smiley, 2006).

Today's clergy stand on the shoulders of giants, even as they face the challenge of preaching in a postmodern world. "Priests today have to compete with a digital media culture where sound bites, tweets and social media updates are the currency of communication," according to John Gering, Catholic program director at the Washington-based advocacy group Faith in Public Life (Montemurri, 2015).

Priests, ministers, rabbis, and imams must proclaim spiritual truths and lead believers. They lead by preaching. Their preaching defines them. Preaching is the single, overarching ministerial act that reaches large numbers of people (often in very large spaces) and makes individuals feel part of a faith community. Those who preach take on the role of messenger for a divine, all-knowing, all-loving being who dignifies life on earth and offers salvation and eternal life to believers, and who lays down the law—a tall order.

In Rome on April 26, 2015, Roman Catholic Pope Francis leveled with a group of newly ordained seminarians, exhorting them not to give boring sermons. Catholic Online reported the full quotation: "Let this be the nourishment of God, that your sermons are not boring, that your homilies reach people's hearts because they come from your hearts, because what you say to them is what you carry in your heart" (Ramos, 2015). If conventional public speaking training and homiletics are the answer, why do most preachers bore their congregations? Why don't they speak from their hearts? Why don't they voice their souls?

Traditional Clergy Training

Conventional clergy training may include a brief brush with public speaking techniques and generally does include a single course in homiletics. An online search of the term *public speaking* conjures thousands of resources designed to improve breathing, clarity, voice projection, and delivery, tools that, though helpful, fall far short of accessing the heart or the soul. "Homiletics," the primary training method for preaching, refers to work that equips clergy to discern, research, and structure a sermon, but not how to communicate it. Even at top flight seminaries a single homiletics course may help tyros prepare a sermon, but, again, not communicate it. In some cases, a single unit on voice and delivery is tacked onto the end of a homiletics course syllabus. Public speaking, though given a nod, is clearly seen as a skill divorced from the content and message it is meant to enhance, referred to on some online preaching resources as "mere" or "secular."

Paradigm Shift in Clergy Training

Richard F. Ward, the Fred B. Craddock Professor of Homiletics and Worship at Tulsa's Phillips Theological Seminary, writes that "the discipline of homiletics is undergoing a radical transformation" (Ward, 1996). Such change is crucial, because the "topical/conceptual" approach to preaching is "critically, if not terminally ill" (Eslinger, 1987, p. 11). Rev. Joseph Byrd's description of a "deductive" sermon illustrates this dry formula: "The major points of the sermon should be developed after the topic has been chosen . . . These major points . . . logically support the proposition . . . The conclusion should summarize the proposition . . . " (Byrd, 1992, pp. 155–156). "Most communication scholars have declared this 'conveyer belt' approach to be 'dead'" (Conquergood, 1983, p. 26), giving rise to a new style of sermon that consists, rather, of "voices, images, ideas, and interpretations woven into some definitive design for speaking" (Ward, 1996).

Aspiring clergy who have not been nourished by the meat-and-potatoes practical tools that are needed to speak from the soul, who have been served only bread-and-water public speaking techniques or pie-in-the-sky homiletics training, can take heart. Ward (1992), having noted the overdue shift in preaching practice, points to visionary training grounded in performance studies theory and best practices in theatre performance, transcending both homiletics and public speaking:

> Preaching is a performance of the sermon, that is, a vocal and physical action through which the form of the sermon becomes sound and image. The sermon becomes transformed from something which is encoded in print on a page into an oral-aural event for both preacher and hearer. (p. 77)

Ward acknowledges that the popular perception of "performance" must be redeemed, citing unsavory descriptors such as "melodramatic, theatrical, stagey, playacting" (Ward, 1992, p. 76). "Star turn," "chew the scenery," and "make a scene" are no more positive. Dwight Conquergood dignifies theatre arts with his view of humankind as "*homo histrio* . . . performing creatures who constitute and sustain their identities and collectively enact their worlds through roles and rituals" (Conquergood, 1983, p. 27). Anthropologist Victor Turner agrees, with his view of humankind as "*homo performans*" (Turner, 1987, p. 12).

According to Childers (1998),

> Preaching and the arts have been making a long slow move in each other's direction . . . Seminaries began to see the value of teaching 'drama skills' to their students. . . . W.J. Beeners . . . of Princeton Theological Seminary . . . began hiring actors from the New York Stage . . . Wayne Rood directed plays at the Pacific School of Religion . . . In New York, Union Theological Seminary hired the accomplished actor Robert Seaver to work with its budding preachers. (p. 10)

Experiential Theatre Voice and Speech Training

> Voice and speech training is a key element of theatre training. Actors must know how to use their voices in many different ways . . . without hurting themselves. They must also be able to express themselves and communicate their thoughts, feelings and emotions through their voice. For most people this requires training. (Verdolini, 1998, p. 60)

"Why is this relevant to people who are not in theatre? Because the material and techniques taught in theatre classrooms are, actually, applicable to anyone who uses her/his voice" (Verdolini, 1998, p. 60). Clergy are an obvious example of voice users who benefit from this approach.

With experiential, hands-on theatre voice training,

> [S]tudents are often able to discover truths about their voice and how to use it through guided explorations, rather than being told what to do. These explorations usually involve attention to physical, sensory information. Increasing awareness of physical sensation is a good tool for actors to learn to focus on the present, and also has the benefit of keeping the analytic mind from interfering with learning a vocal skill. (Verdolini, 1998, pp. 60–61)

The work of the late theatre voice trainer Arthur Lessac, the first to develop and codify experiential training, looms large in these pages, but contemporary creators of other training methods may also find a good home in the therapeutic setting. Whatever the approach, each theatre voice training method and every theatre voice practitioner should be grounded in universal vocal concepts and practices and should remain focused on the client. A seeker is in safe hands with a qualified, experienced trainer. The Voice and Speech Trainers Association's (VASTA, Inc.) maintains on its website (https://www.vasta.org/) an index of professional trainers, alphabetized and arranged by country and state. VASTA, Inc. is a 30-year-old, nonprofit, volunteer-driven, international organization dedicated to serving the needs of the voice and speech profession and to developing the art and science of the human voice.

Theatre Voice Training for Clergy

While Ward and other visionaries who attest to a paradigm shift in clergy preparation have provided persuasive theory underpinning the need for a performance perspective, and suggested useful strategies, the final, crucial pieces of the puzzle wait in the wings: (a) the exploration of the speaking voice in a coherent progression of theatre voice techniques and (b) the exploration of scriptural text in a sequence of theatre text work.

Schneider and Sataloff recommend a team approach to professional voice use. A prominent member of that team is the acting-voice teacher who has two roles. First, to advocate for the repossession of each speaking voice and its unique acoustical timbre and, second, to offer "a means of releasing the words from a text into a lively and expressive form of speech . . . an experience involving not simply the isolation of themes or extraction of ideas but also the engagement of the senses" (Ward, 2001, p. 61). The theatre voice trainer delivers this work in private lessons, a workshop, a course, or a seminar, which can all benefit clergy in different ways, while accommodating schedules and learning styles.

In direct response to Pope Francis's warning about boring sermons, the innovative Sacred Heart Major Seminary in Detroit, Michigan, invites Henry Ford College acting teachers Arthur Beer and Mary Bremer-Beer to conduct 3-week "Preaching Boot Camps" for seminarians (Montemurri, 2015). Participants do physical stretches, hold candles while exhaling slowly (to avoid blowing them out), try tongue twisters, write and deliver speeches about their mothers *to* their mothers, and memorize and deliver theatrical monologues with religious themes.

The False Voice

Why must the speaking voice be repossessed? Humans are born with wondrous speaking voices, fine instruments, and we play them, cooing in our cribs, demanding our needs be met with piercing shrieks and convulsive sobs, and flouting grammar to create breathtaking oral poetry. "Language is a complex, specialized skill, which develops in the child spontaneously, without conscious effort or formal instruction, is deployed without awareness of its underlying logic, [and] is qualitatively the same in every individual" (Pinker, 1994, p. 18). Pinker calls language an "instinct," implying that "people know how to talk, in more or less the sense that spiders know how to spin webs" (Pinker, 1994, p. 18). Where does it all go? Into the unconscious vice grip of habit, according to renowned British voice trainer Patsy Rodenburg: "As life and its pressures infiltrate the infant and then the child, habits grow and take control. The natural voice begins to slip away and is only sometimes rediscovered and remembered in heightened moments" (Rodenburg, 1992, p. 23). "A lifetime of habits can constrict the voice in a way that decreases its flexibility and strength. These constricting habits can come from a variety of sources, be they physical, emotional or even psychological" (Verdolini, 1998, p. 60). Cynthia Bourgeault, Episcopal priest, author, and mystic, maintains that "each of us, in response to perceived threats to our well-being, develops a false self: a set of protective behaviors driven at root by a sense of need and lack" (Bourgeault, 2004, p. 94). Whatever the cause, the free, authentic, and responsive voice flees, leaving the imposter, the false voice, in its place.

Lessac Training Theory: Resonant Voice Therapy

Arthur Lessac's highly developed training system, a "gestalt," is much more than a single training technique, but it is related to Resonant Voice Therapy (RVT). The goal of RVT is "to achieve the strongest, 'cleanest,' possible voice with the least effort and impact between the vocal folds . . . In speech-language pathology, preeminent therapists including Dr. Daniel Boone and Dr. Morton Cooper emphasize 'resonant voice,' sometimes called 'forward focus'" (Verdolini, 1998, p. 34).

In 1960 master voice trainer Arthur Lessac published the first edition of his landmark text *The use and training of the human voice: A biodynamic approach to vocal life.* The work has been used worldwide by theatre voice trainers and SLPs ever since. Lessac's

> approach to voice and speech is . . . based on three concepts: "Tonal action," "Structural action," and "Consonant action." Tonal action refers to resonant voice production, facilitated by what he calls the "Y-buzz." Structural action refers to an inverted megaphone facial posture, that extends to the pharynx and hypopharynx, and may partially account for a slight vocal fold abduction noted in some videoscopic examinations of the larynx. Consonant action . . . refers to the treatment of consonants as instruments in an orchestra, for clean articulation and intelligibility . . . (Verdolini, 1994, p. 14)

Lessac used the spelling "NRG" rather than "energy" and held the view that "our speech and our speaking voice should always be fueled, fed, and supported by an emotivated trinity of NRG qualities: consonant NRG, tonal NRG, and structural NRG" (Lessac, 1997, p. 176). He recommended using "the vocal NRGs as a trinity-NRG experience—as if the consonant, tonal and structural NRGs were moving and functioning arm in arm" (Lessac, 1997, p. 206). Lessac created a series of text explorations designed to identify the optimal, spoken, dynamic opportunities of each NRG. He suggested exploring text by "leading" with each NRG and, finally, switching among the NRGs in a free, spontaneous response to dynamics in the text, a response that varies each time the text is spoken.

The average person attributes acoustics to architecture, assuming that buildings are the only resonating chambers. Lessac investigated human acoustics and the internal, kinesthetic perception of vocal sound waves:

> Vibrating, bony sections of the hard palate, teeth, facial mask and head set up direct and sympathetic vibrations that amplify vocal sounds . . . When your voice functions solely as an inner vibrating current, never pushed and never impeded, you will experience it as a bone-conducted, vibrating feeling . . . that stimulates, energizes and relaxes . . . that transmits its bone-conducted vibrations to the farthest row and corners of the theatre or concert hall. (Lessac, 1997, p. 124)

How liberating to be freed from the microphone as the ultimate means of projection, trusting that the natural amplification system, the bones, will do the work, freeing the proclaimer to look up and out to connect with the congregation.

Consonant sounds are the shapers of vowel sounds, and in an imaginative leap beyond boilerplate, crisp diction, Lessac created the "consonant orchestra," assigning each of the 24 consonant sounds of spoken English to an instrument with similar pitch range, tone color, and action. Consonant sounds become strings, brass, woodwinds, drums, cymbals, whistles, wind machines, and sound effects. Lessac suggests that the speaker:

> Learn the action of each simulated musical instrument and the sensation of that action–this is the actual playing of the instrument, and it is always something that can be physically felt. This instrumental approach is guided by the same principles that guide the musician: when he plays his instrument he does not force, pound, scrape, squeeze, push or tighten . . . Once you learn how to produce the feel of the orchestral consonants, you can focus your attention on playing them lightly, softly, smoothly–musically. (Lessac, 1997, pp. 68–69)

"Structural NRG, Lessac's third vocal NRG, refers to the mold, shape, and size of the human voice and speech instrument and its sound-box structure" (Lessac, 1997, p. 160). This "reverse-megaphone shape" sound-box structure (Lessac, 1997, p. 160) remedies the lateral, tight-lipped speaking habit most adult speakers settle into, which inhibits speech and places it in the back of the mouth and throat, rather than in the front of the mouth and facial mask. Structural NRG relies on a yawn sensation or "yawn energy" to promote a larger oral sound box and optimal, forward "facial posture," allowing vowel sounds room to resonate and magnify. Lips are free to reach forward without tension to create rounded lip shapes that give vowel sounds a visible form and signature. The structural NRG dynamic is arguably the subtlest of Lessac's trinity of NRGs and the hardest to grasp, but the most liberating when mastered. Tonal NRG depends on structural NRG. "Vocal bone resonance without proper form of the oral cavity becomes tinny, shrill and strident" (Lessac, 1997, p. 14).

Lessac's work features so prominently here because in over 40 years of voice training the author has witnessed the work's positive and profound effects on thousands of voices. Lessac de-mystified the production of the human voice in a clear system that allows the speaker to explore, identify, feel, evaluate, and participate in his or her own speaking. He invites every speaker to the feast in his Chapter 2 heading: "Don't envy a good voice . . . You have one!" (Lessac, 1997, p. 9).

How Does Lessac Training Technique Work?

> RV (Resonant Voice) . . . usually refers to *easy* voice associated with *vibratory sensations* in the facial bones. In the Lessac approach, the consonant "y" and nasal consonants ("m," "n," and "ng") are used to facilitate training of this vibratory "resonance." Cooper's

approach utilizes the utterance "m-hmmm" during conversation as a guide post for resonant voice during ongoing speech. (Verdolini, 1998, p. 34)

A study was undertaken

> [T]o test the hypothesis that resonant voice is produced by narrowing the laryngeal vestibule and is characterized by first formant tuning and more ample harmonics . . . Spectral analysis showed that first formant tuning was exhibited during resonant voice productions and that the degree of harmonic enhancement in the range of 2.0 to 3.5 kHz was related to voice quality: non-resonant voice had the least amount of energy in this range, whereas a resonant-relaxed voice had more energy, and a resonant-bright voice had the greatest amount of energy . . . (Smith, Finnegan, & Karnell, 2005)

An offshoot of Arthur Lessac's work is Lessac-Madsen Resonant Voice Therapy (LMRVT):

> LMRVT is unique in that it corrects both hypo- and hyperadducted vocal fold posturing by guiding vocal behavior toward barely-abducted or barely-adducted laryngeal posturing. A study led by Berry indicates that a barely ab/adducted glottal width of .6 mm produces maximum intraglottal pressure while minimizing impact stress to the vocal folds. (Seligmann, 2005, p. 1)

Individual Voice Training for Clergy

Many clergy find their way to theatre voice trainers via word of mouth. If an academic theatre department is within range, clergy sometimes contact that department about training. The author does not advertise services, but clergy who attend the New Lectio Divina sessions described below sometimes request private lessons.

A preliminary meeting with a client gives the trainer evidence of the speaking voice in action and allows for discussion of training goals and expectations. The author listens for breathing, voice placement, the articulation of the 24 English language consonant sounds, the formation and differentiation of parent and neutral vowel sounds, and vocal flow unimpeded by glottal shocks or vocal fry. Training goals once set, a sequence of areas is explored in weekly, hour-long sessions.

The first session begins with a simple warm-up of the body focused on the key area between the base of the nose to just below the shoulders, where muscle tensions manifest. Exercises include a pendulum, side-to-side head swing, a side-to-side looking across an imaginary line on the horizon, a back-of-the-neck stretch, shoulder circles with lip trills, and alternating shoulder circles with tongue tip trills. These are followed by a series of lung vacuums, an actor training exercise of unknown origin. Breath is blown briskly out the mouth, residual air is released in a quick "sh" sound, the mouth is closed, and the nose is held shut while the elbows are raised. After a 10-second wait, the nose is released, the mouth is opened, and a deep, involuntary breath fills the lungs. Warm-up concludes with a gentle yet brisk shaking of the head and face while emitting free-form sound and then a hummed "m."

In a second session the author begins resonance work, using the "m" sound to localize the sensation of vibration and awaken the speaker's kinesthetic sensation of vocal sound waves in the bones of the face and head. The "m" sound is hummed, then sirened in pitch. When comfortable with sustaining the sound, the client is asked to gently press the tragi over the ear openings so the "m" is a felt, inner sensation rather than an external emanation. Most clients are stunned by the effortless magnitude of the vibration. Next, an "m" sound is sustained in a hypernasal, twang focus, which is then transitioned into a balanced, forward focus. Last is the "shaking scale of 'm,'" an exercise created by the author, in which the client hums an "m" sound, gradually rising and then descending in a half-tone scale, gently shaking a different area of the body with each pitch change.

Subsequent sessions are devoted to (a) discovery and refinement of Lessac's "y-buzz," [the long "e" vowel sound, more forwardly placed than the "m" sound]; (b) opening of the mouth, not by dropping the jaw, but by activating the *levator labii superioris* and zygomatic muscles and rounding the lips forward [Lessac's yawned structural action]; (c) cork-in-mouth exploration of Lessac's 10 structure vowel sounds [as in the words "ooze, ode, all, oil, odd, alms, ounce, add, I'd, earth"]; (d) introduction of Lessac's consonant orchestra, including sustainable consonants [n, m, v, z, zh, voiced th, ng, l, s, f, sh and unvoiced th] and tappable consonants [d, t, b, p, g, k, dg, ch, dz, ts, the combination sounds dl and tl]; and (e) free-form exploring of each individual sound which includes [for sustainable consonants] sirening on varied pitch patterns, singing legato melodies in each, creating spontaneous jazz-like improvisations based on a single sound or combinations, and [for tappable consonants] creating percussion solos on each sound or combinations. In each case movement is encouraged to embody the felt sense of a given sound.

Training relies on multiple repetitions and kinesthetic perceptions of the y-buzz, vowel sounds, and consonant sounds and the location and appreciation of the tension-free, fine motor movements involved in producing these sounds: the subtle forward stretching of cheek muscles, the effortless lift of the soft palate in a yawn sensation, the relaxed forward rounding of the lips, the firm but relaxed contact of the tongue tip on the alveolar ridge, and the relaxed tongue resting behind the lower teeth. The trainer listens intently and suggests

Box 8–1

Fr. D.L., a member of the Dominican order, was posted to a Roman Catholic parish in Virginia in the 1990s. While an intelligent, educated, and compassionate priest, his preaching was the subject of complaints to the pastor, who referred Fr. D.L. to the author for training. Quickly apparent was Fr. D.'s tendency to pull his lips into a tense, lateral position. What he intended as a pleasant smile was in fact a rictus more off-putting than a frown. When asked to form and practice Lessac's warm-up sequence "woo, woe, war, wow," he felt keenly his inability to form the "w" sound in the lateral lip position. In repeating, and feeling, the relaxed forward facial posture of the w-word sequence, Fr. D. was able to cultivate and maintain a relaxed, semi-forward, neutral facial posture, between authentic smiles and the active production of the 10 structure vowels. (The author invited him to lightly rest his fingertips on his cheek muscles while speaking the "woo, woe, war, wow" sequence, and he isolated and identified the subtle forward movement of the muscles.) His face became more animated and audience directed, with an affect befitting his utterance, and his resonance intensified, infusing his preaching with warmth and energy.

physical adjustments and images that cultivate and reinforce a keen appreciation of the pleasurable tingling, itching, and vibration felt when vocal sound waves resonate in bone.

Clients are asked to engage in a few 5- to 10-minute exploration sessions each day, in a vocal "studio" that may be the car, the kitchen, or an empty football field, and they are asked to report on their practice at the start of the next session.

Evaluation and Outcomes of "Individual Clergy Training"

"Individual Clergy Training" is undertaken by the author not as therapy measured by scientific research, but as a ministry rooted in service, performed in addition to full-time, academic theatre voice training duties. Since Schneider and Sataloff advocate for a team approach to training professionals, welcoming the acting-voice teacher as an acknowledged and indispensable guest at the table, in this same inclusive spirit the author/theatre trainer offers some in-the-trenches reporting of outcomes with clergy.

Clergy learning to play the instruments of their voices find the exploration of the vibrating human voice to be an intriguing, rather than a remedial, process, although strong egos may need to be checked at the door. The active discovery of universal concepts and principles of voice function is enlightening and freeing: clergy buy into the logic of an economical yet constant outflow of breath that vibrates the vocal cords, producing waves of sound that move forward and up to resonate in the bones of the face and head. They begin to perceive that their vocal sound waves can be projected to congregations in the form of vowel and consonant sounds, that the bones of believers' ears receive the voiced sound waves and vibrate in sympathy, and that congregations feel as well as hear the "shepherd's" voice.

Most clergy are surprised to recognize in themselves habits that can impede the free-flowing voice, although some have experienced tell-tale hoarseness or voice loss. It is a revelation to them that anesthetizing and tense vocal habits stand in the way of bold annunciation, habits that undermine the finest seminary training, keeping the proclaimer/teacher/preacher from being "heard, understood and felt," a phrase spoken by theatre voice trainer Dudley Knight at a VASTA, Inc. conference session.

Accordingly, the most representative outcome of Individual Clergy Training, is the clergy's satisfaction with achieving their goal of bringing the Word of God to life.

Another way of capturing outcomes of the Individual Clergy Training program is through the use of imagery. In *Body Wisdom* Lessac describes the functionality of images in physical training, proposing that "Any conversion or transformation process will . . . hire an image to do the job" (Lessac, 1978, pp. 73–74). The author proposes that clients also hire images to express the felt experience of their own voices, and that such images mark a crucial turning point in the learning process, demonstrating ownership of what has been learned.

Speech pathologist Joanna Cazden addressed the use of images guardedly at the 2005 ASHA convention, presenting on "Imagery in Voice Therapy: Neurolinguistic Rationales and Clinical Guidelines." Cazden proposed that imagery is "not factually accurate, not precise, non-scientific and therefore inferior, but, perhaps, useful anyway. Imagery can describe a desired physiology in a subjective, sensory way, a useful, jargon-free way that may even help clarify a practitioner's own ideas" (Cazden, 2009).

Imagery and metaphor are recognized and respected as traditional components of theatre voice training. Theatre trainers use images to guide speakers to unfamiliar sound placements and varied vocal qualities. Speakers use images to achieve gravity-defying placement of sound, and speakers use language images (read similes and metaphors) to signal and celebrate a vocal sea change, to confirm that a basic training gesture (i.e., Lessac's y-buzz or the chanting of a line of text) has been internalized, felt, and used on the *speaker's* terms. Cazden refers only briefly to images from the speaker's perspective, saying that "imagery offered by the patient is often useful, as a label for new behavior, even if not a precise descriptor, but not a substitute for repetition of new behaviors, for secure motor learning." Plainly, an artful, fresh naming of experience is a signpost, not journey's end. At the outset of training clients' parroting of training vocabulary, a rebounding of terms retained, though dutiful, is a welcome good faith effort. Later in the process, however, images, like tennis serves deftly returned or jazz musician's solo riffs and spins, outstrip good faith effort and become qualitative measurement. Trainers must flag and deploy such images, using them to coach clients on to subsequent vocal discoveries and the fresh images they elicit.

In addition to the feedback testimonials and the use of imagery, five parameters are used by the author to describe the physical outcomes of the Individual Clergy Training Program, evaluating these parameters before and after the completion of the program:

1. consistent forward vocal focus: evaluated by the ability to support sound to the ends of phrases and sentences (poor = limited support, fair = moderate support, good = relatively consistent support, excellent = consistent support);
2. improved articulation: evaluated by use of tapped and sustained consonant sounds

Box 8–2

The following are examples of images used by those receiving Lessac training from the author as well as from other trainers:

Resonance . . . feels like heaven . . . an internal vibration bubbling up from its true source.

. . . resonance in the head makes me think of myself as a monk in a vast, open monastery

My head is a gong.

This clear "EEEEEEEEE" felt like pulling a flower out of the mud by its stem.

The sound I made today came from a bear with a megaphone in (his) liver.

It has this Tibetan monk quality . . . the chant seems to align your body, mind and spirit (and this from a cynic).

Resonance feels like a feather moving back and forth really fast and hard . . .

It's like sliding your sound onto a different shelf, but doing so in the dark.

I . . . had the idea of kissing each word with a baby kiss . . .

I like the [long "o"]. It rushes out of my mouth and hurtles unchecked into the atmosphere.

My voice is a moody anemone . . .

The vibrations send . . . my spirit soaring through a window.

. . . my throat felt like an unclogged drain

. . . my voice no longer cowers behind my uvula . . . .

. . . voice . . . more or less releases the volcano that churns inside all of us.

in speech (poor = some use of initial consonant sounds, fair = some use of initial and medial consonant sounds in speech exercises, good = use of initial, medial and some final consonant sounds when reading aloud, excellent = use of initial, medial and final consonant sounds in all three positions while speaking spontaneously, doing speech exercises, reading aloud and speaking in public);
3. release of tension and relaxation: evaluated by degree of visible muscle tightening, shallow or effortful breathing, and posture (poor = torso tension, mouth breathing, leading with raised chin, fair = some torso flexibility, some nose breathing, moderately raised chin , good = flexible, relaxed torso, equal mix of nose and mouth breathing, excellent = free, energized torso, effortless, efficient, integrated nose and mouth breath, energized elongation of the upper spinal vertebrae); and
4. improved fullness and projection of voice evaluated by ability to reach all listeners in spaces of various sizes (poor = audible in an office setting with some laryngeal strain or breathiness, fair = audible in a classroom with some back placement and minimal consonants, good = audible in a large meeting room with consistent bone resonance and clear consonant sounds, excellent = filling a large ballroom or theatre space with unamplified, bravura resonance and onomatopoeic consonant sounds).

Between 2000 and 2016 the author provided Individual Clergy Training for five clergy from four denominations, between the ages of 28 and 52, including one woman. Training was provided once a week for various time spans, ranging from 3 to 12 weeks. Each session lasted 60 minutes. The program covered the steps described in the section "Individual Voice Training for Clergy," sufficient sessions permitting. Individual training was provided in the author's office and various performance spaces in the University of Virginia Drama Building. By the completion of training, all five clergy reported satisfaction with their training. The author's evaluation revealed that all five improved in consistent, forward vocal focus, three improved in articulation, and in release of tension and relaxation. On the other hand, only two improved in fullness of voice and projection.

The female minister who was trained is an intense introvert. Her full, released voice sounded very loud to her, and she was not able to commit to it. Two other trainees were not able to marshal the confidence required to raise the speaking voice in large spaces. Personality traits can limit the scope of training.

Words in Theatre, Worship, and Life

> Needing words and connecting with them should involve our intellects, our emotions and our very souls . . . The right to speak coupled with the need for words taps into all parts of our mind, body and spirit . . . bubbles up through our voice, until finally, with a sense of relief and release, the words escape us by means of articulation . . . the ancient Greeks and Romans recognized that speaking is a sacred and dangerous act . . . Rituals and prayers are remnants of the word's sacred function as a direct influence over events, a direct communication with something beyond us. (Rodenburg, 1993, pp. 4–8)

It is hard not to overstate the power of speaking scripture *aloud*. There is no substitute for the physical, embodied act of bringing words to life by speaking them. The act of speaking is physical (though not an overt flailing of limbs)—facial and torso muscles are engaged in the process, and the palpable sensation of the acoustical voice unites both speaker and the listener in sympathetic frequency. Such vibration gives words an embodied immediacy, chiming multiple meanings, images, and free associations and inciting physiological reactions such as trembling, deeper breath, temperature swings, goose bumps, tingling, itching, hair standing on end, sweating, "elevator stomach," flowing tears, or laughter. Such reactions are authentic responses to words (and their freight), not forced outward signs of generalized emotion. The physicality, or embodiment, of words transforms speaking into proclaiming, an act which we humans reserve for only the most profound and powerful messages, and no message is more powerful than the Word of God to the ears of devout believers.

The Bible is not only a source of doctrine, but also "a source of story and vision" (Frye, 1991, p. 3). The Bible, while superb literature, is an ancient book. Yet it is timeless.

> . . . text lingers over time in available ways. Out of that lingering, however, . . . words . . . erupt into new usage . . . In that moment of re-utterance, the present is freshly illuminated, reality is irreversibly transformed . . . What has been tradition . . . becomes available experience. In the moment of speaking and hearing, this treasured tradition now becomes present experience, inimitable, without parallel, irreversible. In that utterance, the word does lead reality. (Breuggeman, 1999, p. 1)

In modern translations of the Bible certain passages, such as 1 Corinthians 13 ("If I speak in human or angelic tongues, but do not have love . . . ") are rendered as prose, when in the original text they were "formatted as a hymn, a poetic dance of imagery and language, emotion and linear instruction" (Thompson, 2010, p. 244).

> By activating our sense of rhythm, poetry accesses our right-mode operations and systems. Reading poetry has the effect of catching us off guard. Our imaginations are invigorated when our usual linear expectations of prose . . . don't apply . . . poetry not only appeals to right-mode processing, but to left mode as well, given its use of language. This makes it a powerful integrative tool. (Thompson, 2010, p. 150)

> The moment of speech is a poetic rendering in a community that has come all too often to expect nothing but prose. It is a prose world for all those who must meet payrolls and grade papers and pump gas and fly planes. When the text, too, has been reduced to prose, life becomes so prosaic that . . . a dread dullness besets the human spirit . . . The speaker must truly be a poet. After the scientist and the engineer, finally comes the poet . . . to evoke a different world, a new song, a fresh move, a new identity, a resolve about ethics, a being at home. (Brueggemann, 1989, pp. 9–10)

Given the need for preacher-poets, how can minds and hearts be trained to communicate sacred text with brio? This can happen with theatre text work, which can achieve palpable results in a single session, compared to the repeated sessions required in the Individual Clergy Training process.

Theatre Text Work

General Concept

A graduate student in a Master of Fine Arts Acting Program asked recently, "What *is* text work?" Simply put, text work translates "words on the page into living speech" (R. F. Ward, personal communication, October 7, 2016).

Cicely Berry, Voice Director with Britain's Royal Shakespeare Company, pioneered theatre text work. Patsy Rodenburg, her protégé and now a noted theatre voice trainer, acknowledges Berry's vision; "No one in voice work today can deny the immense contribution that Cicely Berry has made. Almost single-handedly she has made the work both respectable and exciting . . . Now all of us . . . can . . . help people . . . acquire those vocal rights which will change them forever" (Rodenburg, 1992, p. xiii).

Theatre Text Work for Clergy

Development

In the summer of 1993, the author was introduced to RSC text work in an intensive workshop with Berry, and (then) Head of Voice at the RSC, Andrew Wade. In 2000 the author spent a sabbatical leave in Stratford-upon-Avon working with Wade. Witnessing text work in a range of settings and traveling with Wade to Wales, Scotland, Sweden, and India to assist with intensive workshops revealed the scope of text work developed and delivered by the RSC Voice Department to thousands of actors appearing in hundreds of plays over a span of decades. The practical text work revolutionized this author's theatre production coaching and theatre teaching, but a deeper application of the work was to be revealed.

When asked to offer two intensive, day-long voice and preaching workshops to Baptist clergy, the author received a clear call to apply text work to scripture. Clergy were guided through explorations of an extended passage from Ephesians, an unalloyed paean of ecstatic praise and thanksgiving: "God is above every name that is named, not only in this age but also in the age to come . . . " At one point both the ordained participants and the author were struck dumb by the profound words; the physical act of speaking them seemed to forge a direct connection to God. One minister asked "What was *that*?" The author had neither a logical nor a scientific response.

Lectio Divina ["Divine Reading"] (LD)

Traditional *Lectio Divina* (TLD)

"*Lectio Divina*, defined historically . . . is the manner of reading ecclesial texts developed and practiced in Benedictine monasteries" (Casey, 1996, p. vii). " . . . monks tended to read slowly, probably vocalizing the words as they read. Often significant passages would be committed to memory . . . favorite works would be re-read many times . . . " (Casey, 1996, p. 4). *Lectio Divina* is "a simple but comprehensive practice of praying the scripture that leads gradually but steadily from the mind to the heart" (Bourgeault, 2004, p. 65). The four steps of traditional LD are *Lectio, Meditatio*, *Oratio*, and *Contemplatio.*

> A good portion of the preacher's homiletical preparation should involve the ancient art of *lectio divina*. It is imperative . . . that the preacher hear the voice of Jesus himself before he begins to translate that same voice into the language of his post-modern hearers. The given pericope should be read [*Lectio*], meditated upon [*Meditatio*], prayed [*Oratio*] and contemplated [*Contemplatio*], and then read, meditated upon, prayed and contemplated again and again and again . . . the questions to be asking are these: What is Christ saying? What is he saying to me? What is he saying to my people? How can I say what Christ says in a way this post-modern world can "hear" today? (Genig, 2013)

New Lectio Divina (NLD)

NLD Description

Those practicing *New* Lectio Divina, mirroring the steps described above, "Read Aloud, Repeat, Respond, and Proclaim," as detailed below. The process of NLD innovates in that it relies on RSC text work techniques, but this process might be termed "*old* Lectio Divina," since the Desert Mothers/Fathers doubtless possessed only one copy of the Word, and a member of the community read aloud from that copy. Listeners received the Word via the ear, hearing it rather than seeing it in print, in a marked contrast to the modern practice of passive, silent reading (Figure 8–1).

New Lectio Divina (NLD) Training

A typical NLD session begins with participants standing in a circle. A group of less than five, or a senior group, sits. Standing participants are invited to engage in a Wolfson-Hart technique, simply stepping in and out of the circle. After a rhythm is established, the group is invited to proclaim their first names as they step in, and the entire group affirms each individual by echoing the name on the step out. Then the author points to each individual, and that person's name is again repeated by the group.

The ice broken, physical and vocal warm-up begin, followed by voice exercise rhymes such as, "What a to-do to fly today at a minute or two to two, a thing distinctly hard to say but harder still to do, for they'll beat a tattoo at a quarter to two . . . ." Warm-up concludes with a lip-awakening "Whether the weather be cold, whether the weather be hot, whether the weather be fine, whether the weather be not, we'll weather the weather, whatever the weather, whether we like it or not."

The group is now ready to encounter a scripture passage, either by reading it aloud together in the circle or alone walking around the space. The author then asks what stood out in the initial reading—whether a single

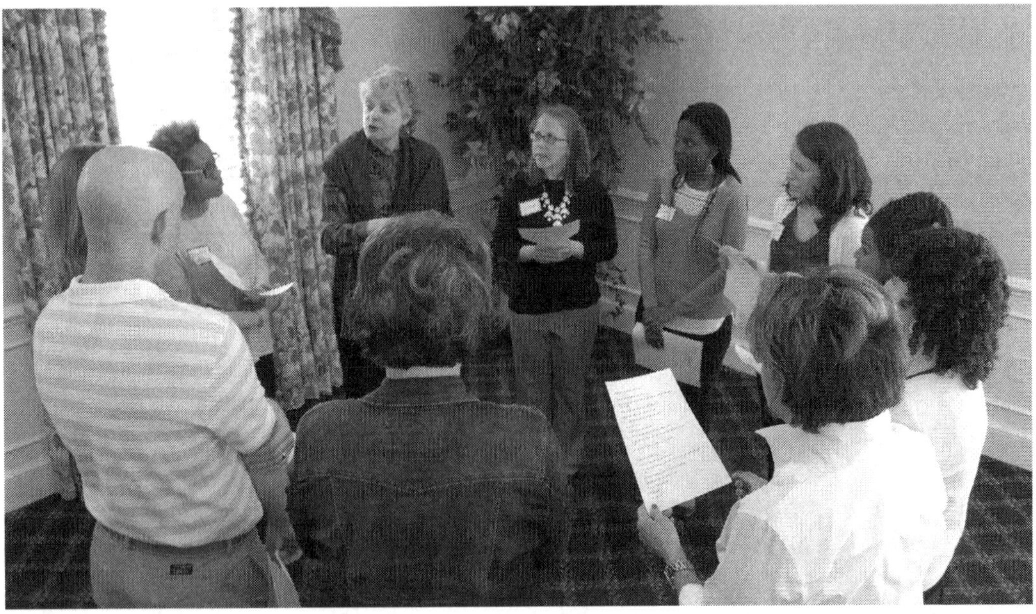

Figure 8–1. *New Lectio Divina session with clergy, Uptick program (premier development track for high-potential leaders offered by the Spence Network) Glenmore Country Club, Charlottesville, Virginia. (Photo credit: Laura McDaniel.)*

word or word sequence, a rhythm or rhyme, a thought, or a free association. Answers to these questions begin a verbal mapping of the text, as words and speech dynamics are singled out and come off the page, alive in time and space, as they are spoken. The text is then deconstructed and reconstructed as it is repeated aloud in many formats, until the action of the words is felt in the mouth. (Scores of text explorations could be done; an hour-and-a-half-session allows for 10 to 12.) Three examples reflect the mode of practice, in the voice of the session leader: read a text in two-word pairs, so that the previous word is repeated (In the . . . the beginning . . . beginning was . . . was the . . . the Word), etc.; read the entire passage aloud, inserting an affirmative "yes!" after key words (In the beginning, [yes!], the Word, [yes!], was made flesh, [yes!], etc., and then read the text without the inserted "yes!," to experience the intensified words as powerful storytelling prompts); on a single pitch chant at full voice through each phrase of the text, take a quick breath, and immediately speak the phrase to feel the residual vocal richness and flow from the chanting. Additional text explorations appear at http://www.NewLectioDivina.com (Burke, 2012). Also valuable is a visual marking of text with highlighters of two colors to reveal opposing dynamics (i.e., single- versus multisyllable words, positive versus negative words, subjects and verbs (primary versus secondary), and vowel and consonant sound opportunities).

An explored text is an owned text. Effortless articulation and projection serve up the words, not because speech skills are promoted by a trainer, but because mapped words "beg" to be spoken, heard, understood, and felt.

Individual clergy are then invited to read the passage. Each reader responds to the words uniquely, giving them a new-minted, three-dimensional quality. The session concludes with clergy processing their "text journey" and articulating take-away points from the experience (Figure 8–2).

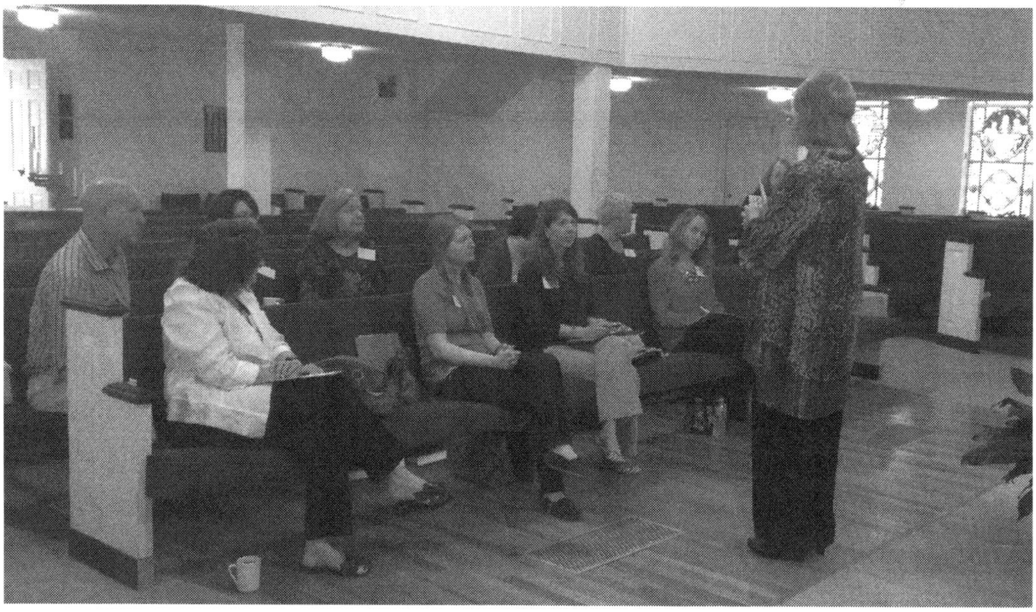

Figure 8–2. *New Lectio Divina session with clergy, Pumps in the Pulpit program, Crozet Baptist Church, Crozet, Virginia. (Photo credit: Laura McDaniel.)*

NLD Evaluation and Outcomes

The author concludes that the NLD program has achieved its goals when the following behaviors are observed in participants: deep and regular breathing, bodies that are more grounded and upright, eyes open wide and looking to other believers in the circle, faces soft, expressive and undefended, focused and intense listening, facial and gestural responses to words and phrases spoken by themselves and others. Clergy are more physically and vocally present, ironically, when connected to a metaphysical deity.

Outcomes are evaluated by clergy members' descriptive feedback regarding their NLD experience either in the form of spoken words at the conclusion of the session. That can be in the form of spoken words at the conclusion of the session or e-mailed testimonials after the fact. Testimonials usually include vivid similes, metaphors, and images. The author proposes this amended echo of Cazden's take on images: [Religion and faith] "are not factually accurate, not precise, non-historical, non-scientific and therefore inferior, but, perhaps, useful anyway." Clergy testimonials are featured on the author's NLD website and on brochures. Clergy reading testimonials from other clergy (whatever the denomination) might hear cues, clues, and connections not captured by scientists' quantitative measures.

Box 8–3 presents a range of testimonials from clergy describing their new found vocal and spiritual experience.

Patricia Raun refers to the product of theatre text work as "transformational identification" (Raun, 2009, p. 320).

Box 8–3

"I have watched Kate Burke lead groups in a masterful and even holy manner. Her comprehensive mastery of her field and her own spirit impart a kind of calm to participants. I am deeply impressed at how she enables even frequent readers of the Bible to experience the presence of God in the Scriptures in fresh and deep ways . . . " (Baptist minister)

"At a session I recently attended, Kate had the group recite nine scriptural verses . . . over and over again. At the beginning of the session we were merely reading the words, albeit with understanding. By the session's end, after employing Kate's simple but powerful techniques, we spoke these same words as if they had claimed us and we were called to proclaim them." (Rabbi)

"The Word came alive." (Deacon)

"Are hugs in order? You took me on a journey from my mind to my heart." (Church elder)

"As if someone walked into the room, unrolled a papyrus and read the text for the first time . . . An extraordinary spiraling down into true Christian unity." (Manager, Christian bookstore)

"I felt myself strangely and wonderfully stirred as I was reading Scripture after Friday's experience with you . . . now the experience is far richer and sometimes even physically moving as my body, mind and spirit all respond to the words . . . You have given me the impetus to speak the words aloud, to experience the sounds, silences, cadences unnoticed in silent reading." (Episcopal Priest)

> As a performer I believe that if I am not transformed by words, and if I do not lead my audiences to transformation, then I am not doing my job . . . I do not use the word "transformation" lightly. There is nothing quick or superficial about the experience . . . It is life changing . . . It is a physical, intellectual, and spiritual feeling of awakening. (Raun, 2009, p. 320)

" . . . Presbyterians wept, Episcopalians clapped, and academicians were speechless," wrote Jana Childers, Associate Professor of Homiletics at the San Francisco Theological Seminary, after hearing a sermon which altered her life and that of her faith community (Childers, 1998, p. 17). "I could not identify the crucial ingredient that made that sermon different from other effective sermons . . . I abandoned homiletical analysis . . . Apparently, the Holy Spirit is much more willing to be stirred up than I had previously believed . . . " (Childers, 1998, p. 17). "Call it passion, life, authenticity, naturalness, conviction, sincerity, or being animated. Call it fire, sparks, electricity, mojo, spiritual lava, or juice. It is what listeners want in a preacher" (Childers, 1998, p. 16).

Conclusion

Theatre voice trainers help clergy cultivate their speaking voices, but "to really train someone's voice we need to help them finish the process. We need to teach them how to enter a text. We need to lead them, through their own bodies and experiences and memories, to the shared space between them and the words they speak" (Raun, 2009, pp. 320–323).

One NLD veteran testified that "the opportunity to proclaim . . . to the group felt like a tremendous privilege. The ancient words of lament and hope—which have been chanted, sung, and proclaimed for millennia in hundreds of languages—had become at

Box 8–4

Maren, a Mennonite minister, first attended an NLD session in April 2009. "The text was from the book of Ephesians, focusing on a call to ministry, since it was a session for clergy. After a few voice warm-up exercises, we got to know each other's names and became comfortable with one another before we entered into an hour of various readings of the text.

Whether we read the whole text as a group, took turns with various lines or words, spoke them to one another or read the text aloud while walking around the room, the text took on its own life and began speaking straight to my heart. It came alive, took on different depth. The words leaped off the page and became 3-D.

I have since then attended and hosted numerous workshops. Something happens to me and my voice in these sessions. The various techniques and exercises get behind the walls in my mind, the walls my senses put up to hem me in, restricting me, inhibiting my speaking voice. New Lectio Divina allows my heart and soul to be vulnerable, to be touched directly by the Word that comes from God. My voice lets the words emerge from deep within and proclaims them with power, grace and clarity" (M. Hange, personal communication, October 1, 2016).

once personal and universal. I stepped out of the church sanctuary . . . with the words . . . reverberating inside my body" (Miska, 2014). Not only had this participant entered God's Word—God's Word had entered her.

References

Baptist Church United States. (n.d.). http://www.pewforum.org/files/2013/05/report-religious-landscape-study-full.pdf

Baptist Church Worldwide. (n.d.). https://www.bwanet.org/

Bourgeault, C. (2004). *Centering prayer and inner awakening*. Lanham, MD: Rowman and Littlefield.

Brueggeman, W. (1989). *Finally comes the poet*. Minneapolis, MN: Fortress Press.

Brueggeman, W. (1999). *Texts that linger, words that explode*. Minneapolis, MN: Fortress Press.

Burke, K. (2012). *Resources, the speaking voice, text work exercises*. Retrieved from http://www.newlectiodivina.com/

Byrd, J. (1992). Methods of preparation. In M. Duduit (Ed.), *Handbook of contemporary preaching* (pp. 155–156). Nashville, TN: Broadman & Holman.

Casey, M. (1996). *Sacred reading*. Liguori, MO: Liguori Publications.

Cazden, J. (2005). *Imagery in voice therapy: Neurolinguistic rationales and clinical guidelines*. Presented at the American Speech-Language and Hearing Association convention, San Diego, CA.

Childers. J. (1998). *Performing the word*. Nashville, TN: Abingdon Press.

Colleges and Universities of the Anglican Communion. (n.d.). Retrieved from http://cuac.anglicancommunion.org/

Conquergood, D. (1983). Communication as performance: Dramaturgical dimensions of everyday life. In J. Sisco (Ed.), *The Jensen lectures: Contemporary studies*. (pp. 24–43). Tampa, FL: University of South Florida.

Episcopal Church. (n.d.) Retrieved from http://www.episcopalchurch.org/page/about-us

Eslinger, R. (1987). *A new hearing: Living options in homiletic method*. Nashville, TN: Abingdon.

Frye, N. (1991). *The double vision: Language and meaning in religion*. Toronto, Canada: University of Toronto.

Genig, J. (2013). Preaching IN and TO a post-modern world. *Homiletic and Pastoral Review*. Retrieved from http://www.hprweb.com/2013/08/preaching-in-and-to-a-post-modern-world

Lessac, A. (1997). *The use and training of the human voice: A biodynamic approach to vocal life*. Boston, MA: McGraw-Hill.

Miska, R. (2014). Celebration of Catholic women's vocations: Kate Burke. *Young Adult Catholics*. Retrieved from http://youngadultcatholics-blog.com/2014/05/30/celebration-of-catholic-womens-vocations-kate-burke/

Montemurri, P. (2015). Hallelulah! Actors help future priests amp up sermons. *Detroit Free Press*. Retrieved from http://www.freep.com/story/news/local/2015/05/17/dfp-catholic-priests-preaching-boot- camp/27494807/

Pinker, S. (1994). *The language instinct*. New York, NY: William Morrow.

Ramos, T. (2015). Pope Francis urges priests to stop giving boring sermons. *Catholic Online*. Retrieved from http://www.catholic.org/news/hf/faith/story.php?id=60026

Raun, P. (2009). Transformational identification: Empathy through poetry and text. In R. Cook (Ed.), *The moving voice* (pp. 320–323). San Diego, CA: University Readers/Voice and Speech Trainers Association.

Rodenberg, P. (1992). *The right to speak*. New York, NY: Routledge.

Rodenburg, P. (1993). *The need for words*. New York, NY: Routledge.

Schneider, S., & Sataloff, R. (2007). *Voice therapy for the professional voice*. Retrieved from https://www.scribd.com/doc/23179261/Voice-Therapy-for-the-Professional-Voice

Smiley, M. (2006). Retrieved from http://www.pbs.org/wnet/religionandethics/2006/01/13/january-13-2006-reverend-mary-jo-smiley/2437/

Smith, C., Finnegan, E., & Karnell, M. (2005). Resonant voice: Spectral and nasendoscopic analysis. *Journal of Voice, 19*(4), 607–622. Retrieved from https://www.ncbi.nlm.nih.gov/pubmed/16301106

Thompson, C. (2010). *Anatomy of the soul.* Carol Stream, IL: Tyndale House.

Titze, I. (1988). The physics of small amplitude oscillation of the vocal folds. *Journal of the Acoustical Society of America, 83*(4), 1536–1552. Retrieved from https://www.ncbi.nlm.nih.gov/pubmed/3372869

Turner, V. (1987). *The anthropology of performance.* New York, NY: PAJ Publications.

United States Religious Denominations. (n.d.). Retrieved from http://www.adherents.com/rel_USA.html

Verdolini, K. (1994). *A vocologist's guide: Voice therapy and training.* Iowa City, IA: National Center for Voice and Speech.

Verdolini, K. (1998). *Guide to vocology.* Iowa City, IA: National Center for Voice and Speech.

Verdolini-Marston, K., Burke, M., Lessac, A, Glaze, L., & Caldwell, E. (1995). Preliminary study of two methods of treatment for laryngeal nodules. *Journal of Voice, 9*(1), 74–85.

Ward, R. (1992). *Speaking from the heart.* Nashville, TN: Abingdon Press.

Ward, R. (1996). Performance turns in homiletics. *Reformed Liturgy and Music, 30,* 2. Louisville: Worship Ministries of the Christian Reformed Church. Retrieved from http://www.religion-online.org/showarticle.asp?title=340

Ward, R. (2001). *Speaking of the holy.* St. Louis, MO: Chalice Press.

Ziegler, A., Gillespie, A., & Verdolini, K. (2010). *Behavioral treatment of voice disorders in teachers.* Basel, Switzerland: Karger. Retrieved from https://www.ncbi.nlm.nih.gov/pmc/articles/PMC2855257/

Index

Note: Page numbers in **bold** reference non-text material.